Latina/o Healing Practices

Latina/o Healing Practices

Mestizo and Indigenous Perspectives

Edited by

Brian W. McNeill and Joseph M. Cervantes

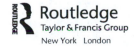

Routledge
Taylor & Francis Group
New York London

Routledge
Taylor & Francis Group
270 Madison Avenue
New York, NY 10016

Routledge
Taylor & Francis Group
2 Park Square
Milton Park, Abingdon
Oxon OX14 4RN

Printed in the United States of America on acid-free paper
10 9 8 7 6 5 4 3 2 1

International Standard Book Number-13: 978-0-415-95420-4 (Hardcover)

Library of Congress Cataloging-in-Publication Data

Latina/o healing practices / [edited] by Brain McNeill & Joseph M. Cervantes.
     p. ; cm.
   Includes bibliographical references and index.
   ISBN 978-0-415-95420-4 (hardbound : alk. paper)
   1. Traditional medicine--United States. 2. Hispanic Americans--Religion. 3.
Hispanic Americans--Medicine. 4. Traditional medicine--Latin America. 5. Latin
Americans--Medicine. 6. Latin Americans--Religion. I. McNeill, Brian, 1955- II.
Cervantes, Joseph Michael.
   [DNLM: 1. Spiritual Therapies. 2. Hispanic Americans. 3. Medicine, Traditional. 4.
Religion. 5. Spirituality. WB 880 L367 2008]

GR105.3.L38 2008
398'.353--dc22   2007048349

Visit the Taylor & Francis Web site at
http://www.taylorandfrancis.com

and the Routledge Web site at
http://www.routledge.com

Contents

An Appreciation of Dr. Michael W. Smith (1960–2006)

LORRAINE GARCIA-TEAGUE

It is with great pleasure that I pay tribute to Michael W. Smith, MD. Although I did not know Dr. Smith as long as others in his field did, he touched my heart in such a short while. He became one of my mentors in August 2005 and on April 17, 2006, he passed away. Although he was battling a chronic illness, you would have never known it because he never complained. In the eight months that I knew him, we worked closely together on several projects and submitted a couple of grants, he as principle investigator and I as one of several co-investigators. He gave me more guidance than I ever imagined and was unselfish in his support of junior investigators. As an RN and PhD, I can attest that he recognized all disciplines, and treated everyone with whom he came in contact with great respect.

Dr. Smith was born on August 18, 1960, and grew up in San Ysidro, California, and in Michigan. He completed his undergraduate degree at Yale University and received his medical degree at the University of Illinois–Rockford School of Medicine. Dr. Smith completed his residency training at Harbor-UCLA Medical Center in Torrance, California where he received several national honors and served as co–chief resident. After completing his residency, he took a position as an associate clinical professor in the Department of Psychiatry at Harbor-UCLA Medical Center. Because he always gave 100 percent to everything he involved himself with, he also served as academic chair of the John F. Wolf, MD, Human Subjects Committee Number 2, and served with distinction as a member and vice chair of the Institutional Review Board of the Los Angeles Biomedical Research Institute at Harbor-UCLA.

He was also the medical director of the Alliance for the Mentally Ill/A Better Life Endeavor Integrated Service Agency at Harbor-UCLA, a challenging program that serves individuals with severe and chronic mental disorders. Dr. Smith gained trust from all patients and had a special talent in treating them. This type of position would in itself be overwhelming for an average psychiatrist, but at the same time, Dr. Smith was also director of the National Institute of Mental Health's Harbor-UCLA Research Center on the Psychobiology of Ethnicity. In all these positions he remained a humble, soft-spoken man. When it came to presentations and public speaking he was a dynamic and interesting teacher. He was both bilingual (fluent in both English and Spanish) and bicultural. He was a sought-after speaker who gave informative domestic and international talks.

He was considered an expert on ethnopsychopharmacology, and on the use of herbal remedies as a supplement to traditional approaches in the treatment of mental illness, particularly as it relates to ethnic minority populations. His research helped introduce the newer antipsychotic medications into the clinics of the Los Angeles County Department of Mental Health. Needless to say, Dr. Smith made profound contributions to the mental health community, both regionally and nationally.

Accomplishing all this at such a young age, you would think he had little time for anything else, but I have come to learn that he mastered balance in life. He was a very dedicated husband, had a close relationship with his only brother, and always made time for his family. He was loyal to his staff and very generous. Being around him was always a celebration of some kind. I have learned so much from him, but most of all, I learned to celebrate and appreciate life, as he did every day.

Contributors

German Ascani was born in Buenos Aires, Argentina. He received a BA in psychology from the University of California–Berkeley, an MS in physiology and biophysics from Georgetown University, and an MD from the University of California–Davis School of Medicine. Dr. Ascani completed his residency in psychiatry at Harbor-UCLA Medical Center in Torrance, California, where Michael W. Smith served as his mentor. Currently, Dr. Ascani works in community mental health in the San Francisco Mission Mental Health Clinic.

Arlene Carrasco is the first in her family to have attained a higher-education degree. In 2005, she completed a BA in psychology with a double minor in Spanish and education at the University of California–Irvine. While at UCI she was involved in leadership, research, and community service positions. In 2005 she was the undergraduate recipient of the National Association for Chicana and Chicano Studies Cervantes Premio, a national and prestigious award, for a paper she wrote as part of the undergraduate research program at Washington State University (WSU). Currently, she is a third-year student in the PhD program in counseling psychology at WSU, where Dr. Brian W. McNeill serves as her mentor. She has presented her previous research at various conferences and was recently invited to present at the Hispanic Mental Health Conference in Saginaw, Michigan.

Jeanett Castellanos currently serves as the director for the Social Science Academic Resource Center in the School of Social Sciences at the University of California–Irvine and as a lecturer for the Department of Social Sciences and the Chicano/Latino studies program. In addition, she has served as a consultant for various higher-education institutions in the area of cultural competency. Her research focuses on the college experience of racial and ethnic minority students and the psychosociocultural factors that affect their retention. Dr. Castellanos has coedited two books, *The Majority in the Minority: Expanding the Representation of Latina/o Faculty, Administrators and Students in Higher Education* (with Lee Jones), and *Pathway to the Latina/o Ph.D.: Abriendo Caminos* (with Alberta M. Gloria), both of which address Latino student experiences in higher education.

Joseph M. Cervantes received his PhD in community clinical psychology from the University of Nebraska–Lincoln in 1977. He is a professor in the Department of Counseling at California State University–Fullerton and maintains an independent practice in child, adolescent, and family psychology. He holds diplomates in both clinical and family psychology from the American Board of Professional Psychology and is licensed in the states of California and Hawaii. Dr. Cervantes's research interests are in the interrelatedness of cultural diversity and indigenous spirituality. He serves on the editorial board for the journal *Professional Psychology: Research and Practice*, and has been a journal reviewer for *Cultural Diversity and Ethnic Minority Psychology,* and the *Journal of Education and Latinos.* Dr. Cervantes also currently serves as the ethics chair for the Orange County Psychological Association, and is a member on the Sexual Misconduct Oversight and Review Board, Diocese of Orange, Office of the Bishop.

Kenneth G. Davis is an associate professor of pastoral studies at St. Meinrad School of Theology in St. Meinrad, Indiana, and has published 12 books and 50 articles in both English and Spanish on the religion of U.S. Hispanics. He has lectured around the United States, as well as in Central America, Europe, and Mexico, and will soon publish the third edition of his *Misa, Mesa, y Musa: Liturgy in the U.S. Hispanic Church.*

Eileen Esquivel is a Cuban American Santera who has been in the Santería religion all her life. She has witnessed more than 50 ceremonies in her time and has taken part in various rituals. A practitioner with many years of experience and knowledge, she guides others in their lives and consults the saints and spirits for guidance.

Alberta M. Gloria received her doctorate in counseling psychology from Arizona State University and is currently a professor in the Department of Counseling Psychology and director of the Chicano/Latino studies program at the University of Wisconsin–Madison. Her primary research interests include psychosociocultural factors for Latinas/os and other racial/ethnic students in higher education. She was awarded the 2002 Emerging Professional Award from Division 45 of the American Psychological Association for outstanding early career contributions in promoting ethnic minority issues in the field of psychology, and in 2003 Dr. Gloria received the Kenneth and Mamie Clark Award from the American Psychological Association of Graduate Students for her contributions to the professional development of ethnic minority graduate students. She recently coedited, with Jeanett Castellanos, *Pathway to the Latina/o Ph.D.: Abriendo Caminos,* which addresses the experiences of Latino students in pursuing higher education.

Karen V. Holliday currently holds the positions of postdoctoral fellow in Psychiatric Genetics at the University of Texas Health Sciences Center at San Antonio, assistant research anthropologist at the Center for Culture and Health at the University of California–Los Angeles, and consultant to the Biomedical Research Institute at Harbor-UCLA Medical Center in Torrance, California. Her research interests include Latino/a identity; mental health; public health; religious healing; psychiatric genetics; ethnography; community consultation and ethical engagement; complementary and alternative medicine in Ecuador, Mexico, and the United States.

Brian W. McNeill received his PhD in counseling psychology in 1984 from Texas Tech University in Lubbock, and is currently a professor and director of training for the counseling psychology program at Washington State University. Dr. McNeill is the coeditor, with Roberto J. Velásquez and Leticia Arellano, of *The Handbook of Chicana and Chicano Psychology and Mental Health,* and is a licensed psychologist in the states of Washington and Idaho, where he practices and consults. He has served on the editorial boards for the *Journal of Counseling Psychology* and *Professional Psychology: Research and Practice.* His current research interests include Latino spirtual healing traditions, issues in Chicano psychology, and the training and supervision of professional psychologists.

Lara Medina holds a doctorate in American history from the Claremont Graduate University in Claremont, California. Her research and publications focus on Chicano religious history, public ritual, and Chicana feminist spirituality, and she is the author of *Las Hermanas: Chicana/Latina Religious-Political Activism in the U.S. Catholic Church.* Other published works include "Chicanos and Religion: Traditions and Transformations" in *Teaching Religion and Healing*, edited by Linda L. Barnes and Inés Talamantez; and "Communing with the Dead: Spiritual and Cultural Healing in Chicana/o Communities" in *Religion and Healing in America*, edited by Linda L. Barnes and Susan S. Sered. Dr. Medina is an associate professor in Chicana and Chicano Studies at California State University–Northridge.

Rosalilia Mendoza is a first-generation Mexican American from a family of eight, born and raised in California's San Fernando Valley. She graduated from the University of California–Irvine in 2006 with a bachelor's degree with honors in psychology/cognitive sciences and a minor in Chicano and Latino studies. She is currently pursuing a master's degree in counseling psychology at the University of Wisconsin–Madison. Her research interests include Latino psychological well-being and college experiences. Several of her research activities include investigating Mexican American and Latino college students' help-seeking behavior and attitudes toward mental health, Latinas'/os' college adjustment, graduate school aspirations, and psychological well-being.

Sandra Nuñez, BA, MA, enjoys being a freelance writer and traveling to distant lands. She grew up in California's Imperial Valley, and credits her sensitivity of cultural competence and tolerance to this experience. Her degrees from the University of California–Irvine and the University of California–Los Angeles, with majors in anthropology, social science, and Latin American studies, she credits to her husband, Joe. She has collaborated on several books, including *The Encyclopedia of Multicultural Psychology*, edited by Yo Jackson.

Fernando A. Ortiz is currently an assistant professor at Alliant International University's California School of Professional Psychology in San Diego, where he specializes in personality assessment, multicultural competencies, and clinical skills. He received his PhD in counseling psychology at Washington State University, specializing in cross-cultural research and Mexican ethnopsychology. He completed a postdoctoral internship at the University of California–Santa Barbara Counseling Center with a specialization in multicultural clinical training. His research interests include minority personality assessment and cross-cultural issues, Mexican ethnopsychology, and indigenous healing modalities. He has worked extensively with ethnic minorities in the California mental health system.

Michael W. Smith, (deceased), received his BA in psychology from Yale University and his MD from the University of Illinois–Rockford. He completed a residency in psychiatry at Harbor-UCLA Medical Center in Torrance, California, where he also served as the medical director of the Alliance for the Mentally Ill/A Better Life Endeavor Integrated Service Agency at Harbor-UCLA Medical Center. As a resident he was awarded an American Psycological Association Minority Fellowship and a DISTA Fellowship. In addition, he served on the Expert Committee of Psychiatric Medications for the Los Angeles County Department of Health Services. Dr. Smith was also an associate professor of psychiatry at the University of California–Los Angeles School of Medicine, and director of the National Institute of Mental Health's Harbor-UCLA Research Center on the Psychobiology of Ethnicity. His primary focus was in research exploring the mechanisms involved in determining ethnic, gender, and individual variation in response to psychotropic medication. He was the principal investigator on a number of studies of alcoholism, bipolar disorder, depression, schizophrenia, and smoking cessation for patients with schizophrenia. Dr. Smith published numerous articles, book chapters, and abstracts on ethnopsychopharmacology.

Lorraine Garcia-Teague was born and raised in San Bernardino, California. Aside from devoting 22 years of her life to nursing, in 2005 she completed a two-year postdoctoral training program at the University of California–Los Angeles in the field of pharmacogenetics in the Mexican population. Prior to her postdoctoral study, she was a research assistant and part-time coordinator at UCLA, where she assisted with the development of a human immunodeficiency virus (HIV) education adherence program and ran several of its education classes. She is currently working at the National Institute of Mental Health's Harbor-UCLA Research Center on the Psychobiology of Ethnicity in Torrance, California. The majority of her time is spent on an international project on the genetics of bipolar disorder in Latino populations, which is funded by the National Institute of Mental Health.

Introduction

Counselors and Curanderas/os—Parallels in the Healing Process

BRIAN W. MCNEILL AND JOSEPH M. CERVANTES

Contrary to the popular notions espoused in almost every introductory psychology textbook, the applied practice of psychology did not begin with the work of Sigmund Freud and his followers. It is now increasingly acknowledged that psychotherapy as a healing practice has been a long-standing culturally embedded tradition, separate from modern medicine and the medical model of diagnosis and treatment of various maladies and diseases (Wampold, 2001a). While spirituality has long been ignored within the psychological literature, it is currently recognized that the spritual dimension of peoples' existence is part of a needed and more comprehensive approach to understanding mental health and mental illness, especially for culturally diverse individuals (Cervantes & Parham, 2005). Our purpose in this volume is threefold. First, there is a need to present the variety of contemporary mestizo and indigenous healing practices that have manifested in spiritual traditions across the variety of Latina/o cultures in the United States. This need has become more relevant given the increased presence of several distinct Latina/o immigrant populations in communities throughout this country. Second, knowledge of these practices has a direct relationship to personal and professional awareness of how they contribute to the belief systems, attitudes, and behaviors of individuals. This awareness will inevitability play a salient role in the development of effective interventions within these populations. Third, the recognition of culturally distinct healing practices has a direct relationship to nontraditional psychological methods that have historically not been acknowledged nor valued as relevant techniques and procedures that may be important in working with Latina/o families. Consequently, the professional practice of psychology may be challenged with regard to the inclusion of novel methods and processes that go against the grain of traditional counseling and psychotherapy, yet provide meaningful and effective work within these populations. Further, the issue of ethical practice is a subsequent consideration related to what is appropriate to use when a traditional psychotherapy relationship is integrated with healing practices consistent with that of a healer, or *curandera/o*.

An earlier development that has lead to a discussion of contemporary mestiza/o healing practices is the history of psychotherapy and indigenous healing systems that has come to be known as *mestiza/o psychology* (Ramirez, 1983, 1998). This conceptual and sociohistorical backdrop will provide the needed understanding for contemporary applications that have been related to this important dialogue. We now examine the history of the amalgamation of psychological systems leading to the creation of a mestiza/o psychology.

THE MIX OF HISPANIC, INDIGENOUS, AND "NEW WORLD" PSYCHOLOGIES

In the landmark volume, *Chicano Psychology,* Padilla (1984) has reviewed the Hispanic origins of psychology in Spain, indigenous psychology prior to the Spanish conquest in the so-called New World, as well as postconquest psychology in Mexico. Noting that the history of psychology in Spain coincided with the development of medicine, Padilla documents the establishment of the first medicinal hospital in Spain in 580 at Mérida, followed by numerous medical and psychiatric advances from the 11th to 15th centuries, resulting in Spain being referred to as the "cradle of psychiatry." These developments led to the establishment of the first hospital for the mentally ill in Valencia—which, Padilla notes, is an event hardly recognized outside of the Spanish-speaking world.

When Hernán Cortes and the Spanish conquerors encountered the tribal people known as the Mexica or Aztecs, they discovered a highly developed civilization, advanced not only in the areas of farming, architecture, and medicine, but also with a sophisticated system of public health including mental illness, along with a library of medicinal herbs and their uses. The Mexica divided insanity into two main categories. According to Schendel (1969, cited in Padilla, 1984), the first, so-called active insanity (*xolopeyotl*), was believed to be due to the abuse of narcotic and/or poisonous green plants and fungi such as jimson weed, peyote, and hallucinogenic mushrooms. Remedies included herbal antitioxins, purgatives, and withdrawal. As Padilla points out, such remedies are not so different from those performed by contemporary practitioners for the use of alcoholism and drug addiction. Passive insanity (*tlahuiliscayotl*) included illnesses that resemble what we pesently know as mania, schizophrenia, and depression (Belasso, 1969, cited in Padilla, 1984), and were treated by special healers known as *tonalpouohqui* who used techniques of catharsis, dream interpretation, and psychotherapy.

According to Padilla, the Mexica conception of psychopathology consisted of social, physiological, and psychological elements. Relevant to the social component, the presence of a disturbed person was viewed as a disruption of the normal equilibrium of a community and as something that affected the entire community through bad weather resulting in the loss of crops or by an invasion from an enemy. It was thus important to cure patients not only for their own sake, but also to restore equilibrium to the community. Physiologically, the Mexica identified the heart as the origin of feelings, passions, and emotions, and therefore responsible for the affective and behavioral functioning of the person. One who was severely emotionally disturbed was said to have lost his heart. In terms of psychological problems, the tonalpouhqui was the sanctioned healer with the knowledge and moral authority to assist patients by means of lengthy conversations to cure a person from an evil sprit that might possess her. The personal characteristics and language of the tonalpouhqui were responsible for a favorable outcome. As we will see, these characteristics of healers hold true across time and culture.

Another Spanish explorer, Álvar Núñez Cabeza de Vaca, who was in 1535 shipwrecked for eight years among the various indigenous groups of present-day northern Mexico and southern Texas, also described the systems of herbal remedies and practices involved in healing with various groups (Cabeza de Vaca, 2003; Krieger, 2002). Based on the shamanistic practices he observed, and his own Christian practices, Cabeza de Vaca and his compatriots engaged in spritual healing ceremonies in the form of rituals for members of tribes; they became known for their curative powers, thus gaining the trust of the native peoples:

> The manner in which we performed cures was by making the sign of the cross over them and blowing on them, and praying a Pater Noster and an Ave Maria, and as best we could, beseeching our Lord God that he grant them health and move them to treat us well. Our Lord God in his mercy willed that all those on whose behalf we made supplication, after we had made the sign of the cross over them, said to the others that they were restored and healthy, and on account of this they treated us well, and refrained from eating in order to give their food to us, and they gave us skins and other things. (Cabeza de Vaca, 2003, p. 94)

As Torres (1996) and Galante (2000) note, these practices may represent one of the earliest examples of the mestiza/o tradition of syncretism in the fusing of European and indigenous spiritual practices. Curanderismo, or folk healing, within Latina/o communities remains an extension of these early practices.

Psychology continued to develop in Mexico and other Latin American countries with the establishment of facilities for the mentally ill at Acapulco, Jalapa, Oaxaca, Oaxtepec, Puebla, and Veracruz, Mexico, as well as in Havana, Cuba, and Guatemala in the 1500s. Yet it was not until 1751 that the first hospital for the care of the mentally ill was established in the United States (Rumbaut, 1971, cited in Padilla, 1984). Padilla (1980) documents the numerous contributors from Argentina (e.g., Rodolfo Rivarola), Cuba (e.g., Alfredo Aguayo), Puerto Rico (e.g., Carlos Albizu-Mirandna), and Spain (e.g., Juan Luis Vives) in both the applied and experimental areas of psychology. This development continued through the teaching of psychology in Mexico in the 1800s through the work of Esequiel Chávez and the establishment of the first psychological research lab by Enrique Aragon in 1916 to the eminent work of Rogelio Díaz Guerrero (1975, 1977). From Mexico to the United States, contributions from forerunners and elders such as Marta Bernal, Alfredo Castañeda, John Garcia, Amado Padilla, Manual Ramirez III, and George Sánchez continued, leading to the development of a contemporary Chicana/o mestiza/o psychology (see Velásquez, Arrellano, & McNeill, 2004).

CHICANA/O MESTIZA/O PSYCHOLOGY

According to Ramirez (1998, 2004), a Chicana/o mestiza/o psychology is derived from the knowledge and experience of the mestiza/o or mixed-race peoples in the Americas, including those of African American, American Indian, Asian American, and European heritages. Seven major principles underlie the mestiza/o worldview:

1. *The person is an open system.* In the mestiza/o worldview, the person is an open system interacting and deriving knowledge from others, the environment, and the universe in order to achieve harmony with one's surroundings and understand the meaning of life.

2. *The spiritual world holds the key to destiny, personal identity, and life mission.* In this way, the spiritual world is the source of power and knowledge. Individuals believed to have special knowledge, access to supernatural powers, or possession of such powers influence personality development and psychological functioning. "Special persons" within the community, including such traditional healers as curenderas/os, espritistas, shamans, and clergy, as well as contemporary counselors and psychologists who may assist people in their search for self-knowledge and identity, provide treatment, and advise individuals experiencing personal conflicts, existential crises, or adjustment problems. Ramirez emphasizes that "temporary" healers such as counselors and psychologists may be viewed as possessing magical, spiritual, or psychological powers. A strong sense of spirituality can also play an important role in achieving harmony and protection against negative supernatural forces. Religion (e.g., Catholicism) and indigenous beliefs can define this sense of spirituality.

3. *Community identity and responsibility to the group are of central importance in development.* In mestiza/o communities, the individual is socialized to develop a strong sense of responsibility to the group, including close ties to homeland and extended family, and a strong identification with the family and community. Individuals view themselves and are always viewed by others as representative of the group. Cultural traditions and rituals provide this socialization. The cultural value of *familismo* (familism) in Chicana/o culture and

the powwow held by Native American groups in North America serve this purpose.

4. *The foundations of good adjustment to life (mental health) are liberation, justice, freedom, and empowerment.* The historical realities of mixed ethnic peoples include struggles against political, social, and economic oppression. Poverty, human misery, racism, linguistic barriers, repression of individual rights, state sanctioned brutality and inequality of opportunity continue. These realities form the socialization of mestiza/o people, as heroes of the struggles are looked upon with esteem and admiration.

5. *Total development of abilities and skills is achieved through self-challenge.* Indigenous peoples of North America believe that self-challenge, endurance of pain, hardship, hunger, and frustration encourage the development of the individual's full potential. In this manner, one learns self-control and self-discipline. Coping with life's environmental, social, and personal challenges and problems serves to form the mestiza/o worldview and personality.

6. *The search for self-knowledge, individual identity, and life meaning is a primary goal.* The Mayas and the Nahuatl-speaking peoples of the Valley of Mexico believed that an individual comes to earth without a face and without an identity. Identities were achieved through socialization and education. In order to develop an identity, a person had to learn self-control and personal strength, which led to the development of free will.

7. *Duality of origin and life in the universe and education within the family play a central role in personality development.* The psychological concept of the duality of origin and life emerged from the cultures of the indigenous peoples of Central and South America and the Caribbean. Polar opposites including male and female, religion and war, poetry and math were fused in the cultures of the Nahuas and Mayans. These cultures also viewed education as the key to development of personality and free will. Parents educated their children up to about age 15, when they entered a school to be taught by the philosophers (*tlamatinime*). In addition, education was formal and mandatory.

In Ramirez's (1998) concept of "mestizoization," the openness to experience and diversity reflected in the mestiza/o worldview made indigenous peoples receptive to other ways of life and philosophies, while the concept of duality allowed them to combine opposites, and encouraged incorporation of other peoples' philosophies and ways of life. In the search for self-knowledge, every culture, person, and worldview was believed to reflect knowledge necessary to understand the mysteries of life and the self. Thus, diversity was accepted and incorporated into the self through both genetic and cultural amalgamation. Consequently, the genetic mestiza/o represents the mix of European and native cultures and ideologies. Cultural mestizoization forms the basis for the works collected in this volume as the result of the variety of spiritual philosophies and religions among the mix of African Americans, Europeans, Latinos, and native peoples.

Indigenous healing systems have historically been part of every ethnic and cultural group (Wampold, 2001a). A principle outcome of the dynamic intermingling between the Spaniard and the Indian of the old world was the development of a system of healing known as *curanderismo*. This set of beliefs based on a model of holistic health has been studied exclusively over the last several decades (Keefe, 1981; Kiev, 1964, 1968; Martinez & Martin, 1966; Padilla & Salgado de Synder, 1988; Rubel, 1960; Torrey, 1983). We now turn to a more detailed description of curanderismo as a critical link to understanding the mestiza/o perspective and the indigenous healing paradigm.

CURANDERISMO AS A MESTIZA/O PSYCHOLOGICAL SYSTEM

As summarized by McNeill (2005), in all civilizations, traditional or indigenous healers have existed and worked within the realm of physical/psychological/spiritual medicine. Similarly, in every Mexican barrio, someone knows of a healer traditionally referred to as a curandera/o. Curanderismo is a mestiza/o folk healing practice and tradition that represents a fusion of Judeo-Christian religious beliefs, symbols, and rituals along with indigenous herbal knowledge and health practices. Curanderas/os are believed to have supernatural power or access to such power, and their abilities are perceived as *el don*, a gift from God. Curanderas/os treat a variety of physical ailments and social problems.

For Latinas/os, and specific to Mexicans and Mexican Americans, knowledge or exposure to the practice of curanderismo may vary with upbringing, degree of acculturation and/or ethnic identity, social class, and geographic location. As Harris, Velásquez, White, and Renteria (2004) note, forth- or fifth-generation Chicanas/os may not possess a complete knowledge of curanderismo, but may have knowledge of beliefs most salient to their families of origin and acquired through the socialization process. Indeed, it may be rare that most Chicanas/os do not practice some aspect of curanderismo, whether it is the use of teas, herbs, or foods for the treatment of physical, mental, or spiritual illness (Harris et al., 2004). Epidemiological studies on curenderas/os indicate a wide range of their usage, varying from 1% to 54% depending on the sample and study (see, e.g., Mayers, 1989). As such, the healing process evidenced in the use of curanderismo is grounded in psychological/spiritual paradigms that share common characteristics. This point has been repeatedly made by Frank & Frank (1991), Torrey (1983), and Wampold (2001a), who point out the fact that mental health professionals employ a belief system and therapeutic process that articulate assessment and treatment phases relative to how new learning is to occur. In addition, the use of ritual is not a unique or innovative process, as family therapists have utilized these interventions for decades in their work with a variety of diverse clients (Imber-Black, Roberts, & Whiting, 2003). Consequently, as contemporary healers working with Latina/o populations, we need to not only understand the role and functions of traditional healers and their methods, but also understand why their methods work, and how they may not be all that different from the procedures and rituals we employ as psychologists.

Curenderas/os are typically known individuals in the community who share their clients' experiences, geographic location, socioeconomic status, class, language, religion, and beliefs regarding the causes of pathology (Trotter & Chavira, 1997). It is this shared worldview between patient and healer that explains why Mexican Americans seek help from curanderas/os and why they are effective (Harris et al., 2004). Thus, curenderas/os are respected for their role as healers, spiritual advisors, and counselors, and for their lengthy training and education in both indigenous and religious beliefs, practices, and rituals. As a result, the curendera/o is often the first person an individual will turn to in times of need, prior to seeking treatment with a physician or psychologist, or when a family's attempts at conventional treatment fails (Harris et al., 2004; Keefe, Padilla, & Carlos, 1979).

Curenderas/os take a holistic orientation, valuing good relations among the physical and social environments and the supernatural. According to Ramirez (1998), curative activities typically fall into four categories:

1. Confession, atonement, and absolution to rid the body of sin and guilt that can cause illness and maladjustment. Healing occurs through prayer, or *limpias* (ritual cleanings) in which the body is sprinkled with holy water.
2. Restoration of balance, wholeness, and harmony through self-control. Illness and maladjustment are viewed as a lack of self-control as a person allows feeling, emotions, or desires to run unchecked, and is viewed as being out of balance or of fragmented spirit. Curative rituals may consist of ridding the person's body of negative elements or confronting the evil sprit that has possessed the person or taken his or her soul.
3. Involvement of family and community in treatment occurs as family members and close friends may accompany the patient to the home of the curendera/o and make a commitment to support the reintegration of the patient into the family, community, and culture. In these ways, wholeness and harmony of the family and community are restored.
4. Communication with the supernatural sets curenderas/os apart from others, as they are believed to be able to communicate with the sprit world directly or to facilitate communication between the person who needs help and the supernatural world.

Similarly, Trotter and Chavira (1997) describe healing activities of curenderas/os in south Texas in terms of the three treatment levels that include the *nivel material* (material level), the *nivel espiritual* (spiritual level), and the *nivel mental* (mental level).

Curenderas/os diagnose and treat within the realm of their expertise, referring to others (e.g., a physician) when necessary. There are various types and specialty areas of curanderas/os including *parteras* (midwives), *sobadores* (those who treat muscle sprains), and *yerberos* (herbalists). Harris et al. (2004) note that spiritual healing, massages, tea, and prayer are prescribed by curanderas/os for emotional conditions or cultural syndromes such as *susto* (extreme fright or fear), *mal puesto* (hexes), *mal de ojo* (the evil eye), and *envidia* (envy or extreme jealousy). Professional curanderas/os also address physical ailments (e.g., diabetes); social problems (e.g., marital conflicts, family disruptions); psychological disturbances (e.g., depression); changing peoples' fortunes in love, business, or home life; and removing or guarding against misfortune or illness (Trotter & Chavira, 1997).

COUNSELORS AND CURANDERAS/OS

Why is the curandera/o often effective? Torrey's *The Mind Game* (1983), first published in 1972, studies curanderismo in Santa Clara County, California, as well as healing traditions in other cultures including Borneo and Ethiopia. Torrey concludes that the differences between psychiatrists and so-called witchdoctors may not be so great, citing common components in all healing traditions. These components include a *shared worldview*, the *personal qualities* of the therapist, *patient expectations*, and use of *techniques*. Over a number of years Jerome Frank (Frank, 1961; Frank & Frank, 1991) has argued that all healing practices share (1) an emotionally charged, confiding *relationship* with a healer; (2) a *healing context* in which the therapist has the power and expertise to help and a *socially sanctioned role* to provide services; (3) a *rationale or conceptual schema* to explain problems, and (4) a *ritual or procedure* consistent with the treatment rationale.

More recently, Fisher, Jome, and Atkinson (1998) expanded upon and reviewed the evidence supporting what they term "universal healing conditions" in a culturally specific context that includes four common components. First, it is now widely accepted across all therapeutic orientations or approaches to psychotherapy that the *therapeutic relationship* serves as a base for all therapeutic intervention across cultures. Second, a *shared worldview* or conceptual schema or rationale for explaining symptoms provides the common framework through which the healer and client work together. Third, *client expectations* in the form of faith, or hope in the process of healing, exist across cultures. These three factors set the stage for the *therapeutic ritual or intervention* that all healing shares in the form of a procedure that requires the active participation of the client and therapist that is believed by both to be the means of restoring the client's health.

Recent research in common factors associated with psychotherapy effectiveness by Wampold (2001a, 2001b) supports the view that all healing traditions share common healing factors responsible for effectiveness. In his impressive review and analysis of the research on the efficacy of psychotherapy, Wampold (2001b) presents a strong case for the lack of evidence supporting the medical model of psychotherapy where specific therapeutic treatments or "ingredients" (e.g., empirically supported treatments) are assumed to be primarily responsible for the effectiveness of psychotherapy. Wampold concludes that all treatments intended to be therapeutic are equally efficacious. Attempts to identify specific effects have not produced consistent findings. In contrast, the *therapeutic relationship or working alliance* has consistently been demonstrated to be related to outcome across various treatments. Interestingly, allegiance to the specific therapy investigated has also been shown to be related to outcomes, as therapeutic allegiance results in effects larger than treatment effects. Adherence to treatment delivered with manuals is not superior to treatment delivered without manuals. Finally, *therapist effects* in the form of the personal qualities of the therapist account for about 9% of the variance in outcome, and the typical research design that ignores therapist effects results in an overestimation of treatment effects. Perhaps for these reasons, curanderismo continues to survive, and serves a vital function in Mexican American communities.

Consequently, as practitioners, it is vital that we not engage in what Torrey (1983) terms "psychiatric imperialism," through which we assume that our contemporary Western therapeutic approaches are good, and that what we do not know or understand, or what is different to us, is therefore deficient. We need to open up our own worldviews to appreciate and understand why our mestiza/o clientele may turn first to a curendera/o or priest in times of need, and that referral to or consultation with a traditional healer may often be the best therapeutic decision. A connecting link has been the identity of the term *indigenous*, which is a theme that is interwoven throughout this volume. The idea of identifying with a mind frame that incorporates traditional healing methods and communication with a spiritual dimension as the foundation to emotional, mental, and psychological well-being is a significant factor in the psychotherapeutic process, and one that is that is especially highlighted in this book.

THE ORGANIZATION OF THIS BOOK

In this volume we will attempt to provide examples of the array of both historical and contemporary mestiza/o perspectives and healing practices, as well as their connection to spiritual practice. In order to reflect these multiple perspectives and capture the essence of spirituality in a multidisciplinary fashion, we have drawn upon the expertise of a wide range of scholars whose training and background include psychology, ethnopsychiatry, spiritual and religious studies, anthropology, and higher education. Cervantes (2004) describes the indigenous perspective as one that underscores an understanding to one's sociohistorical identity and helps to capture a spiritual reference point that is affirming and supportive of one's humanistic agenda and the unveiled opportunity to be of service to one's community. All of the chapters contained in this volume reflect the openness to experience and diversity that characterizes the mestiza/o worldview. While these collected essays share in common the view of healing from the mestiza/o perspective, we have attempted to organize these works into three sections consistent with three major themes.

In section 1, "Mestiza/o and Indigenous Perspectives," Joseph M. Cervantes's "What Is Indigenous About Being Indigenous: The Mestiza/o Experience," describes the indigenous viewpoint that comprises a piece of the mestiza/o worldview or consciousness, highlighting the fact that an indigenous state of being is in fact the opportunity to own a deeper sense of self-empowerment, develop an awareness and appreciation for the feminine, and initiate a sociopolitical consciousness about responsibilities to one's communities. The long mestiza/o tradition of life meaning provided by devotional spirituality through popular folk saints as related to healing is reviewed by Fernando Ortiz and Kenneth G. Davis in "Latina/o Folk Saints and Marian Devotions: Popular Religiosity and Healing," demonstrating the healing power associated with devotional behaviors related to veneration of the saints. Brian W. McNeill, Eileen Esquivel, Arlene Carrasco, and Roslilia Mendoza's "Santería and the Healing Process in Cuba and the United States," examines the views of psychological healing associated with this Afro-Cuban religion from the perspectives of both traditional healers and their clientele.

In section 2, "Indigenous and Mestiza/o Healing Practices," the variety of traditions is explored. In "Herbal Remedies in Psychiatric Practice," Michael W. Smith and German Ascani extend the literature dating back to the Mexica by reviewing the use of current herbal medications in relation to psychological illness, symptomatology, and contemporary psychiatric practice with mestiza/o peoples. Smith and Ascani's discussion of herbal remedies specific for Latina/o groups is crucial, as many families from this sector of the community often times present with nontraditional remedies or pharmacological agents that they have received from a *farmacia, botanica,* or their own local healer source. Nuñez's chapter addressing *Brazil's Ultimate Healing Resource: The Power of Spirit,* demonstrates the early influence of Afro-Yoruban civilization on the syncretism between indigenous African religion and Catholicism present in the traditions of Candoblé and Santería, along with the later influence of *kardecismo* (kardecism), culminating in modern spirtualist healing movements. This work is especially relevant in noting how the belief in a higher power or healing source can be a potent factor in the credibility of patients' emotional belief systems and their subsequent healing processes. A similar theme is highlighted in Karen V. Holliday's "La Limpia de San Lazaro as Individual and Collective Cleansing Rite." While a *limpia* or cleansing is an individual ritual conceptualized as a therapeutic process, Holliday also demonstrates its social or communal relevance through an anthropological understanding of the role of emotion in the healing process. Alberta M. Gloria and Jeanette Castellanos's *"Rese un Ave María y ensendi una velita: The Use of Spirituality and Religion as a Means of Coping with Educational Experiences for Latina/o College Students,"* illustrates how many university students, often assumed to be assimilated into the dominant culture, continue to maintain the importance and credibility of an indigenous spiritual perspective passed on by previous generations. In addition, the authors highlight the role of spiritual practices or rituals that play an important part of these young adults' everyday routine in developing coping responses to educational experiences and challenges, and developing a sense of self as cultural and spiritual beings.

Chicanas/os are increasingly returning to and reclaiming their cultural roots, which include the indigenous influences, practices, and consciousness that have often been hidden, internally and externally oppressed, or viewed as primitive. For many, these traditions (e.g., *Los Días de los Muertos*, or Days of the Dead) have never been lost and provide strength, resilience, and comfort during difficult times and life transitions. Such traditions represent a spiritual practice responding to the history of colonization; displacement from land, language, and religion; class stratification; and efforts to assimilate a distinct ethic population (Medina & Cadena, 2002). As demonstrated by the chapters contained herein, similar trends are also apparent in the resurgence of other Latina/o spiritual healing traditions such as *Santería* and *Espiritismo* in Cuban American and Puerto Rican communities, respectively.

Thus, in section 3, "Contemporary Aspects of Mestiza/o and Indigenous Healing Practices: Reclamation and Integration," we see how these traditions survive and flourish today. Lara Medina's "Los Espírítus Siguen Hablando: Chicana Spiritualities," demonstrates the multiple ways Chicanas reclaim, explore, and express their spirituality through ceremony or ritual and adds a critical dialogue to the process of creating emotional and psychological space for expressing a mestiza-inspired spirituality that can promote the transformation of one's perspective and provide an alternative way to examine female gender. Medina highlights the importance of reclaiming one's indigenous values and spirituality and how this process can unify communities and bring about a relevant consciousness that can inform various levels of human development. While she does not state it directly, her writing implies that the formation of an indigenous consciousness adds to the evolution in one's emphasis on social justice, consequently augmenting personal responsibility in caring for the home community. The mestiza/o view of spirituality and religiousness is throughly explored within the continuing context of Fernando Ortiz, Kenneth G. Davis, and Brian W. McNeill's "Curanderismo: Religious and Spiritual Worldviews and Indigenous Healing Traditions." The authors demonstrate the contemporary relevance of an understanding of curanderismo through a case example and conceptual framework for practice. The spiritual practices of Santería, spiritism, and spiritualism are presented as viable alternatives in Karen V. Holliday's "Religious Healing and Biomedicine in Comparative Context." These systems of "folk medicine" are then compared to the dominant biomedical model and conceptualized as counterhegemonic religions that allow participants to address health and life problems that are not addressed through mainstream biomedicine.

Consequently, we now move on to the variety of Latina/o healing practices. Indeed, as the practitioners of Santería often say, *Hay muchos caminos* (there are many roads), and those diverse roads lead to an essential dimension of our psychospiritual "beingness," our connection to each other, and our connection to a supreme healing source.

The interest of this book has been fermenting in the editors of this volume for a few years, particularly as the rise in Latina/o immigration has become an increased reality in the United States. There is little doubt that this reality will impact all sectors of the community including business, education, health, and psychological wellness. It is in this regard that health, psychological wellness, and well-being are fundamental issues especially relevant to practitioners who work with Latina/o populations. Providing a relevant conceptual and practice base for psychological issues that are generated by and within this population is a significant dimension in the publication of this book. The role of healing practices, psychological process, and culturally appropriate ethical behavior are all fundamental themes that need be dealt with in the treatment of indigenous, immigrant families. It is hoped that the writings herein will provide a significant backdrop and resource toward that effort.

REFERENCES

Belsasso, G. (1969). The history of psychiatry in Mexico. *American Journal of Psychiatry, 101*, 731–738.

Cabeza de Vaca, A. N. (2003). *The narrative of Cabeza de Vaca.* Edited and translated by R. Adorno & P. C. Pautz. Lincoln: University of Nebraska Press.

Cervantes, J. M. (2004). Mestizo spirituality: A counseling model for Chicano and Native/Indigenous peoples. Manuscript submitted for publication.

Cervantes, J. M., & Parham, T. H. (2005). Toward a meaningful spirituality for people of color: Lessons for the counseling practitioner. *Cultural Diversity and Ethnic Minority Psychology, 11*, 69-81.

Díaz-Guerrero, R. (1975). *Psychology of the Mexican: Culture and personality.* Austin: University of Texas Press.

Fischer, A. R., Jome, L. M., & Atkinson, D.R. (1998). Reconceptualizing multicultural counseling: Universal healing conditions in a culturally specific context. *Journal of Counseling Psychology, 26*, 525–588.

Frank, J. D. (1961). *Persuasion and Healing: A Comparative Study of Psychotherapy.* New York: Schocken Books.

Frank, J. D., & Frank, J. B. (1991). *Persuasion and Healing: A comparative study of psychotherapy* (3rd ed.). Baltimore: Johns Hopkins University Press.

Galante, P. (2000). *Cabeza de Vaca: The rider on the psychic borderlands in Nicolas Echevarria's Cabeza de Vaca.* Retrieved October 10, 2006, from http://www.lehigh.edu/~ineng/pag2/pag2-issue.html.

Harris, M., Velásquez, R. J., White, J., & Renteria, T. (2004). Folk healing and curanderismo within the contemporary Chicana/o community: Current status. In R. J. Velásquez, L. M. Arellano, and B. W. McNeill (Eds.), *The handbook of Chicana/o psychology and mental health.* Mahwah, NJ: Erlbaum.

Imber-Black, E., Roberts, J., & Whiting, R. A. (2003). *Rituals in families and family therapy.* New York: Norton.

Keefe, S. E. (1981). Folkmedicine among urban Mexican Americans: Cultural Persistence, change and displacement. *Hispanic Journal of Behavioral Sciences, 3,* 41–58.

Keefe, S. E., Padilla, A. M., & Carlos, M. L. (1979). The Mexican-American extended family as an emotional support system. *Human Organization, 38,* 144–152.

Kiev, A. (1962). *Magic, Faith, and Healing: Studies in Primitive Psychiatry Today.* New York: Free Press.

Kiev, A. (1968). *Curanderismo: Mexican-American folk psychiatry.* New York: Free Press.

Kriegar, A. D. (2002). *We came naked and barefoot: The journey of Cabeza de Vaca across North America.* Edited by M. H. Krieger. Austin: University of Texas Press.

Martinez, C. and Martin, H. W. (1966). Folk Diseases among urban Mexican Americans. Journal of *American Medical Association, 196,* 161–164.

Mayers, R. S. (1989). Use of folk medicine by elderly Mexican-American women. *Journal of Drug Issues, 19,* 283–295.

McNeill, B. W. (2005). Curanderismo in la comunidad. *La Comunidad: Newsletter of the California Latino Psychological Association.*

Medina, L., & Cadena, G. (2002). Días de los muertos: Public ritual, community renewal, and popular religion in Los Angeles. In T. Matovina and G. Riege-Estrella (Eds.), *Horizons of the sacred: Mexican traditions in U.S. Catholicism* (pp. 69–94). Ithaca, NY: Cornell University Press.

Padilla, A. M. (1980). Notes on the history of Hispanic psychology. *Hispanic Journal of Behavioral Sciences, 2,* 109–128.

Padilla, A. M. (1984). Synopsis of the history of Chicano psychology. In J. L. Martinez & R. H. Mendoza (Eds.), *Chicano psychology* (2nd ed., pp. 1–23). Orlando, FL: Academic Press.

Padilla, A. M. & Salgado de Synder, U. N. (1988). Psychology in Pre-Colombian Mexico. *Hispanic Journal of Behavioral Sciences, 10,* 55–66.

Ramirez, M. (1998). *Multicultural/multiracial psychology: Mestizo perspectives in personality and mental health.* Northvale, NJ: Aronson.

Ramirez, M. (2004). Mestiza/o and Chicana/o psychology: Theory, research, and application. In R. J. Velásquez, L. M. Arrellano, & B. W. McNeill (Eds.), *The handbook of Chicana/o psychology and mental health* (pp. 3–22). Mahwah, NJ: Erlbaum.

Robel, Arthur J. (1960). Concepts of disease in a Mexican-American community in Texas. *American Anthropologist, 62,* 966–977.

Rumbaut, R. D. (1971). Bernardino Alvarez: New World psychiatric pioneer. *American Journal of Psychiatry, 127,* 137–141.

Schendel, G. (1968). *Medicine in Mexico.* Austin: University of Texas Press.

Torres, E. (1996). *Curenderos and shamans in the Southwest: Response to Cabeza de Vaca's narratives in regard to healing methods and his role as a folk healer as compared with three curanderos (a position paper).* Retrieved October 11, 2006, from http://www.hartford-hwp.com/archives/41/251.html.

Torrey, E. F. (1983). *The mind game: Witchdoctors and psychiatrists.* New York: Jason Aronson.

Trotter, R. T., & Chavira, J. A. (1997). *Curanderismo: Mexican-American folk healing* (2nd ed.). Athens, GA: University of Georgia Press.

Velásquez, R. J., Arrellano, L. M., & McNeill, B. W. (Eds.) (2004). *The handbook of Chicana/o psychology and mental health.* Mahwah, NJ: Erlbaum.

Wampold, B. E. (2001a). Contextualizing psychotherapy as a healing practice: Culture, history, and methods. *Applied and Preventive Psychology, 10,* 69–86.

Wampold, B. E. (2001b). *The great psychotherapy debate: Models, methods, and findings.* Mahwah, NJ: Erlbaum.

Part One

MESTIZA/O AND INDIGENOUS PERSPECTIVES

Chapter One

What Is Indigenous About Being Indigenous? The Mestiza/o Experience

JOSEPH M. CERVANTES

The rise in immigrant populations over the past ten years has caused an increase in awareness of the differences in values, beliefs, health style patterns, religions, and spiritualities of several distinct ethnic and cultural groups (Carmarota, 2001; U.S. Census Bureau, 2000; Yeh, Hunter, Madan-Bahel, Chiang & Arora, 2004). Incorporated within these differences is a growing familiarity with the term *indigenous*. The term indigenous is a reference to those populations who, by historical origin, were the original inhabitants of a designated land or nation. As such, indigenous healing is defined as those beliefs, traditions, and strategies that originate within a culture or society and are designated for treating members of a given cultural group (Helms & Cook, 1999). In addition, indigenous will refer to a state of consciousness and personal awareness that views life as cyclical, interconnected, and interlingual. Consequently, this recognition and/or development of an indigenous attitude suggest that life events evolve and transform yet maintain a critical relationship to one another (Bezanson, Foster, & James, 2005). In addition, these life events have particular meaning and a communication pattern that respects human spirit and elemental forces (earth, water, fire, air; see Cohen, 1998; Kremer, 1997; Torrey, 1972; Yeh, Hunter, Madan-Bahel, Chiang & Arora, 2004). Among Latinas/os, (in particular, Mexicans and Mexican Americans) ancestral histories are embedded in the mestiza/o experience—namely, the forging of several different racial and ethnic backgrounds that have contributed to their unique identity (Cervantes & Ramirez, 1992; Morones & Mikawa, 1992). The mestiza/o experience and the indigenous backdrop are interrelated, and consequently form an essential basis toward a critical identity for many Mexican and Mexican-American groups.

This chapter will explore the indigenous nature of Mexican Americans and why this understanding and awareness may be an important aspect of personal and cultural identity. Consequently, the term *mestiza/o* will be used herein to designate the unique interrelationships among identity, indigenousness, and spirituality. A philosophical and psychospiritual understanding of what it means to be indigenous is the primary intent of this chapter. It will begin with an overview of history relevant to the understanding of indigenousness, followed by a discussion of the Mesoamerican worldview. The relevance of mestiza/o spirituality and indigenous knowledge will then be discussed), as will the role of indigenous wisdom, a relevant epistemology, and the indigenous paradigm for the new millennium. The chapter will conclude with specific directions for the counseling professional.

WHAT DOES *INDIGENOUS* MEAN, AND WHY IS IT RELEVANT?

The term *indigenous* refers generally to those who were born in their country of origin and whose ancestors were native to their land. However, more particularly, the term refers to those groups of people or communities who have been designated as of the *First Nations*, or the people who originally inhabited the land before colonization (Costantine, Meyers, Kindaichi, & Moore, 2004; Yeh, Hunter, Madan-Bahel, Chiang, & Arora, 2004). As Maybury-Lewis (2002) has noted, indigenous peoples maintained their own languages, cultural and tribal histories, and a distinct spirituality that was non-Christian. In addition, indigenous people have historically been viewed as subordinated and marginalized, and often dominated by domineering or conquering groups that claimed jurisdiction over them. Acuña (1988, 1996) discusses the history for the indigenous people of the Americas and the exploitation that was involved in their loss of language, culture, and way of living. These populations, now referred to as communities of Mexican origin—or, simply, Mexican Americans—come with centuries-old histories that were long ago embraced by their ancestral families. Duran and Duran (1995) have commented on how native peoples have suffered a 500-year history of forced colonization and genocide. In brief, wars, geographic relocations, boarding schools, and disease have all contributed to the decimation of American Indian communities and the subsequent impact of intergenerational trauma. Similar observations have been made by León-Portilla (1972), Montoya (1992), Tello (1998), and countless others regarding mestiza/o peoples, most of whom have their origins in Mesoamerican ancestry regardless of which side of the borderlands of the Americas they are from (Anzaldúa, 1987).

The concepts of *indigenousness* and *healing* have characteristically been used interchangeably, with each defining the other relative to ethnicity, health status, well-being, and the allegiance to a group's spirituality (Koss-Chioino & Hefner, 2006; Moodley & West, 2005). This chapter advocates the idea that indigenousness is a state of mind that is typically learned as part of socialization and cultural referencing; continuous exposure to select attitudes, behaviors, and relational style; and an internalized belief in an "Old World" (i.e., precolonial) culture. An added perspective is provided by Kremer (1997), who states:

> Recovering indigenous mind is, actually, the development of the social imagination of sustainability in places where the connections with the ancient indigenous understandings of sustainability have been severed... an integration of the past for the sake of the future, not for the sake of the re-creation of the past or going back to it in some way. (P. 32)

In brief, the understanding of what it means to be indigenous involves the weaving of present knowledge into the past in order to develop a broader perspective relative to one's existential space within one's community.

Being indigenous implies the role that generational stories serve in acknowledging the relationship of one to the larger whole, highlighting the relevance of prayer and ceremony, and understanding one's connection to nature and to the earth. Other writers, like Cohen (1998), comment on the necessity of Native American medicine to facilitate the significance of prayer, ritual, meditation, and relationship to the earth, thus bringing healing to communities and advancing relevant changes in one's consciousness. Bastien (2003) provides an additional perspective indicating that the meaning of life is rooted in experiences grounded in the sacred relationships of alliance. Her ideas reflect a belief that the identity of people and the role of human development are based on a framework of moral and ethical relationships. In similar fashion, the concept of relational consciousness proposed by Hay and Nye (1998), while not employing a reference to indigenousness, ascribes to related ideas in social awareness and responsibility to others. Hay and Nye make reference to critical connections among the embracing of one's spirituality, a groundedness in one's being, and a desire to serve others. Consequently, a psychology of social justice is a natural extension of the development of indigenousness that leads invariably to the protection of the earth and its resources (Duran, 2006; Garrett & Wilbur, 1999; Rodriguez, 2002).

It is proposed herein that being indigenous incorporates the embodiment of an earth-based spirituality—namely, the recognition that all life is interconnected, and that this awareness influences and guides responsible action toward appropriate moral and ethical behavior and a commitment to the well-being of others (Cohen, 1998; Krippner, 1995). The recovery of past cultural history is less relevant than the incorporation of spiritual tools and appropriate ritual that can increase personal awareness and highlight prayer and ceremony in one's development (Kremer, 1997). Being indigenous serves as the necessary platform toward becoming a person of integrity and wisdom (Montoya, 1992; Poonwassie & Charter, 2005).

THE MESOAMERICAN INDIGENOUS WORLDVIEW

The exploration and "discovery" of the Western Hemisphere, later to be called the Americas, has been the subject of many texts, commentaries, and histories (Barreiro, 1992; Josephy, 1991; León-Portilla, 1972, 1973; Wolf, 1982). The view from the other side—namely, the varied perspectives of indigenous people from the Americas—has historically understood that the 1492 invasion by Christopher Columbus promoted 500 years of myth-making and the creation of mixed-race people who long after continued to live in cultural repression and internalized psychological rejection. The "discovery of America" set a foundation for how the continent would think about its people and their respective interrelationships, and whose voices and narratives should be listened to and whose ignored.

(Barreiro, 1992) However, this "discovery" led to a lost spiritual awareness of the continent as "Mother Earth—she who gives life" (Duran & Duran, 1995).

It is against this historical background that Mexican Americans arose as a unique blend of several ethnic and racial groupings, but primarily the intermingling of the Spaniards and native, indigenous peoples. Cervantes and Ramirez (1992), Morones and Mikawa (1992), and Ramirez (1983, 1998) describe this syncretic process of merging values, religious and spiritual beliefs, worldview perspectives as resulting in the personality character of the mestiza/o. Ramirez (1983) refers to the mestiza/o perspective as a dynamic, synergistic process developed from the amalgamation of peoples, philosophies, and cultures bridging the European continent and the Americas: the intermingling of physical, psychological, cultural, and spiritual ties between the Spaniard and the Indian. As noted by Ramirez (1983) and others (see, e.g., Carrasco, 1990; Ortiz de Montellano, 1990; Vasconcellos, 1925; and Vigil, 1998), the indigenous people of Mexico responded to this tension through dynamic adaptation; however, they did not yield their central core beliefs about spiritual presence. This blending and amalgamation of genotypical and sociocultural dimensions did not come without religious and political struggle, a struggle initially evident in the conquest history of the Americas (Carrasco, 1990; Todorov, 1985; Ortiz de Montellano, 1990; Menchu, 1985), and in the significant psychological and spiritual upheaval that was to impact future generations of indigenous and mixed-race communities residing in the Americas who were attempting to incorporate a common identity (Acuña, 1996; Anzaldúa, 1987; Garcia, 1998; Goizueta, 2002; Mirandé, 1985; Paz, 1961).

Mestiza/o Identity

The incorporation of a mestiza/o mind set and the subsequent identity that this label held prompted a need to effectively navigate the multilayered and racially stigmatizing contexts of being mestiza/o (Paz, 1961; Ramirez, 1983). Acuña (1996) and Vigil (1998) have described this racial grouping as an intermixture of Spanish, Indian, and African peoples with underlying psychodynamics that emphasize oppressive life narratives and psychological inferiority. Morones and Mikawa (1992) highlight religion, spirituality, and philosophical belief systems as characterizing this population. Ramirez (1983) discusses the *mestizoization* process as one strongly influenced by Native

American beliefs, which reflect themes of the earth as interconnected, sensitivity to all levels of life and their dependence
on each other, and as a perpetual search for self-knowledge
and life mission. Paz (1961) characterizes the mestiza/o as the
"sons of La Malinche," the result of the *chingada*—meaning one
who has been violated and has lost one's spiritual essence. For
Falicov (1998), the term *mestiza/o* implies those who represent
a mixture of indigenous and Spanish blood and culture, and
struggle with internalized oppression and a historical sense of
the conquered. Montoya's (1992) description of soul loss, a continuous search for one's indigenous heritage, and reconnec-
tion with the sacred captures a predominant theme in these
multiple narratives of being mestiza/o—or, in other commonly
used terms for this population, Chicana/o or Mexican American (Acuña 1988, 1996; Garcia, 1998; Mirandé 1985; Vigil,
1998). This soul loss theme has been further defined within
a psychological and clinical perspective by Duran and Duran
(1995) and Duran (2006).

Viewing *mestizaje* ("mestiza/o-ness") as both a gift (Vasconcellos, 1925, 1927) and a curse (Paz, 1961) has long defined a
contradictory and unsettled discourse for the Mexican American who has historically enacted narratives of psychological
wandering and soul loss (Acuña, 1988; Anzaldúa, 1987; Garcia, 1998; Montoya, 1992). At the psychological level, Todorov
(1984) suggests that the mass destruction of families, community systems, reigning hierarchies, and physical structures
contributed to the initial crumbling of a national consciousness. With those life events came the subjugation, exploitation,
and slavery of people. No longer were the People of the Sun, as
described by Anzaldúa (1987), the holders of their own physical and spiritual destinies, but now forced to learn the rules
of enslavement, and a new ethnic label, the *conquered* or the
mestiza/o, for generations to come. Current psychological perspectives would describe this generational insult on the psyche
as psychological trauma and a long-established pattern of post-
traumatic stress disorder (Duran, 2006). Five hundred years of
psychological invasion has had a salient impact in the development of this labyrinth of shame, and an inability to reintegrate
the indigenous birth right that long predated Columbus and
the Spaniard influence (Josephy, 1991; Wolf, 1982).

The Religious and Spiritual Backdrop

The more insidious assault on the Mexican/indigenous psyche
was the destruction of the religious/spiritual framework that was

the essence of the life cycle (Avila, 1999; Carrasco, 1990; Ortiz de Montellano, 1990; Todorov, 1984). Paz (1961) eloquently comments on this process, referring to the conquest as a violation of the psychological womb, a great rupture with the Mother, and a spiritual depression and moral suicide resulting in a systematic repetition of historical and generational failure. In Mexican celebrations, when Mexicans and Mexican Americans alike exclaim, "Viva Mexico, hijos de la chingada," Paz (1961, p. 74) refers to the "chingada" as the violated mother, and the "hijos" as bad Mexicans, our enemies,... but not us." As such, subjugation and psychological imprisonment of communities from Mesoamerica initiated a cataclysm of events that contributed to ensuing wars, rivalry, and battles among brothers and sisters and their communities—and ultimately, the denial of indigenous roots, and earth spirituality as the great teacher.

It is the search for this indigenous spirituality, referred to as mestiza/o spirituality (Cervantes, 2007; Cervantes & Ramirez, 1992), is suggested as a critical link to the rediscovery of indigenous/spiritual beliefs. It is this return of the soul and the indigenous mind to the awareness of the mestiza/o that is a vital connection to the healing of many Latina/o communities. A summary of a mestiza/o spirituality perspective emphasizes the following philosophical concepts:

- awareness, respect, kindness, and inner responsibility for the sacredness of one's life journey and its interconnectedness to the larger cosmic reality;
- review and renewal of one's religious/spiritual beliefs, rituals, and traditions;
- rediscovering and re-remembering the lost traditions, ceremonies, and prayers of the ancient ones;
- forgiveness of one's past wrongdoings and reaffirmation of one's connection to a larger cosmic reality;
- learning to become a person of knowledge/becoming impeccable;
- realization that service to others is the natural order of things.

This psychospiritual healing paradigm suggests that the cultural identity of being Mexican American is grounded not in the historical realities of conquered status, internalized racism, and oppression, nor in acculturation and bilingual language abilities. Rather, this ethnic and cultural label is embedded within centuries-old beliefs that have embraced indigenous/shamanic roots and have continued to survive in spite of the conquest (Acuña, 1996; Avila, 1999; Falicov, 1998; Matovina & Riebe-Estrada, 2002).

Anzaldúa (1987), Avila (1999), Duran and Duran (1995), and Montoya (1992) are a few of the isolated voices who advocate the regaining of ancestral spiritual beliefs in order to reaffirm an existential purpose and address the continued destruction of Mother Earth. The challenge for the Mexican American will not only be in the resolution of the "chingada" syndrome commented on by Paz (1961), but in the rebirth of an ancient wisdom that could have relevance and meaning in the new millennia.

THE RELEVANCE OF A MESTIZA/O SPIRITUALITY AS RELATED TO INDIGENOUS KNOWLEDGE

It is advocated herein that knowledge, wisdom, and spirituality are interconnected dimensions that characteristically form the core to the perspective of life for aboriginal or indigenous peoples (Poonwassie & Charter, 2005). In similar voice, Cohen (1998) highlights the connection related to beliefs about healthy living, causes of disease, and the spiritual principles that affirm or restore balance. For this author, as for many others who write about healing traditions (Moodley & West, 2005), indigenous knowledge is embedded within the concept of *wholeness,* as in the notion that all things are interconnected and that everything is part of a single whole that is greater than the sum of its parts. This knowledge is then understood as an awareness of self in relation to the balance of life energy in the body; the balance of ethical and just behavior; the balance of relationships within family and community, and a harmony with nature. It is this level of salient interplay among physical, sociointerpersonal, psychological, and environmental aspects that define the spiritual principles and provide the backdrop to indigenous knowledge.

A similar, philosophical outline is provided by several other mestiza/o writers who ascribe to the significance of this theme. Anzaldúa (1987), Cisneros (1991, 1994), Montoya (1992), and Quiñonez (1998), all prominent Chicana/o and Latina/o poets and writers, each articulate the impact of soul loss and generational trauma on the psyche of mestiza/o people, and the need to restore balance and a relevant spirituality toward individual and community healing. Cisneros's (1991, 1994) now classic stories of growing up Chicana/Latina and her insightful commentary on the spirituality of being Mexican captures a power and validated humor about the mestiza/o experience. Poetry by Quiñonez (1998) reflects on the often truncated experience of being Mexican American while still searching for a more complete spiritual essence lost centuries ago. It is Anzaldúa (1987) and Montoya (1992) who described a fundamental understanding of the essence of an indigenous spirituality that is exclusively mestiza/o. Anzaldúa writes that:

> la Virgen de Guadalupe is the single most potent religious, political and cultural image of the Chicano/Mexicano... is a synthesis of the old world and the new, of the religion and culture of the two races in our psyche, the conquerors and the conquered. (P. 30)

Montoya highlights this internal conflict, which, while giving homage to La Virgen, our Earth Mother, focuses on the continuing struggle toward the incorporation of the indigenous for the mestiza/o. "So today," he writes, "the struggle within our Mejicanidad es una lucha antigua entre lo Indio y lo Europeo—and from there the struggle/joda vacillates entre Chicano/Hispano, Mejicano/Indio y hasta Latina/o eres tu, bruto! Quo Vadis, Chicano? [Who are you, Chicano?]" (p. 232).

Suggested in the preceding discussion is the proposition that the mind set of being indigenous is intimately interwoven with one's spirituality and the sociocultural realities of one's human experience. This point is highlighted in writing by Cervantes & Parham (2005), who posit that a relevant spirituality for people of color is sculpted from the sociopolitical experience and sociohistorical backdrop of a particular community. As such, there is a significant interplay between the maintaining of one's historical and ancestral background and the intuitive dimension of one's consciousness. Arredondo (2002) addresses eloquently the intuitive dimension of the mestiza in her discussion of gender and ethnic identity conflicts for contemporary Latinas. Her description of three significant and powerful, female icons—La Malinche, La Virgen de Guadalupe, and Sor Juana Ines de La Cruz—are models of how to, "transcend gender politics and be cultural brokers and social change agents..." (p. 313). In brief, the incorporation of the feminine within the context of being indigenous promotes the emergence of empowering mestiza/o images that enhance the experiences of love, security, and healing of relationships.

Additional writers, all Chicana feminist theologians, similarly agree that a more relevant spirituality for those of mestiza/o origin should incorporate the historical feminine images from Malintzin (often referred to as La Malinche) and La Virgen with the language of the heart, *flor y canto.* (Flower and song refers to a lightness of being and an indigenous approach to accessing one's spirituality.) This commentary is understood as the acknowledgment of creativity, intuition, and spirit becoming an equal partners with rationality. Loya (2002) argues that a spirituality for the mestiza must include the owning of one's indigenous history with a sense of empowerment and deeper appreciation for the feminine, which has become forged from the cultural backdrop of oppression, poverty, and discrimination. Added to this dialogue is the development of a sociopolitical consciousness that considers the dimensions of race, class, and sexual orientation as important organizing principles that can incorporate a stronger sense of community among its members (Pineda-Madrid, 2002). This writer also advocates that an understanding of *carnalismo*, the expression of deep loyalty to one's community of family, becomes a relevant theme in this narrative of mestiza/o spirituality. Consequently, the spirit of brotherhood and sisterhood widens the significance of *la familia*, which affirms a presence of unity, strength, and struggle within adversity. Rodriguez (2002) reflects on the power and wisdom of flor y canto—namely, music, poetry, and song—as a pre-Colombian perspective on how to arrive at one's truth. She writes that knowledge intuited through a nonrational base enriches understanding about one's existence as *self in community*, which becomes a primary and fundamental highway toward greater awareness of others. It is suggested in her writing that service, leadership, and an embodied spirituality is created, and she emphasizes an indigenous heritage that is affirming and provides a guided hope for the future.

A final commentary on the relevance of a mestiza/o spirituality and the relationship to the indigenous is provided by Arredondo (2002), who describes the importance of understanding the life stories of others from a sociopolitical and sociocultural background. She argues that it is from this vantage point that we gain an acute awareness of human survival despite prejudice, oppression, and colonization and consequently become a more vibrant community that affirms the past and allows one to be present and resourceful for the future. A full circle is made with Kremer (1997), who states that the recovery of the indigenous mind is the healing that comes through the remembering of the original instructions that provide for a healing of the heart through song, dance, ceremony, stories, and music. The feminine incorporates the mestiza heritage, better known as flor y canto, which provides a relevant spirituality as the foundation for the essence of being indigenous in the modern world (Garrett & Wilber, 1999).

THE ROLE OF INDIGENOUS WISDOM

The "wisdom keeper" in a community has often been referred to as the individual who has managed successfully to survive various life learning conflicts and challenges to the human condition (Ardelt, 2004, 2005; Sternberg & Jordan, 2005; Wall & Arden, 1990). Conceptually, wisdom has been described in several ways, which include acts of transformation, engagement, discernment, nonjudgmental respect, and the inculcation of gratitude and community involvement. There is a similarity between these descriptions of wisdom and mestiza/o indigenousness, which has been illustrated as an acknowledgment of one's ancestral roots and a related set of behaviors about how to engage meaningfully with self and one's community. Hay and Nye's (1998) discussion of *relational consciousness* in their dialogue of children's spirituality approximates this notion of connectedness with self and others and is also described by Rodriguez (2002) as *self in the community*. Indigenous wisdom is the outcome of learning from one's past, recovery of one's ancestral/generational stories, and a creative engagement toward the transformation of one's community.

This quality of wisdom refers to the idea of wholeness— namely, that all things are interconnected and that consequently whatever contribution or destruction one cause in the web of life one does to oneself. A Nahuatl term from the language of the ancient Maya nation from Mexico captures the essence of this relationship. The phrase *en la ke'ch* is roughly translated as you are my other me or in Spanish *tu eres mi otro yo*. The phrase makes reference to a world view that everything in the universe is intertwined with the same life-giving spirit that permeates all creation (Menchu, 1985: Montoya, 1992). In essence, the creator or life force is within and evident among all living beings, whether animate or inanimate. Similarly related is the notion of balance—that is, the maintenance of a physical and a psychological equilibrium in all relationships toward harmony in one's actions with others, all other living beings, and the earth.

This evolved understanding also engages one to promote flor y canto (i.e., laughter and song) and a willingness not to take oneself seriously. Cisneros (1989, 1994), in each of these writings, provides a meaningful example of how her Mexican Catholicism shaped her beliefs of contradiction and subtleties of religious hypocrisy through her story of virgin motherhood as modeled through the generational stories of La Virgen de Guadalupe. For Cisneros (1994), the Spanish phrase *aguantate* (endurance and survival at all costs) means putting up with unmerited and chronic suffering, domestic violence, and other physical, mental, and psychological abuse. As a result, being able to laugh at one's life circumstances without falling victim to them is the intended message.

It is advocated herein that one's search for personal identity should also include some understanding of one's Mesoamerican roots. Broadening one's circle of awareness relative to the cultural and historical backdrop of indigenous background can serve as a salient element to the discovery of a deeper layer of one's sense of personhood. In the reclamation of an ancestral history, it may be recognized that the brownness of one's skin, whether apparent on the outside or simply captured in one's ethnic awareness, is no accident. Darker skin serves as a reminder of the "original people," the First Nations, who had their own creation stories, ceremonies, and psychological and spiritual frameworks through which to understand life.

The meaning of indigenous wisdom focuses especially on Mexican Americans with the discussion of two religious/historical icons, (La Virgen de) Guadalupe and Malintzin (La Malinche). These two female icons underscore the strength of the feminine, the creative and empowering force that is a cultural gift for mestiza/o communities. In the case of Guadalupe, she is revered as the patron saint of the Americas, the protector of families and communities and a psychological and spiritual symbol of universal love and healing. Malintzin, historically often viewed as the traitor to her indigenous community, actually models a loyalty to family at the expense of her demise. Her voice is one that beckons one's truth and ability to speak what needs to be spoken. Compassionate wisdom is the gift that is a salient part of the mestiza/o legacy (Leon, 2002; Rodriguez, 2002).

This quality of compassionate understanding has been sculpted from the contextual realities of oppression, poverty, class, racism, and subjugation. It is this wisdom that needs to rightfully reclaim its place in the larger human collective, and be recognized as a cultural endowment for the mestiza/o. A meaningful and inclusive understanding of one's people and community must also incorporate an awareness and concern for the poor and the oppressed (Freire, 1970). This inclusively permits an opportunity for the care of others who experience misfortune, have limited resources, or have been ravaged by generations of poverty and social disease. A sense of carnalismo, a brotherhood and sisterhood mentality, are fundamental markers in the strength and unity of family and community.

Indigenous wisdom reminds us of the relevance of the life story that is framed within contextual identities and provides a deeper meaning toward understanding one's cultural reality and significance (Arredondo, 2002; Ramirez, 1998). This is a contribution of strength for the future while reclaiming the past to set the standard and the stage for the future (Kremer, 1997).

TOWARD AN INDIGENOUS EPISTEMOLOGY

An epistemology for descendants of Mesoamerican communities has been a primary focus in this writing. It is a promotion of harmony among the physical, mental, social, and spiritual dimensions of the human experience, often referred to currently as *holistic health*. As such, the term *indigenous* implies a more comprehensive understanding to the concept of a web of life. Further, this perspective for the mestiza/o worldview embodies an awareness in which the individual views oneself as part of a relational network (Hay & Nay, 1998; Rodriguez, 2002). This observation, further clarified by Goizueta (2002), provides culturally symbolic celebrations such as *El Día de Los Muertos* (the Day of the Dead), communal procession on Good Friday, and the use of altars as highlighting the fact that one's family, one's barrio, one's ancestors, and God exist in relationship. A similar perspective is noted by Yeh and Wong (2000), who state that individuals from interdependent and collectivistic cultures view selfhood as being relational and contextually driven: "In other words, personhood has meaning and relation to others in a social situation in which one interacts" (p. 412).

The integration of an indigenous perspective provides several distinct characteristics. Initially, this knowledge base makes available a portal into the intuitive/creative flow of life given that there is increased openness to various dimensions of human experience. As a result, there is less distinction between what is pertinent to the mind versus the body (Cohen, 1998; Lee & Armstrong, 1995). Secondly, this perspective provides structure to affirm one's spiritual awakening and a more appropriate order of transpersonal experiences. As noted by Lee and Armstrong (1995), there is a unique difference between linear thinking, which is the dimension of modernism, and circular thinking, which is characterized by intuitive reasoning and less concern about causality. A similar understanding is noted by Assagioli (1991), who comments that the psychospiritual realm permits the human experience to be viewed as a larger whole, interconnected through a life force that is binding of all living entities.

Further, recognizing the indigenous in oneself affirms the relevance of spirituality in one's being, which is not cast off in second or third place but is viewed as a primary dimension to one's existence. Third, the indigenous gives permission to own and discover one's ancestral roots and what implications this may prove for one's past learning as it provides a focus on informing the present and future. Loya's (2002) commentary on the need to own one's indigenous history is understood as providing the relevant backdrop to an increasing self-awareness of social injustice issues that may be impacting one's communal responsibilities. This opportunity to "wake up" can alert an individual toward increased self-empowerment and a determination to change one's life circumstances—that is, learning to effectively manage the various social and economic life forces that are immediately challenging.

Finally, an indigenous understanding allows for a personal, historical/collective healing that can help recognize and "own" one's own cultural woundedness. Duran (2006) discusses this woundedness as generational with native people relative to the destruction of language, culture, and spirituality. As noted by several authors, in particular Anzaldúa (1987), Montoya (1992), and Quiñonez (1998), the psychospiritual issues of generational trauma have impacted mestiza/o people, particularly from Mexican, Mexican American, and Central American communities. The ability to own one's full spectrum of human experience allows for a deeper healing to occur and the immergence of a subsequent internal revolution that can galvanize one's emotional and psychological intentions in life (Assagioli, 1991).

An epistemology of indigenousness provides a larger perspective to hold the rational, empirical world while feeling in harmony with one's intuitive and transpersonal awareness. As noted by Goizueta (2002), this perspective can balance an interconnection of the magical and spiritual dimensions of reality while managing logical and empirically verifiable experience. This integration creates a perspective in the beauty of all things, which highlights an awareness that the divine or spiritual is evident in all creation. Wilber (1996, 1998) offers an additional look at this integration of religion, science, and ancient wisdom that resonates with this discussion of indigenousness.

Ultimately, an indigenous perspective highlights a belief that we are brother and sister to each other, as noted in the Mayan phrase *(en la ke'ch tu eres mi otro yo)*, which provides a bridge of connection to all beings. This understanding leads to the natural consequence of increased enlightenment and tolerance for diversity, which promotes a different set of voices and dialogue in the attainment of peace for self and others.

THE INDIGENOUS PARADIGM
IN THE NEW MILLENIA

An indigenous mind set has historically been viewed as a perspective that has both ancestral and antiquated roots (Lee, Oh, & Mountcastle, 1992). Implied in this definition is that this conceptualization does not fit into a modern environment in which the reigning paradigm of linear thinking, empiricism, and subsequent research methodologies that utilize quantitative approaches have long been the approved ways to search for knowledge (Ramirez, 1983; Wampold, 2001). This chapter has argued that indigenousness provides an understanding that is more detailed and far reaching with regard to its fundamental base. In brief, an indigenous attitude and the rediscovery of one's place in the collective can serve many distinct opportunities for the advancement of a humanistic science and perspective. As already indicated, an indigenous way of life is consistent with the inclusion of spirituality in one's beliefs. As such, this relationship between a holistic worldview in concert with a spiritual mind frame gives one permission to become more authentic and fully aware of the human experience while recognizing the fragileness of the human condition. Further, this paradigm provides more creative outlets for one's actions and interrelationships with others and views the social and physical environment as significant context toward the integration of harmony and balance (Koss-Chioino & Hefner, 2006).

Further, relational tools begin to emerge as there is an increased room for social networking without impairing agendas, the facilitation of ceremony that can alleviate mental health problems and affirm one's existential place, and the development of a unique perspective that enhances the quality of one's life (Garrett & Wilbur, 1999).

The indigenous paradigm may be rightfully called the development of *peacekeepers*—that is, individuals who are increasingly committed to the social, economic, and well-being of their communities. This level of regard is fundamental toward affirming a community of peace that can heighten appropriate sensitivities among people, the initiation of relevant spiritualities that are communal and collaborative, and the welcoming of creativity and renewed energy to assist with the evolution of humanistic agendas.

What is indigenous about being indigenous is the development of an attitude, a commitment toward the understanding of one's ethnic, cultural, and ancestral background. A willingness to bring forward this knowledge toward the healing of one's community and subsequently, the healing of all nations is the anticipated vision as we look toward the creation of harmony and a renewal integration of the spirit in one's life journey. Spirit-giving awareness, ceremony, healing, wisdom, mutual respect are the cultural gifts of being indigenous and a significant, cultural reference point toward the more focused vision of peace for one's community.

IMPLICATIONS FOR THE
COUNSELING PROFESSIONAL

The acknowledgment of an indigenous mind set and the related integration into the counseling process has some distinct responsibility for the counseling professional (Yeh, Hunter, Madan-Bahel, Chiang, & Arora, 2004). Each of the principle observations that follow are intended to promote ethical and professional guidance relative to utilization of an indigenous perspective that is clinically useful and psychologically appropriate to the client populations that one is treating.

1. Mestiza/o families, emphasized especially in this chapter with regard to Mexican, Mexican American, and Central American peoples, have historically integrated a strong spiritual base in their lives (Carrasco, 1990; León-Portilla, 1972, 1973; Ramirez, 1983). Whether an

indigenous perspective is appropriate or not, the role of spirituality remains a relevant and critical focus in the psychological care for this community (Cervantes & Ramirez, 1992; Matovina & Riebe-Estrella, 2002). Consequently, exploration of the religious and spiritual beliefs of an individual or family should be viewed as a important aspect in the initial assessment. This inquiry could provide relevant detail and information about presenting problems and the subsequent design of an appropriate treatment plan.

2. As in any ethnic or cultural identity, this dimension can have significant psychological and behavioral implications for individuals (Phinney, 1990). It is incumbent on the psychotherapist that there be objectivity and appropriate respect for the ethnic identification of the client (Sue & Sue, 2007). Consequently, should the therapist maintain and/or integrate an indigenous orientation to one's role as a professional, this perspective should be carefully evaluated relative to counseling practice. In brief, the expectation that the therapist not impose one's beliefs on the client is the expected standard of care. Failure to recognize this would lead the professional's belief system to become self-serving and not attend to the well-being of the client.

3. Be aware of the power of ritual and ceremony if it is to be utilized in treatment (Cole, 2003; Imber-Black, Roberts, & Whiting, 2003). The use of any process that heightens emotion can have profound implications in the counseling process. It is recommended that any procedure that varies from accepted psychological practice be disclosed to the client such that this individual can be informed about the strengths, benefits, and implications of utilizing nontraditional approaches in the counseling process. Examples of indigenous clinical work where ritual and ceremony can play a role are:
    - conducting a blessing to initiate closure on a psychological process or achieved goal;
    - use of prayer to invoke the four directions in preparation for a counseling session;
    - calling out spirits and ancestors to bear witness to one's emotional/psychological pain;
    - the use of sage to cleanse the energy of a client who has experienced trauma;

int.

- supporting the immergence of visionary experience both in and outside the counseling session in order to promote spiritual insight and awareness.

    Each of these clinical techniques and interventions must be embedded within a theoretical framework that is consistent with the needs of the client and his/her belief system.

4. The counseling professional should be aware of any nontraditional methods or procedures that are being utilized and are not part of the expected arsenal of accepted psychological techniques and interventions (Moodley & West, 2005; Lee, Oh, & Mountcastle, 1992). Aside from the previous discussion of ritual and ceremony, should there be other procedures that would be more appropriately identified with an indigenous belief system, several issues should be considered:

    - The client should be provided formal consent relative to the psychological process that is being conducted.
    - The professional should develop a peer support group to review and receive feedback relative to nontraditional techniques and methods that have been incorporated as part of psychological care.
    - The professional should seek training, education, and supervision as needed regarding the alternative practice arena that one is incorporating (Moodley & West, 2005).
    - The professional should distinguish between psychological counseling, spiritual counseling, and the degree to which there is an integrated approach to one's work. It will be significant that the professional maintain one's identity as a mental health provider (i.e., as a psychologist) and a practice that is consistent with appropriate ethical guidelines and state licensure.

5. Visionary experience can be generally a common observation with Mexican American clients (Cervantes & Ramirez, 1992; Falicov, 1998; Matovina & Riebe-Estrada, 2002). It may not be unusual to have a client indicate that he has been visited by the Virgin Mary, the angels, or some other transpersonal experience that has been an aspect of his cultural belief system (Cardeña, Lynn, & Krippner, 2000). The understanding of visions with mestiza/o communities is an important one to distinguish from a psychotic process. As noted earlier in this chapter, the role of the intuition, creativity, and transpersonal phe-

nomena are closely tied together, which suggests that having visionary experiences is not unusual (Cardeña, Lynn, & Krippner, 2000). It is recommended that the professional be aware of this issue and evaluate symptoms and problems within the appropriate context.

6. The integration of an indigenous perspective for the mental health professional is an emerging competency that seeks to incorporate a more complete spectrum of the human condition for Mexican and Mexican American populations. There is some caution with respect to one's practice as a mental health professional. It is suggested that this caution be supported with regular dialogue with other professional peers who can provide the necessary feedback and supervision for treatment of this client population. This specialty is unique, given the combination of several dimensions that are commonly present with these communities. These include: distinct culture and ethnicity; a Mesoamerican/indigenous historical perspective; the interplay of spirituality and various other factors that have not been identified in this writing (e.g., language and socioeconomic status; see Falicov, 1998; Paniagua, 2005; Sue & Sue, 2007).

7. The incorporation of an indigenous epistomology implies a spiritual framework that has direct implication for the practitioner (Cervantes, 2007). Familiarity with themes of spiritual literacy in counseling will be important in order to appropriately contextualize the professional relationship between client and therapist (Miller, 1999; Morgan, 2007; Richards & Bergin, 1997). However, just as relevant is the recognition that the practitioner be internally aware and accepting of her own spirituality and how this dimension has been integrated into practice with mestiza/o populations. It is recommended that just as one recognizes one's own psychological triggers and emotional vulnerabilities, the practitioner evaluate and "own" her understanding of spirituality and the implications this awareness has for selfhood.

REFERENCES

Acuña, R. (1988). *Occupied America: A history of Chicanos* (3rd ed.). New York: Harper and Row.

Acuña, R. F. (1996). *Anything but Mexican: Chicanos in contemporary Los Angeles*. London: Verso.

Anzaldúa, G. (1987). *Borderlands/La Frontera: The new mestiza.* San Francisco: Spinsters/Aunt Lute.

Ardelt, M. (2004). Wisdom as expert knowledge system: A critical review of a contemporary operationalization of an ancient concept. *Human Development, 47,* 257–285.

Ardelt, M. (2005). How wise people cope with crises and obstacles in life. *Revision, 284,* 7–19.

Arredondo, P. (2002). Mujeres Latinas—santas y marquesas. *Cultural Diversity and Ethnic Minority Psychology, 8,* 308–319.

Assagioli, R. (1991). *Transpersonal development: The dimension beyond psychosynthesis.* London: Crucible.

Avila, E. (1999). *Woman who glows in the dark.* New York: Tarches/Putnam.

Barreiro, J. (Ed.) (1992). *View from the shore: American Indian perspectives on the quincentenary.* New York: Akwekon Press.

Bezanson, B. J., Foster, G., & James, S. (2005). Herbalistas, curandeiros, and bruxas: Valuable lessons from traditional systems of healing. In R. Moodley & W. West (Eds.), *Integrating traditional healing practices into counseling and psychotherapy* (pp. 305–315). Thousand Oaks, CA: Sage.

Blatner, A. (2005). Perspectives on Wisdom-ing. *Revision, 28,* 29–33.

Cardeña, E., Lynn, S. J., & Krippner, S. (Eds.). (2000). *Varieties of anomalous experience: Examining the scientific evidence.* Washington, DC: American Psychological Association.

Carrasco, D. (1990). *Religions of Mesoamerica.* New York: Harper and Row.

Cervantes, J. M. (2007). Mestiza/o spirituality: A Mesoamerican counseling epistemology and model for psychological intervention. Manuscript submitted for publication.

Cervantes, J. M., & Parham, T.A. (2005). Toward a meaningful spirituality for people of color: Lessons for the counseling practitioner. *Cultural Diversity and Ethnic Minority Psychology, 11,* 69–81.

Cervantes, J. M., & Ramirez, O. (1992). Spirituality and family dynamics in psychotherapy with Latina/o children. In L. Vargas & J. Koss-Chioino (Eds.), *Working with culture: Psychotherapeutic interventions with ethnic minority children and adolescents* (pp. 103–128). San Francisco: Jossey-Bass.

Chevez, L. G. (2005). Latin American healers and healing: Healing as a redefinition process. In R. Moodley & W. West (Eds.), *Integrating traditional healing practices into counseling and psychotherapy* (pp. 85–99). Thousand Oaks, CA: Sage.

Cisneros, S. (1991). *Woman hollering creek and other stories.* New York: Vintage Books.

Cisneros, S. (1994). *Loose Women.* New York: Knopf.

Cohen, K. (1998). Native American medicine. *Alternative Therapies, 4*, 45–57.

Cole, V. L. (2003). Healing principles: A model for the use of ritual in psychotherapy. *Counseling and Values, 47*, 184–194.

Constantine, M. G., Myers, L. J., Kindaichi, M., & Moore, J. L. (2004). Exploring indigenous mental health practices: The roles of healers and helpers in promoting well-being in people of color. *Counseling and Values, 48*, 110–125.

Duran, E. (2006). *Healing the soul wound: Counseling with American Indian and other native peoples.* New York: Teachers College Press.

Duran, E., & Duran, B. (1995). *Native American postcolonial psychology.* Albany: State University of New York Press.

Falicov, C. J. (1998). *Latina/o families in therapy: A guide to multicultural practice.* New York: Guilford Press.

Freire, P. (1970). *Pedagogy of the oppressed* (Trans.). New York: Seabury Press.

Garcia, I. M. (1998). *Chicanismo: The forging of a militant ethnos.* Tucson: University of Arizona Press.

Garrett, M. T., & Wilbur, M. P. (1999). Does the worm live in ground? Reflections on Native American spirituality. *Journal of Multicultural Counseling and Development, 27*, 193–206.

Goizueta, R. S. (2002). The symbolic world of Mexican American religion. In T. Matovina & G. Riebe-Estrada (Eds.), *Horizons of the sacred: Mexican traditions in U.S. Catholicism* (pp. 119–138). Ithaca, NY: Cornell University Press.

Hay, D. and Nye, R. (1998). *The Spirit in the Child.* London: HarperCollins.

Helms, J. E. & Cook, D. A. (1999). *Using Race and a Culture in Counseling and Psychotherapy: Theory and Process.* Needham Heights, MA: Allyn & Bacon.

Imber-Black, E., Roberts, J., & Whiting, R. A. (Eds.). (2003). *Rituals in families and family therapy.* New York: Norton.

Isasi-Diaz, A. M. (2004). *La lucha continues: Mujerista theology.* New York: Orbis Books.

Josephy, A. M. (Ed.) (1991). *America in 1492: The world of the Indian peoples before the arrival of Columbus.* New York: Vintage.

Koss-Chioino, J. D., & Hefner, P. (Eds.). (2006). *Spiritual transformation and healing: Anthropological, theological, neuroscientific, and clinical perspectives.* Lanham, MD: Altamira Press.

Kremer, J. (1997). Recovering indigenous mind. *Revision, 19,* 32–46.

Krippner, S. (1995). A cross-cultural comparison of four healing models. *Alternative therapies, 1,* 21–29.

Lee, C. C., & Armstrong, K. L. (1995). Indigenous models of mental health intervention: Lessons from traditional healers. In J. G. Ponterotto, J. M. Casas, L. A. Suzuki, & C. A. Alexander (Eds.), *Handbook of multicultural counseling* (pp. 441–456). Thousand Oaks, CA: Sage.

Lee, C. C., Oh, M. Y., & Mountcastle, A. R. (1992). Indigenous model of helping in nonwestern countries: Implications of multicultural counseling. *Journal of Multicultural Counseling and Development, 20,* 3–10.

Leon, L. D. (2002). "Soy una Curandera y soy una Catolica": The poetics of a Mexican healing tradition. In T. Matovina and G. Riebe-Estrella (Eds.), *Horizons of the sacred: Mexican traditions in U.S. Catholicism* (pp. 95–118). Ithaca, NY: Cornell University Press.

León-Portilla, M. (1972). *The broken spears: The Aztec account of the conquest of Mexico.* Boston: Beacon Press.

León-Portilla, M. (1973). *Time and reality in the thought of the Maya.* Boston: Beacon Press.

Loya, G. I. (2002). Pathways to a mestiza feminist theology. In A. P. Aquino, D. L. Machado, & J. Rodriguez (Eds.), *A reader in Latina theology* (pp. 216–240). Austin: University of Texas Press.

Maryboy, N. C. (2004). A native woman's views of the language of spirituality. *Revision, 26,* 11–12.

Matovina, T., & Riebe-Estrada, G. (Eds.). (2002). *Horizons of the sacred: Mexican traditions in U.S. Catholicism.* Ithaca, NY: Cornell University Press.

Maybury-Lewis, D. (2002). *Indigenous peoples, ethnic groups, and the state.* Boston: Allyn and Bacon.

McCormick, R. (2005). *The healing path: What can counselors learn from aboriginal people about how to heal?* In R. Moodley & W. West (Eds.), *Integrating traditional healing practices into counseling and psychotherapy* (pp. 293–304). Thousand Oaks, CA: Sage.

Medina, L., & Cardena, G. R. (2002). *Dias de los muertos:* Public ritual, community renewal and popular religion in Los Angeles. In T. Matovina and G. Riebe-Estrella (Eds.), *Horizons of the sacred: Mexican traditions in U.S. Catholicism* (pp. 69–96). Ithaca, NY: Cornell University Press.

Menchu, R. (1985). *I, Rigoberta Menchu: An Indian woman of Guatemala.* New York: Routledge, Chapman, and Hall.

Miller, W. R. (Ed.). (1999). *Integrating spirituality into treatment: Resources for practitioners.* Washington, DC: American Psychological Association.

Mirandé, A. (1985). *The Chicano experience: An alternative perspective.* Notre Dame, IN: University of Notre Dame Press.

Montoya, J. (1992). *Information: Twenty years of Joda.* San Francisco: Chusma.

Moodley, R., & West, W. (Eds.). (2005). *Integrating traditional healing practices into counseling and psychotherapy.* Thousand Oaks, CA: Sage.

Morgan, O. J. (Ed.). (2007). *Counseling and spirituality: Views from the profession.* Boston: Lahaska Press.

Morones, P. A., & Mikawa, J. K. (1992). The traditional Mestizo view: Implications for modern psychotherapeutic interventions. *Psychotherapy, 29,* 458–466.

Ortiz de Montellano, B. R. (1990). *Aztec medicine, health, and nutrition.* New Brunswick, NJ: Rutgers University Press.

Paniagua, F. A. (2005). *Assessing and treating culturally diverse clients: A Practical Guide.* Thousand Oaks, CA: Sage.

Paz, O. (1961). *The labyrinth of solitude.* New York: Grove Press.

Phinney, J. (1990). Ethnic identity in adolescents and adults: a review of research. *Psychological Bulletin, 108,* 499–514.

Pineda-Madrid, N. (2002). Notes toward a Chicana feminist epistomology. In M. P. Aquino, D. L. Machado, & J. Rodriguez (Eds.), *A reader in Latina feminist theology* (pp. 241–266). Austin: University of Texas Press.

Poonwassie, A., & Charter, A. (2005). Aboriginal worldview of healing. In R. Moodley & W. West (Eds.), *Integrating traditional healing practices into counseling and psychotherapy* (pp. 15–25). Thousand Oaks, CA: Sage.

Quiñonez, N. H. (1998). *The smoking mirror.* Albuquerque, NM: West End Press.

Ramirez, M. (1983). *Psychology of the Americas: Mestizo perspectives on personality and mental health.* Elmsford, NY: Pergamon Press.

Ramirez, M. (1998). *Multicultural/multiracial psychology.* Northvale, NJ: Aronson.

Richards, P. S., & Bergin, A. E. (1997). *A spiritual strategy for counseling and psychotherapy.* Washington, DC: American Psychological Association.

Rodriguez, J. (2002). Latina activists: Toward an inclusive spirituality of being in the world. In M. P. Aquino, D. L. Machado, & J. Rodriguez (Eds.), *A reader in Latina feminist theology* (pp. 115–130). Austin: University of Texas Press.

Sternberg, R. J., & Jordan, J. (Eds.). (2005). *Handbook of wisdom.* New York: Cambridge University Press.

Sue, D. W., & Sue, D. (2007). *Counseling the culturally different.* New York: Wiley.

Todorov, T. (1985). *The conquest of America* (Trans.). New York: Harper Perennial.

Torrey, E. F.(1972). What Western psychotherapists can learn from witchdoctors. *American Journal of Orthopsychiatry, 42,* 69–76.

U.S. Census Bureau. (2000). *U.S. population estimates.* Washington, DC: U. S. Government Printing Office.

Vasconcellos, J. (1925). *La raza cosmica: Mision de la raza iberoamericana.* Barcelona, Spain: Agencia Mundial de Libreria.

Vasconcellos, J. (1927). *Indologia: Una interpretacion de la cultura iberoamericana.* Barcelona, Spain: Agencia Mundial de Libreria.

Vigil, J. D. (1998). *From Indians to Chicanos: The dynamics of Mexican American culture.* Prospect Heights, IL: Waveland Press.

Wall, S., & Arden, H. (1990). *Wisdom keepers: Meetings with Native American spiritual elders.* Hillsboro, OR: Beyond Words.

Wampold, B. E. (2001). Contextualizing psychotherapy as a healing practice: Culture, history, and methods. *Applied and Preventive Psychology, 10,* 69–86.

Wilber, K. (1996). *Eye to Eye: The Quest for the New Paradigm.* Boston: Shambhala.

Wilber, K. (1998). *The marriage of sense and soul: Integrating science and religion.* New York: Random House.

Wolf, E. (1982). *Europe and the people without history.* Berkeley: University of California Press.

Yeh, C. J., Hunter, C. A., Madan-Bahel, A., Chiang, L., & Arora, A. K. (2004). Indigenous and interdependent perspectives of healing: Implications for counseling and research. *Journal of Counseling and Development, 82,* 410–419.

Yeh, C. J., & Wang, Y. W. (2000). Asian American coping attitudes, sources, and practices: Implications for indigenous counseling strategies. *Journal of College Student Development, 41,* 93–104.

Chapter Two

Latina/o Folk Saints and Marian Devotions
Popular Religiosity and Healing

FERNANDO A. ORTIZ AND KENNETH G. DAVIS

INTRODUCTION

A cada santo su día—to every saint his day, so the Spanish proverb goes. Indeed, Latina/o spirituality and religiousness are deeply influenced by the recurring presence of saints and confidence in them is symbolically and ritualistically expressed through images, popular devotions, and pilgrimages (Figueroa-Deck, 1994; Pineda, 2004). The Catholic Church officially venerates and celebrates saints based on ancient traditions and a liturgical calendar. Likewise, in traditional Latina/o communities, saints' days can be marked with *fiestas patronales* that involve food, music, ritual, and dancing (Gudeman, 1976; Woodward, 1990).

In this chapter we examine the importance of folk saints in the Latina/o community, their veneration and mythologies, as well as their purported supernatural and religious powers within the context of indigenous healing epistemologies. First, we note the cross-cultural salience of the folk saint phenomenon, and highlight some institutional and historical aspects of its development. We then introduce the concept of canonization and some basic concepts to appreciate the differences between officially canonized saints and folk saints. We include a comprehensive review of the most important folk saints, and representative Marian devotions in Latina/o religiosity.

Finally, due to the limited, almost nonexistent, research on devotional behaviors and healing attributed to the intercession of saints and the Virgin Mary, we develop a conceptual model with specific dimensions derived from our understanding of the role of devotions and venerations in the process of faith-based healing.

CROSS-CULTURAL EXEMPLARS OF FOLKLORISTIC SANCTITY

Every culture since the beginning of human history has had mystics, visionaries, healers, prophets, and saints (Kieckhefer & Bond, 1988). Some have been romanticized and admired for their virtues or exemplary lives, and now stand on the pedestals and altars of churches (Kelly & Rogers, 1993). Others have been idealized and venerated for their status as bandits, revolutionaries, heroes, villains, or outlaws, and have earned a place in the hearts and minds of many believers (Klapp, 1949; Macklin & Margolies, 1988; Romano, 1965). Religious establishments have deplored some folk saint cults and viewed them as "superstitious extrasacramental beliefs," but the folkloric imagination of their followers continues to immortalize their memory by erecting roadside memorials and household shrines with distinctive iconographies (Macklin, 1988; Pineda, 2004).

This universal phenomenon of saint veneration, especially in its popular form, is found in both monotheistic and polytheistic religions (Ben-Ami, 1998). Although Christianity has one of the most sophisticated concepts of saintliness (Kieckhefer, 1988), one finds saintlike manifestations in folkloristic religious traditions in Judaism (e.g., the *tsaddiq*, "just man"; the *talmid hakham*, "scholar"; and the *hasid*, "enthusiast"; see Cohn, 1988); in Islamic mysticism, or Sufism (e.g., *walīs*, "protector, helper"; see Denny, 1988); in Moroccan maraboutism (e.g., *murabit*, "holy man"; *siyyid,* "just man"; see Cornell, 1998); in Hinduism (e.g., *rsis*, "seer"; *śrāmanas* and *munis*, see White, 1988); in Theravāda Buddhism (e.g., the *arahant*, "saint"; see Bond, 1988); in Mahāyāna Buddhism (e.g., the *Bodhisattva*, "being seeking enlightenment"; see Lopez, 1988); and in Confucionism (e.g., *sheng*, "sage"; see Taylor, 1988).

INSTITUTIONAL SAINTS VERSUS
SAINTS OF THE POPULACE

Veneration (Latin *cultus*) of saints plays an important role in the liturgical and pastoral life of the Catholic Church (George & George, 1955). This veneration of saints in Christianity began with the honor paid to martyrs (Tilley, 1991), although earliest reverence was for the Apostles and the Virgin Mary. However, a public *cultus* of saints appears in the second century, in connection with the death and burial of martyrs (Douillet, 1960). The martyrdom of a saint was remembered and celebrated with joy, for this day marked his *dies natalis*, his "real" birthday into heavenly existence (Macklin, 1988).

The prominence of Mary is acknowledged since the first century C.E. and the development of a devotion to her seems to have originated around the second century (Graef, 1985). The cult of Mary has been based on her powers of intercession and supernatural intervention due to her unique role in the life of her savior son (Brownson, 1963).

Official church teaching prescribes that God should receive *latria*, or adoration; that the saints should receive *dulia*, or veneration; and that Mary is worthy of *hyperdulia*, or superior veneration (Hamington, 1995).

An understanding of the communication with saints, at least in the Catholic worldview, presupposes an appreciation of some basic anthropological (how the human person is conceptualized) and eschatological (how the end of human earthly existence is understood) beliefs (Ludlow, 2001).

In general, Catholicism believes in the existence of the soul (Latin *anima*, Spanish *alma*), its distinction (but not dichotomy) from the body, and its immortality or existence after death (Bynum, 1990). *The tem spirit* (Latin, *spiritus*) refers to the principle of life, and it stands for the unseen mysterious force behind the vital, visible processes, and is often used to signify a living, intelligent, incorporeal being, such as the soul, or to signify a universal vital force (Binde, 2001).

Veneration of the saints is based on the Catholic doctrine of the Communion of Saints, which refers to the spiritual solidarity that binds the faithful on earth, the souls (animas) in purgatory, and the saints in heaven (Jeske, Root & Smith, 2004). This solidarity implies a variety of interrelations: (1) *within the church* the faithful participate in the same faith, sacraments, and government, but also a mutual exchange of examples, prayers, merits, and satisfactions; 2) *between the church on earth on the one hand, and purgatory and heaven on the other,* which imply suffrages, invocation, intercession, veneration (Garijo-Guembe & Madigan, 1994).

Purgatory (Latin, *purgare,* "to make clean, to purify") is a place or condition of temporal punishment for those who, departing this life in God's grace, are not entirely free from venial faults, or have not fully paid the satisfaction (i.e., *satis facere* "to make enough"—i.e., to make amends) for their transgressions (Schouppe, 1983). Although the church has not definitely taught the power of intercession of souls in purgatory, some believers in popular devotion direct their prayers in supplication to the souls (animas) of the deceased (Martin, 2006). Most devotees believe that saints have immediate access to God as powerful advocates (Hahn, 1997). Saints bridge human and divine relations between the living and the dead in heaven, purgatory, and on the earth. This type of saintly supernatural advocacy is a meaningful construct in the understanding of intercessory healing (Brown, 1981).

The anthropological and eschatological belief system on folk saint veneration is not necessarily or exclusively Catholic and it often incorporates spiritualism (Walliss, 2001), which believes in the notion of "continuing bonds" and methods whereby the living may maintain bonds with the deceased. Of special relevance is Mexican spiritism (Finkler, 1985), a dissident religious movement that gained popularity in the 1920s, which employs therapies derived from general Mexican traditions of folk healing and spiritualism (Kearney, 1978, 1980). Spiritualism reached prominence as a religious movement from the 1840s to the 1920s, primarily in English-speaking countries and some of its characteristic beliefs include (1) communication with the spirits; (2) that the spirits are closer to God than living humans; (3) that spirits continue to evolve in the afterlife; and (4) that spirits can be consulted for spiritual guidance and healing (Macklin, 1974, 1978). The zeitgeist for some specific folk saint movements (e.g., El Niño Fidencio, Terresa Urrea) was spiritualism, or Mexican spiritism (Macklin & Crumrine, 1973). For example, El Niño Fidencio taught his followers that he would communicate with them through spirit mediums after his death. Mediumship, or "channeling" of the spirit of El Niño Fidencio, is a common practice for healing (Farfan-Morales, 1997; Zavaleta, 1998) and *materias* are the individuals through whom Fidencio manifests himself (Griffith, 2003).

Hagiography, or the study of saints, has generally focused on canonical saints—that is, the imitators of Christ (*Alter*

Christus) who have been canonized or officially recognized as holy by the Christian churches (Kieckhefer, 1988). *Saint* is the title properly given to those human members of Christ recognized by the church, either traditionally or by formal canonization, as being in heaven and thus worthy of honor (Brown, 1981). The Catholic Church has instituted a rigorous process of canonization or official investigation and recognition of someone's sainthood. Prior to the institutionalization of this long and arduous process, all saints were technically folk saints in that the initiative in matters of sainthood came from *vox populi*, the voice of the people (Macklin, 1988). The first officially ratified canonization by a pope was that of Saint Udalricus (Ulric) in 993 C.E. (Griffith, 2003).

However, even today the initiative often arises from the people, as in the case of Mother Theresa. If the candidate for sainthood passes the first investigative phase, he or she may be called Servant of God; the process proceeds to the stages of the Venerable, the Blessed, and, finally, Saint.

In order to be the Blessed and a Saint, it must be proven that several miracles have taken place by his or her intercession.[1] These miracles are usually miraculous cures (Woodward, 1990). This experience of sickness and miraculous healing has been intrinsically related to the phenomenon of saint veneration in Catholicism (Orsi, 2005). Turning to officially canonized saints in times of sickness has been a popular religious practice dating to the patristic era in Christianity (roughly 200–500 C.E.; see Wilson, 1983). Some saints are believed to specialize in specific cures, often ones with which they were associated in life. For example, of special significance in the devotional practices of Latinos/as, Saint Blase, a physician, is the patron saint of throat diseases; Saint Roch is the patron saints of "invalids"; Saint Jude Thaddeus is the patron saint of desperate situations, and Saint Teresa of Avilais the patron saint of headaches (Griffith, 2000; Orsi, 1998). Often, official iconography depicts symbols associated with their intercession.

Folk saints, on the other hand, do not go through any institutional process of canonization; rather, the faithful find some individuals worthy of veneration, respect, and celebration (Griffith, 2003). Without the endorsement of the official Catholic establishment, the populace of Latin America, and people of Latina/o ancestry in the United States, have canonized their own saints (Low, 1988b). Some, in fact, have entered the pantheon of Santería as *orishas* (deities).

Due to the lack of ecclesiastical and institutional recognition, some have considered the spirituality of folk saint veneration a devotion of the marginalized and thus not worthy of study (Griffith, 2000). But folk saints have recently received more attention in hagiographical research.

Marceron (2002) recently cataloged all of the folk saints of France in his *Dictionnare des saints imaginaries et facétieux* [A dictionary of imaginary and humorous saints]. This is the only hagiographical research work that has attempted to catalog the folk saints of a country. Graziano (2006) has completed the most comprehensive study on folk saints in Latina/o America. He offers an in-depth view of the beliefs, rituals, and devotions surrounding some of the most representative folk saints in Latin America.

Whether it is the European folk saints of Scandinavian and German legends (e.g., Santa Claus, Hildegard von Bingen) or of British and Celtic origin (e.g., Saint Corentin), countries with a strong Catholic influence have been the major sources of saint folklore. Some of the saints and their heterogenous folklore in Latin America include the following:

Argentina
  Difunta Correa (Aguilar, 1977, Alvarez, 1967; Anzo-átegui, 1975; Chertudi & Newberry, 1978; Massolo, 1995; Pérez-Pardella, 1975; Torre, 1973)
  Enrique Gómez (Graziano, 2006)
  Gaucho Gil (Graziano, 2006)
  José Dolores (Graziano, 2006)
  María Soledad (Graziano, 2006)
  Miguel Angel Gaitán (Graziano, 2006)
  Nicolas Florencio Caputo, "Taxista Caputo" (Graziano, 2006)
  Pedro Palaitá (Graziano, 2006)
  Pedro Sangueso (Graziano, 2006)
  San La Muerte, "Holy Death" (Thompson, 1998)
Bolivia
  Che Guevara, "San Ernesto de la Higuera" (Graziano, 2006)
Costa Rica
  Doctor Ricardo Moreno Cañas (Low, 1988a)
Guatemala
  Senor Maximón (Chicas-Rendón, 1995, 2001; Nájera, 1993; Pédron-Colombani, 2004; Pieper, 2002)

Mexico
  El Niño Fidencio (Macklin & Crumrine, 1973)
  El Niño Perdido (Graziano, 2006)
  Pancho Villa (Klapp, 1949)
Mexico/United States Borderlands
  Don Pedro Jaramillo (Dodson, 1994; Romano, 1965)
  Jesús Malverde "the Narco-Saint" (Edberg, 2001)
  Los Tiraditos (Griffith, 1992)
  Juan Soldado (Vanderwood, 2001, 2004).
Panama
  Father Guembe (Gudeman, 1988)
Peru
  Sarita Colonia (Johann, 2003),
  El Niño Compadrito (Graziano, 2006)
Venezuela
  Doctor José Gregorio Hernández (Low, 1988; Margolies,
    1988)
  Simón Bolívar (Pollak-Eltz, 1988a)

Latin American cult movements around folk saints emphasize the complexity of popular religious phenomena in these
countries (Macklin & Margolies, 1988). Often, folklore and devotional practices surrounding the veneration of folk saints coexist with the faith and reverence of officially canonized saints
such as Saints Jude and Teresa of Avila, as well as other figures
of popular religiosity (e.g., the Sacred Heart of Jesus, el Santo
Niño de Atocha (Pineda, 2004)). A dialectical process combining iconography, ritual, and religious expression from "official
Catholicism" and "folk Catholicism" are evident in the cults
honoring folk saints (Macklin, 1988). Some argue that this hagiographic fusion created by popular religiosity is a pragmatic
reaction to a perceived hegemonic monopoly of official Catholicism, primarily of European stock, on the canonization process
(Macklin & Margolies, 1988). Originally, saint cults originated
with the Spanish conquest of the New World and they can be
traced back to the local worship of Catholic saints in 16th-
century Spain (Watanabe, 1990). Sixteenth-century patterns of
Iberian Catholicism, with beliefs expressed primarily through
symbols, rites, devotions and liturgical practices (Goizueta,
2004), constituted a local—as opposed to universal—Catholicism concerned with the welfare of relatively small agricultural
communities afflicted by epidemics, pests, droughts, and tem-
pests, and which often necessitated covenants with the saints
through vows, shrines, and pilgrimages (Christian, 1981).

Klapp (1949) studied the universal archetype of folk hero and found that every culture has idealized personages around specific individual traits (e.g., feat, contest, test, quest, clever hero, uncompromising hero, or Cinderella) or altruistic roles (e.g., defender, deliverer, benefactor, and martyr). Latin American and Latina/o folk saints are characterized by extraordinary power, as evidenced by their often heroic and frequently miraculous feats. They are habitually tested by temptation to prove their devotion, and they have been assigned special protective status over certain groups (i.e., patron saints).

Since their deaths, some of these folk saints have earned a Robin Hood image. That outlaw image has especially appealed to certain groups that have adopted them as protectors. For example, Jesús Malverde (Edberg, 2001) and the Santa Muerte (Thompson, 1998) are two patron saints of drug traffickers in Mexico. Jesús Malverde (the "Bad Green One"), whose birth name is Jesús Juárez Maso, is believed to have been a "generous bandit" who served the poor and still intercedes for the marginalized (López-Sánchez, 1996).

The anima of José Cristol Somoza, also known as Comandante Contenegro, is venerated at his grave in Venezuela (Pollak-Eltz, 1988). Reportedly, he became a guerilla leader and fought the authorities. According to legendary accounts, he robbed from the rich and gave to the poor. He was killed in 1970 by the government. Soon people started visiting his tomb and a new cult emerged with a large number of devotees praying at his tomb for all kinds of healing favors.

Juan Soldado, whose real name is Juan Castillo Morales, was a 24-year-old army private who was killed in 1938 in Tijuana, Mexico, after being accused of raping an eight-year-old girl named Olga Camacho (Griffith, 2003). This accused murderer, a victim and now martyr figure in the minds of his followers, has been popularized into a folk saint.

Pancho Villa, whose birth name was Doroteo Arango, and Che Guevara, or Ernesto Guevara de la Serna, are two examples of historical and legendary individuals who, in the eyes of their followers, challenged the status quo or the establishment and gave voice to the injustices, oppression, and concerns of the poor and marginalized (Graziano, 2006).

In Venezuela, the statue or picture of Simón Bolívar is found in private household shrines and on altars. His followers call upon his anima to solve family problems and pray to him for healing (Lecuna, 1987). In his detailed analysis of five folk saints (Juan Soldado, Teresita Urrea, Jesús Malverde, Pancho Villa, and Don Pedrito), Griffith (2003) has extracted several similarities shared by these folk figures. He found that most folk saints existed outside of the religious system and were marginalized from mainstream society. Some experienced dramatic and violent deaths at the hands of a hostile establishment. Followers usually drew parallels between folk saints and Jesus Christ or other orthodox saints. Griffith (2003) also noted the pragmatism that characterized the healing attributed to the intervention of the folk saints.

Yronwode (1995) has classified folk saints into three categories: legendary saints, not yet saints, and mythical saints. She defines *legendary saints* (e.g., Saint Christopher) as Catholic saints that were downgraded by the church to the status of legends due to lack of historical documentation. Such was the case of Saint Christopher. The *not yet saints* status refers to noncanonical figures (El Niño Fidencio in Mexico or Doctor José Gregorio Hernandez in Venezuela) who have earned the veneration of laypeople who lobby for their canonization through the accumulation of miracle stories and the popular religiosity in the form of novenas, statuary, amulets, and candles. The *mythical saints* are those who in the eyes of the church have never existed (e.g., San Lazaro or Santa Muerte).

Romano (1965) developed a healing hierarchy and placed folk saint healers at the top of this healing order. It is based on the sphere of influence that a folk healer has popularly had during his or her earthly existence (e.g., as a brother, daughter, then as a town healer, etc.), and it is often manifested by the number of followers, with the following echelons: (1) daughter/son; (2) mother/father; (3) grandmother/grandfather; (4) experienced neighbor, incipient full-time healer, male or female; (5) village or neighborhood healer; (6) town or city healer; (7) regional healer; (8) international healer; (9) international religious folk saint; and (10) international religious formal saint. Most folk saints began their healing career or vocation within their families and gradually achieved wider recognition.

Macklin and Crumrine (1973) studied the development of three folk saint movements in North Mexico (Teresa Urrea, Damian Bohoroqui, and El Niño Fidencio) and found that these mediumistic and healing cults underwent a four-stage transformation:

1. The "call" by means of a supernatural experience or "vocational struggle" occurs in the future folk saint's life and initiates his or her career.
2. Offering a practical religion with solutions to physical and personal problems, the saint attracts individuals who are seeking such solace and remedy. Common purpose, journey, and encampment near the curer foster group identity.
3. Myths about the miracle worker grow in the group and circulate abroad, intensifying group solidarity and attracting new adherents. Administrators and would-be exploiters enter. A transcendent ideology is introduced with social, political, and religious ramifications. These may be at once restorative and innovative. The success of the folk saint spawns other saints who also attract followers.
4. External, traditional power structures are threatened, and retaliate by applying political pressure so that the last stage sees the decline and eclipse of the movement, and the loss of its innovative elements. The saint, no longer a potential secular power, devotes himself or herself to curing, thus reemphasizing the culturally defined, traditional role of *curandero* (folk healer) or *hitolio* (spiritual healer). (p. 105)

In these three hagiographic accounts, Macklin and Crumrine (1973) found that the folk saints suffered from depression and helplessness, came from relatively low socioeconomic backgrounds, and evolved from an ill-defined, illegitimized, marginal role to a clearly defined traditional and prestigious role as curers. Usually, the childhood of the folk saints was popularized as full of wisdom and insight, prodigious, and many miracles were attributed to them before the age of 10.[2] Invariably, the folk saints had a "separation experience" and went through a transitional liminal period in which they came into contact with supernatural beings and were conferred powers to heal. They were subsequently reincorporated into the secular world already transfigured with a divine mission and curing power. It is at this point that the collectivity or the people popularize their healing powers.

Pollak-Eltz (1988) makes a distinction between a folk saint and anima cults, also called *muertos milagrosos* (miraculous dead), which concern the devotion to the souls in purgatory of persons who died under peculiar circumstances or who for some unknown reason are considered miracle workers by the faithful.

Shrines for saints and animas are decorated similarly with symbols on altars (crosses, holy water, and images) and the same kind of offerings (candles, flowers, plates, ex-votos, and medals).

LATINA/O SPIRITUAL WORLDVIEWS AND POPULAR RELIGIOSITY

In order to fully understand the salience of saint veneration in Latina/o spirituality, one must place it in the context of "popular religiosity." Sociologists of religion differentiate popular religion from "rationalized religion," which usually has a systematized worldview (i.e., theology), division of labor (i.e., priest, intellectuals, and congregation), routinized practices (i.e., prayers and services), and institutionalized (ecclesial) structures (i.e., the church; see Mejido, 1999). Moreover, as popular religion is home based, it is dominated by women.

Popular religion refers to those religious beliefs and practices that differ from the "orthodox," or "official" religious expressions (Bock, 1966). In the case of Latinas/os, popular religiosity did not develop within a social vacuum; rather, these spiritual practices are directly connected to their historico-sociocultural context (De la Torre & Aponte, 2001). Popular religious practices often enable people express their faith in an oppressive and marginalized world, and the tools to negotiate and secure a religious identity (Espin, 1995).

Goizueta (1996) asserts that popular religiosity, which includes veneration of the saints, is a *locus theologicus* for Latinas/os. That is, the saints—whether officially acknowledged by the church or "hidden" in their families and communities— "embody" a dynamic and living faith and can be regarded as a valid theological source, along with Scripture, tradition, and magisterial instruction, in the practice and understanding of the devotees' faith. Contrasted with a Catholicism experienced as alien, oppressive, foreboding, unenthusiastic, uninspired, and sullen, Latina/o theologians conceptualize popular religiosity and faith in popular saints as expressions of a liberating and deep faith handed down through generations of *abuelitas* and *abuelitos*, grandparents (Espin, 1997). Latina/o spirituality is highly affective and symbolic, which contrasts with the often dry, analytical, philosophically oriented discourse of mainline Nordic, Euro-American, Protestant theology and spirituality (Figueroa-Deck, 1994).

This trait of Latina/o popular religious expressivity is typically found in folk saint veneration. Saint folklore is embedded in linguistic expressions through *dichos* (sayings), *refranes* (folk proverbs), *cuentos* (narratives), *leyendas* (legends), and *corridos* (stories). We identified many sayings in a popular collection of proverbs of vernacular expressions encoding popular devotional attitudes and beliefs toward the saints (Appendini, 2001). The *narcocorrido* (narco-story) has become a musical folkloric genre celebrating folks saints such as Jesús Malverde and the Santisima Muerte (Wald, 2001). Other eclectic artistic creations include *retablos* (altarpieces), *reredos* (murals), paintings, plaques, flower arrangements, *papel picado* (perforated paper), *veladoras* (lit votive candles), *capillas* (decorated shrines), *oratorios* (prayer sanctuaries), *altarcitos de casa* (home altars), and *escapularios* (scapularies). At shrines, devotees typically express their petitions on scraps of paper, on the backs of photos, and on the walls of the shrines (Pineda, 2004). It is not unusual to find such tokens as the crutches of the once physically handicapped who now walk, the symbolic eyeglasses of the blind who now see, or the baby clothes of a child born to a couple formerly thought infertile. These votive offerings left with images of saints are called *milagros* (miracles) (Oktavec, 1995). Petitioners pray for favors such as health, a good marriage, a safe passage into the United States, and for the peaceful repose of animas. It is not uncommon to see believers fulfilling a *manda* (vow) or promise made to the folk saint in exchange for a favor received— for example, a person painfully crawling on his or her knees.

This highly sensory involvement with popular saints, images, and rituals represents a visual aesthetic realism that is characteristic of Latina/o spiritualities and it represents an "alternative epistemology of the sacred" (Wedig, 2001). The kissing and touching at the shrines of popular religion, the lighting of candles to pay homage to the Virgin and the folk saints highlight the ocular aesthetic foundations of Latina/o spirituality that differs from the formal, abstract, and tamed aesthetic formulations of Euro-American, modern, and iconoclastic spiritualities (Mejido, 2001).

FOLK SAINTS AND HEALING

In the Judeo-Christian tradition, sickness is sometimes seen as a consequence of sin associated—if not personally— through the universal, original Fall (i.e., biblical transgression committed by Adam and Eve). In addition to medical care, Christians have always believed in petition, intercession, and religious blessings for healing.

In the Old Testament, the faithful sought cure of sickness through prayer and sacrifice, and often sick persons would seek the blessings of priests or prophets. There are several accounts of miraculous cures credited to the intercession of prophets and "men of God" (e.g., Elisae curing Naaman of his leprosy). Sickness was often attributed to the devil.

In the New Testament, miraculous healing was one of the signs of the messianic times. Faith or trust on the part of the sick was often required as a condition for the cure, as it is the case of multiple healings performed by Christ. The practice of praying for the recovery of sickness in private and liturgical prayer has consequently been a part of Christian devotions. The church sanctioned prayers and blessings for the alleviation of sickness, whether preventive or curative. Christians gradually resorted to patron saints to intercede for particular illnesses (Galanter, 1999).

The presence of the charism of healing in the church was attested by the miraculous cures attributed to the saints. The Catholic Church distinguishes three types of healing: (1) miraculous healing by supernatural intervention as duly authenticated by miracles; (2) sacramental healing through the Sacrament of Anointing, which is believed to increase sanctifying grace, faith, trust and spiritual comfort; (3) healing through the sacramentals (prayers or blessings) that provides spiritual comfort, trust, and fortitude (Marsch & Maloney, 1989).

Faith in folk saints lends meaning to illness and recovery (Galanter, 1999). Miraculous healing due to the intercession of folk saints could be considered faith healing (Kaptchuk & Eisenberg, 2001). Healing has been a pervasive theme in the history of Christianity, beginning with its forefather, Jesus Christ, whose ministry included the miraculously healing of spiritual and physical ailments.

Throughout Christian history many people have reported dramatic and miraculous cures. Most of these healing testimonials are attributed to the agency of God, Christ, the Virgin Mary, and the saints. In this way, Christianity and medicine have been deeply intertwined. The images of saints have figured prominently in Christian healing and the faithful often resort to the intercession of saints for particular needs. The connection between saint veneration and the concept of healing is traced back to the veneration of relics (i.e., objects associated with a saint). Christians have venerated saints for a variety of reasons, which include requests for protection from the devil, for agricultural miracles, for military victories, and for personal salvation. However, the most common reason for saint veneration has been healing. After investigating 3,000 miracles in medieval England and France, Finucane (1977) found that 90 percent were related to healing.

Talbot (2002) has researched hagiographical records that recount numerous posthumous miraculous cures attributed to the intercession of saints as well as the types of afflictions cured. She found an intimate association between patterns of miraculous healing and the visitation of tombs and the cult of relics. Miracle narratives include the healing of ailments believed to result from demonic possession (e.g., dementia, nymphomania, obsessive-compulsive behaviors, and phobias). Other afflictions included physical ills such as epilepsy and strokes. Talbot (2002) has categorized the healing attributions or beliefs of the devotees to (1) touch and proximity to the saints' relics; (2) anointing with a substance (e.g., oil) exuded from the saint; (3) touching a piece of clothing or personal possession from the saint; and (4) distance healing through "pious souvenirs" (e.g., amulets, garb).

MARIANISM: DEVOTION AND VENERATION OF THE VIRGIN MARY

The Virgin Mary plays a profound role for Latinas/os, especially those who are Catholic (Taylor, 1987). Appearances of Mary and miraculous cures attributed to her in Latin America are numbered in the thousands (Gebara & Bingemer, 1987). These miracles are often linked to local apparitions, the most important of which include the Virgen de la Caridad del Cobre in Cuba and Our Lady of Guadalupe and Virgin of Solitude in Mexico (Maynard, 1988).

Three important elements enter into Marian devotions: (1) veneration, or the reverent recognition of the dignity of Mary, who is considered an unparalleled intercessor as well as patroness of many Latin American countries; (2) invocation or the calling upon her motherly and protecting role; and (3) imitation or dedication and consecration to her. Every Latin American country has shrines dedicated to her, and she is venerated under multiple titles (i.e., Marian avocations):

Inmaculado Corazón de María (Mexico)
Nuestra Señora de Altagracia (Chile)
Nuestra Señora de Chiquinquira (Colombia)
Nuestra Señora de la Paz (El Salvador)

Nuestra Señora de la Presentation del Quinche (Ecuador)
Nuestra Señora del Rosario (Ecuador)
Nuestra Señora de Suyapa (Honduras)
Nuestra Señora del Valle del Espíritu Santo; Virgen de Coromato (Venezuela)
Virgen de la Caridad del Cobre (Cuba)
Virgen de Copacabana (Bolivia)
Virgen de Lujan (Argentina)

In almost all shrines and places of pilgrimage, one finds votive offerings to symbolize gratitude for healing miracles. These include photos, crutches, clothing, parts of the human body carved out of wood or wax, manacles, chains, and other artifacts as symbols of the restoration of life obtained through the influence of Mary (Stevens-Arroyo, 1998).

So far we have reviewed the historical and religious aspects of folk saint and Marian devotions. We will now apply our psychological understanding of devotional practices and their importance in healing. We offer some practical suggestions on how to conceptualize religious devotional expressions and how to use them in counseling.

A PSYCHOLOGICAL UNDERSTANDING OF HEALING MEDIATED BY DEVOTIONAL PRACTICES

The scientific study of the phenomenon of saints, especially in psychology, is limited to a few studies. Haidt and Algoe (2003) have investigated moral appraisals and emotions associated with a "good event condition" (i.e., saints or people demonstrating humanity's higher or better nature), a "bad deed condition" (i.e., demons and villains, someone demonstrating humanity's lower or worse condition) and found that participants in the good event condition reported feeling happy, wanting to celebrate, and wanting to tell others about their good fortune or good feelings. The authors called this "elevation and admiration toward saints and heroes" (p. 330) and defined elevation as a broader emotion than simply awe—specifically awe at a display of moral beauty. Conversely, the bad deed condition reported a mix of self-labeled anger and disgust. White (1982) has examined extrasensory perception (ESP)—which has implications for healing powers—among 2,532 Catholic saints and found that ESP phenomena among the saints was no different from what is reported in modern cases of saintly figures, and that most of the historical saints reported telepathy, clairvoyance, precognition, and out-of-body experience. White also found that saints had some degree of volitional control of ESP and that this may have been associated with the degree to which they had advanced in their mystical lives. These studies are peripheral to the purposes of this chapter, but suggest the need to further research the relationship between devotion to the saints and psychological well-being and health. Surprisingly, given the importance of saint veneration in faith healing, we did not find studies investigating the psychological variables influencing the healing process.

Our theorizing has lead us to believe that significant psychological concepts, which include constructs studied by positive psychology (e.g., hope, optimism, perseverance, humility, forgiveness, peace of mind, trust), the role of prayer (e.g., prayer of gratitude, supplication, adoration), locus of control (i.e., belief in powerful others) may have healing promoting effects in devotees to the saints and the Virgin Mary. Based on our extensive analysis of the literature on saint veneration and popular Marian devotions, and due to the lack of psychological research on this important topic, we have created eight domains of folk saint devotion to give expression to what we believe are the main multidimensional characteristics of devotional practices. These domains may be helpful when working with individuals and families who identify their religious and devotional practices as an important dimension of their life. Taken together, these domains provide a nice structure with which to build a better understanding of devotional practices and the client's issues. See Table 2.1 for a summary of the main hypothesized dimensions of devotional practices and psychological constructs likely influencing the healing process.

FOLK VENERATION AND DEVOTION ORIENTATIONS

Intercessory Communalism

Veneration of the saints and the Virgin Mary is based on the belief of intercession (Latin *intercede*, "to interpose"), which refers to going or coming between two parties, to pleading before one of them on behalf of the other. Intercession fosters a sense of community and fellowship. Psychological research on the benefits of spirituality and religiousness has found that believers benefit from a sense of community and

Table 2.1 Hypothesized Salutogenic Components of Folk Saint Veneration and Marian Devotion

Characteristics	Healing Promoting Psychological Constructs
Intercessory communalism	Sense of community; locus of control (Fiori, Brown, Cortina, & Antonucci, 2006; Jackson & Coursey, 1988); prayer (Byrd, 1988); optimism (Salsman, Brown, Brechting, & Carlson, 2005)
Promissory fideism	Reciprocity; trust (Village, 2005); gratitude (Emmons & McCullough, (2003)
Folkloric devotionalism	Devotion (Curlin & Moschovis, 2004); respect; faith (Chirban, 1991)
Experiential sacramentalism	Public experiential religiosity (Husaini, Blasi, & Miller, 1999)
Aesthetic pietism	Awe (Keltner & Haidt, 2003)
Magic realism	Cognitive flexibility (Gaynor, 1999); holistic worldview (Peng & Nisbett, 2000)
Spiritual syncretism	Openness to religious experience; receptivity to pluralistic therapies (Belliard & Ramirez-Johnson, 2005)
Liberative ritualism	Hope (Snyder, 2002); spiritual surrender (Cole & Pargament, 1999); meaning in life (Steger & Frazier, 2005)

social support. Devotees to the saints have often expressed a strong spiritual bonding with supernatural companions and guardians, especially in times of distress and sickness. They optimistically place their faith in external sources of strength and support. From the perspective of positive psychology, this may bring about healthful and psychologically beneficial effects.

A client may benefit from perceived support of the saints or the Virgin Mary, and reverential practices can also benefit family cohesion as they join to participate in ceremonies and traditions associated with various holy days (Wolf & Stevens, 2001). Highlighting the importance of the communalism experienced among humans ("horizontal mutuality") and between humans and the divine ("vertical mutuality"), Davis has described devotional practices as "rites of revitalization" because "they revitalize a relationship to the holy patron involved, and they revive human bonds because these rites are familial or communal" (1992, p. 147).

Promissory Fideism

Often faith (Latin *fides*) in the supplication for the intercession has the form of a transactional, contractual, and reciprocal relationship between the saint and the faithful. The supplicant is aware of his dependence on the intercessory advocacy of the saint and makes a promise (*manda*) to the saint in an exchange for a favor. Mandas are initiated for events and circumstances over which humans are thought to have no control (Gudeman, 1988). Most devotees experience an indeptedness and fulfill their promises through pilgrimages to a shrine, the offering of ex-votos (votive offerings), and amends (moral or behavioral commitments). The supplicant is usually aware of the obligatory aspect of the relationship, and willingly enters into a covenant with the saint or with Mary. Several psychological variables play a role in the execution of a manda, including personal determination of need, form of request, choice of saint, selecting of offering, dependence upon faith, personal assessment of success and use of cultural skills (Gudeman, 1988).

Folkloric Devotionalism

Curlin & Moschovis (2004) have recommended engaging in a dialogue with religiously devout patients and find that for the devout, no dimension of life is unaffected by religious and devotional beliefs. They emphasize the salutary effects of devotions. Processions, pilgrimages, novenas, private household shrines, and other religious expressions are often imbued with a spirit of profound faith, hope, respect, veneration, self-surrender, and celebratory joy. Devotionalism ascribed to the saints is characterized by ritualistic ceremonies that are highly conducive to the expression of emotions.

Experiential Sacramentalism

The believer or follower of folk saints experiences and sees the world through sacramental "templates." Veneration practices often include vocal, visual, and tactile involvement in both the articulation of prayers and interaction with symbols and statues. Octavec (1995) has attributed beneficial effects to devotional practices involving saint veneration (e.g., invocations, processions, and milagros). She notes that devotees experience healing results because they perceive devotional practices as efficacious. Saint veneration helps sick people to integrate into their communities, resulting in social approval that enhances their feelings of self-worth. They are able to strengthen family

ties through celebration of saints when they engage in pleasant conversations and festive activities. Some people report a
feeling of self-mastery because it fulfills their emotional need
to do something to try to effect a cure. Most people have a
feeling of spiritual partnership with powerful partners (i.e.,
saints) responsible for bringing the cure that lightens their
emotional and psychological burdens. Most important, they
report a strengthening of their faith by witnessing saint statues covered with symbolism that often has a tremendous emotional impact that instills hope.

Aesthetic Pietism

We use the term *pietism* to highlight the piety, reverence,
or devoutness invested in the expressive "visual rhetoric"
(Pineda, 2004, p. 366) found in the art associated with saint
veneration. Anyone who has been exposed to the veneration
of folk saints at public shrines or private home altars immediately notices the emphasis placed on the aesthetics surrounding this devotional practice. Historically, intricately
artistic detailed work has been consecrated to the veneration
of saints. For example, the *plateresque* and *churriqueresque*
baroque style is the apotheosis of aesthetic pietism in Latin
America, with elaborate frontispieces and highly decorative
entablatures and altars to honor the saints and Mary. Plaster
statues are very realistic, with detailed facial features and, in
the case of crucifixes, with artificial blood dripping from gap-
ing wounds.

The importance of awe has been researched by psychologists in relation to the experience of the supernatural. Religious
awe seems to reprogram people, making them more pious and
more prosocial, with little concern for material wealth, reputation, or other petty concerns of daily life (Keltner & Haidt,
2001). Researchers have also found that religious aesthetic
awe helps one to transcend the self and become absorbed in
something larger than oneself. Grundler (1922, cited in Wulff,
1997) discussed classes of art that often facilitate religious
transcendence, and included religious art and the testimony
of people—particularly saintly people—as occasions of religious awe.

Hahn (1997) studied shrines and iconographic representations of sanctity and coined the expression "rhetoric of
sanctity" to describe visual and verbal hagiographic constructions of holiness and their intended effect on the faithful.
Ornamentation of shrines (lamps, altars, vessels, draperies and

cloths, frescoes, marble columns, and reliquaries of precious materials) and everything associated with them is carefully orchestrated because they represent a saint's connectedness and presence in the midst of the community. The tangible representation invites intimacy and touch.

Magic Realism

We have adopted the term *magic realism* for our description of one of the dimensions of the saint veneration phenomenon for several cultural reasons. This term has a prominent cultural significance for Latinas/os and their worldview as expressed in art and literature; after all, some of the main literary masterpieces in Latina/o culture (Cervantes's *Don Quijote*, Marquez's *One Hundred Years of Solitude*, the works of Rulfo) used magic realist techniques. Contrasted with realism (empiricism, logic, naturalism, rationalization), *magic realism* relies on myth and legend, fantasy, mysticism, magic, meta-narration, romanticism, and imagination. Magic realism involves "the fusion of the real and the fantastic." It offers a worldview that is not limited to natural or physical laws nor only understood through empiricist, mechanistic, objective, and positivist notions. The world of the magic realist is mysterious and enchanted with the presence of saints, angels, and miracles. Magic realists find the transformation of the common and the everyday into the awesome and the unreal (Flores, 1955). It refers "to the occurrence of supernatural, or anything that is contrary to our conventional view of reality" (Chanady, 1985, p. 16). Magic realism "naturalizes the supernatural; that is to say, a mode in which real and fantastic, natural and supernatural, are coherently represented in a state of rigorous equivalence—neither has a greater claim to truth or referentiality" (Warnes, 2005, p. 2). In the magic realist world, time is not linear, causality is subjectively experienced, and the magical and the ordinary are one.

Spiritual Eclecticism

Through a creative and dialectical process, the faith of believers in folk saints has created an eclectic and inclusive devotional worldview in which the saints of official Christianity mingle with the outlaws who champion the populace. One can surmise cognitive flexibility that allows the coexistence of otherwise incompatible belief systems. The invocation of supernatural helpers, whether saints or villains, is equally permissible and the spiritual boundaries that traditionally separated the earthly from the spiritual, the physical from the supernatural, can be easily crossed, as in the case of miraculous healing. Likewise, the supposed moral boundaries of systems of law or economics thought unjust are equally permeable. An intimacy can be established with spirits through mediumship and the souls of the departed can be experienced emotionally and psychologically (e.g., visitation dreams).

Liberative Ritualism

Griffith suitably notes the liberative character of folk saint veneration because:

> traditional folk or popular Catholicism, with its daily and seasonal rituals, its multitude of saints upon whom one may call, and its means of coping with the results of human nastiness, provides many working-class people with what they feel they need... folk Catholicism, with its decidedly pragmatic nature and its wealth of potential Heavenly helpers, serves this purpose. (2003, p. 11)

Devotion and confidence in folk saints provides a source of hope and meaning in people's lives. Religious rituals can facilitate psychological healing and personal integration.

With sound clinical judgment, the counselor can support the client's participation in moving and reassuring rituals, the practice of private devotions and meditative exercises. To the extent that these reverential practices facilitate subjective well-being, the counselor can support and foster spiritual growth (Helminiak, 2001).

Finally, saints are cultural heroes. Their lives and legends are sources of a particular society's teaching about the archetypal man or woman as well as proper relationships within families and communities. Devotees look to the struggles of their favorite saints for examples. It is not difficult for a therapist to question a client about what she thinks a patron saint might have done under similar circumstances, or what favorite stories from the saint's lives may illuminate the client's present situation.

WORKING WITH A DEVOTEE

Miguel is a 45-year-old Mexican American man recently diagnosed with cancer. He was referred to counseling because he has been experiencing considerable distress. In counseling sessions he reports feeling fearful, worried, and panicky. He mentions that he has been unmotivated to pursue his medical treatment. He has been praying to the ánima of El Niño Fidencio and has made a *promesa* (*promise*) to the saint that if he gets better he will make a pilgrimage to El Ezpinazo, a famous Mexican pilgrimage shrine dedicated to El Niño. Recently he prayed to El Niño in the presence of a *materia* (medium) and reported having a beatific vision. Miguel reports that he saw El Niño in the presence of angels, other saints, and the Virgin. At one point, the Virgin reportedly gave El Niño a bowl of water for Miguel to drink. Miguel reports that the water made him feel better (e.g., less tired, less painful in the area of the tumor, and more alert). He indicates that he prays to El Niño every Sunday at the local church, though the chaplain has tried to dissuade him from "worshiping idols" and from believing in "superstitions."

Though he expresses feeling irritated at what he considers insensitivity by church officials, he mentions that he will continue to participate in the *Fidencista* (belivers in El Niño) group rituals because this is very uplifting for him. In one counseling session he showed the counselor a prayer card he carries with him (and the prayer he recites several times a day) along with a blessed scapular to invoke the presence of El Niño.

An informal assessment of the eight veneration and devotion orientations can be obtained by listening and by asking specific information.

1. *Intercessory Communalism.* Listen for the sense of rapport and community with the saints and the Virgin Mary and be aware of the client's hope and optimism attributed to the intercessory power of saints. Adopt an open attitude toward the client's identification with specific features of the saint's patronage (e.g., power to heal a particular ailment) and explore the therapeutic value of this devotional relationship.

2. *Promissory Fideism.* Listen to the sense of trust that is placed in the religious interaction with supernatural beings. Appreciate the level of reciprocity, faith, and gratitude involved in the devotional practice and how these generalize in other domains of the life of the devotee. Pay close attention to the cognitive dynamics of agency, causality, and animacy expressed in the relationship between devotee and saint or supernatural being.

3. *Folkloric Devotionalism.* Listen for specific metaphors or linguistic expressions and devotional behaviors used to

connect and express reverence to the saints (e.g., prayer cards, incantations, medals, and scapulars).

4. *Experiential Sacramentalism.* Listen to how the client describes his experience of devotion. Facilitate the client's participation in visual and tangible devotional practices that involve the transcendent and divine.

5. *Aesthetic Pietism.* Listen for how the devotee expresses awe, piety, and deep emotion related to saint veneration. Note how this piety is aesthetically expressed, and acknowledge the emotional impact and meaning of religious artistic expression (e.g., statues and images).

6. *Magic Realism.* Listen to how the person relates to the supernatural and the powers attributed to the miraculous, the sacred, or the divine. Be aware of references to mystery (e.g., apparitions, dream visitations) and appreciate the use of intuition, imagination, and the possibility of the extraordinary.

7. *Spiritual Eclecticism.* Listen to how the person makes sense of the interrelationships between the different planes of reality (celestial, spiritual, corporal, divine, and human). Attend to how the client integrates different theologies and belief systems to describe devotional experiences.

8. *Liberative Ritualism.* Listen to how God and the saints are depicted. Recognize that some clients may identify with a particular altruistic and humanitarian attribute of a saint. Are the saints and heavenly helpers depicted as kind, gracious, and benevolent beings who faithfully and lovingly get involved in human affairs to heal and to liberate, or to punish and to avenge? How affectively laden are the client's rituals and devotional practices? How did the venerated person deal with similar situations in his life, and what can the client learn from his hero's behavior under similar circumstances?

CONCLUSION

Our review of the literature on saint veneration indicates that miraculous healing has been attributed to the saints and the Virgin Mary since Christian antiquity. Given the importance of this phenomenon in the Latina/o community, and in multicultural populations, it is surprising that more psychological research has not been conducted on this topic. There is a need for interdisciplinary research to study the relationship between devotional practices and health and healing.

The Catholic Church, with its long history of canonization and official investigations into claims of miraculous healing, has rigorously researched the scientific and medical aspects of healing attributed to "official" saints. Similar studies and investigations into popular claims of healing mediated by folk saints could potentially advance our understanding of the role of faith, prayer, hope, and other important psychological concepts in healing.

From a psychological perspective, we suggest that some psychological variables linking the devotional spiritualities may have salutogenic effects on devotees. These potential relationships deserve additional research. Faith-based healing seems to be viewed as increasingly relevant in psychological and psychiatric settings. Recent resurgence of interest in religiousness and spirituality has contributed to a growing body of empirical research examining the connections between religious faith and healing. For instance, higher levels of religious commitment are generally associated with lower levels of depression, anxiety, suicidality, and substance abuse, as well as higher levels of self-esteem, marital satisfaction, hope and meaning, social support, life satisfaction, and positive coping strategies for stress (Ferraro & Albrecht-Jensen, 1991).

We hypothesize that a genuine religious devotion, with internalized attitudes of faith, forgiveness, trust, reciprocity, acceptance, optimism, and hope in the saints and the Virgin Mary, may be related to healthy experiences among Latinas/os.

NOTES

1. A miracle is defined as "an extraordinary event, perceptible to the senses, produced by God in a religious context as a sign of the supernatural" (Pater, 1967, p. 890). Miracles constitute a strong proof of someone's sanctity, and the rigorous process of canonization includes theological, juridical, historical, and scientific verification to ensure that miracles are only explained through supernatural causes. In the cases of prodigious healing or miraculous medical recoveries, medical experts are consulted (Carter, 1959; Hardon, 1954).

2. The theme of the *puer senex*, or aged youth, is recurrent in hagiographic texts, in which the alteration of the normal *cursus aetatis* (stages of life), or *aetatis hominis* (ages of man) has its origin in divine intervention. Often a divine

power to heal is conferred; Kieckhefer & Bond (1988) note
that "there were saints who cried out from the womb, stood
upright at birth, jumped to the baptismal font and dipped
themselves in the water, learned the basics of writing in
three days, were born with monastic tonsures, or toddled
off to monasteries as soon as they learned to walk" (p. 23).
Turner and Turner (1978, p. 71) have found that a *cultus*
or veneration of *Niños* (the Child Jesus under different
avocations) abound in Latin American Catholicism and
that people often kiss and touch images and statues of the
Child Jesus, suggesting a belief in "the tactile transmission of grace" and healing.

REFERENCES

Aguilar, A. (1977). *Miguel Martos y la difunta Correa*. San Juan,
   Argentina: Editorial Sanjuanina.
Alvarez, F. R. (1967). *Una nueva versión sobre la Difunta Cor-
   rea* [A new version of La Difunta Correa]. San Juan: Edito-
   rial Sanjuanina.
Anzoátegui, Y. (1975). *Difunta Correa: devoción, milagros y ora-
   ciones* [Difunta Correa: Devotion, miracles, and prayers].
   Buenos Aires: Editorial S.A.G.A.
Appendini, G. (2001). *Refranes populares de México* [Popular
   proverbs of Mexico]. Mexico City, Mexico: Editorial Porrúa.
Belliard, J. C., & Ramirez-Johnson, J. (2005). Medical plural-
   ism in the life of a Mexican immigrant woman. *Hispanic
   Journal of Behavioral Sciences, 27*, 267–285.
Ben-Ami, I. (1998). *Saint-veneration among the Jews in Morocco*.
   Detroit, MI: Wayne State University Press.
Binde, P. (2001). Nature in Roman Catholic tradition. *Anthro-
   pological Quarterly, 74*, 15–27.
Bock, E. W. (1966). Symbols in conflict: Official versus folk
   religion. *Journal for the Scientific Study of Religion, 5*,
   204–212.
Bond, G. D. (1988). The Arahant: Sainthood in Theravāda Bud-
   dhism. In R. Kieckhefer & G. D. Bond (Eds.), *Sainthood: Its
   manifestations in world religions* (pp. 140–171). Berkeley:
   University of California Press.
Brown, P. (1981). *The cult of the saints: Its rise and function in
   Latin Christianity*. Chicago: University of Chicago Press.
Brownson, O. A. (1963). *Saint-worship: The worship of Mary*.
   Patterson, NJ: Saint Anthony Guild Press.

Bynum, C. W. (1990). Material continuity, personal survival, and the resurrection of the body: A scholastic discussion in its medieval and modern contexts. *History of Religions, 30*, 51–85.

Byrd, R. C. (1988). Positive therapeutic effects of intercessory prayer in a coronary care unit population. *Southern Medical Journal, 81*, 826–829.

Carter, J. C. (1959). The recognition of miracles. *Theological Studies, 20*, 175–197.

Chanady, A. B. (1985). *Magical realism and the fantastic. Resolved versus unresolved antimonies.* New York: Garland.

Chertudi, S., & Newbery, S. J. (1978). *La difunta Correa.* Buenos Aires, Argentina: Editorial Huemul.

Chicas-Rendón, O. (1995). *Recetario y oraciones secretas de Maximón* [Recipes and secret prayers of Maximón]. Guatemala City, Guatemala: Author.

Chicas-Rendón, O. (2001). *Maximón: testimonios de fe* [Maximón: Testimonials of faith]. Guatemala City, Guatemala: Ediciones Ebano.

Chirban, J. T. (1991). *Health and faith: Medical, psychological and religious dimensions.* Lanham, MD: University Press of America.

Christian, W. A., Jr. (1981). *Local religion in sixteenth-century Spain.* Princeton, NJ: Princeton University Press.

Cohn, R. L. (1988). Sainthood on the periphery: The case of Judaism. In R. Kieckhefer & G. D. Bond (Eds.), *Sainthood: Its manifestations in world religions* (pp. 43–68). Berkeley: University of California Press.

Cole, B. S. S., & Pargament, K. I. (1999). Spiritual surrender: A paradoxical path to control. In W. R. Miller (Ed.), *Integrating spirituality into treatment: Resources for practitioners* (pp. 179–198). Washington, DC: American Psychological Association.

Cornell, V. J. (1998). *Realm of the saint: Power and authority in Moroccan Sufism.* Austin: University of Texas Press.

Curlin, F. A., & Moschovis, P. P. (2004). Is religious devotion relevant to the doctor-patient relationship? *Journal of Family Practice, 53*, 632–636.

Davis, K. (1992). A return to the roots: Conversion and the culture of the Mexican-Descent Catholic, 40, 3, 139–158.

De la Torre, M. A., & Aponte, E. D. (2001). *Latino/a theologies.* Maryknoll, NY: Orbis Books.

Denny, F. M. (1988). "God's friends": The sanctity of persons in Islam. In R. Kieckhefer & G. D. Bond (Eds.), *Sainthood: Its manifestations in world religions* (pp. 69–97). Berkeley: University of California Press.

Dodson, R. (1994). *Don Pedro Jaramillo: "curandero."* Corpus Christi, Texas: Henrietta Newbury.

Douillet, J. (1960). *What is a saint?* New York: Hawthorn Books.

Edberg, M C. (2001). Drug traffickers as social bandits: Culture and drug trafficking in northern Mexico and the border region. *Journal of Contemporary Criminal Justice, 17,* 259–277.

Emmons, R. A., & McCullough, M. W. (2003). Counting blessings versus burdens: Experimental studies of gratitude and subjective well-being in daily life. *Journal of Personality and Social Psychology, 84,* 377–389.

Espin, O. (1995). Tradition and popular religion: An understanding of the Sensus Fidelium. In A. J. Bañuelas (Ed.), *Mestizo Christianity: Theology from the Latino perspective* (pp. 148–176). Maryknoll, NY: Orbis Books.

Espin, O. (1997). *The faith of the people: Theological reflections on popular catholicism.* Maryknoll, NY: Orbis Books.

Farfan-Morales, O. (1997). *El Fidencismo: La curación espiritista* [Fidencism: Spiritualist healing]. Monterrey, Mexico: Archivo General del Estado.

Ferraro, K. F., & Albrecht-Jensen, C. M. (1991). Does religion influence adult health? *Journal for the Scientific Study of Religion, 30,* 193–202.

Figueroa-Deck, A. (1994). Latino theology: The year of the "boom." *Journal of Hispanic/Latino Theology, 1,* 51–63.

Finkler, K. (1985). *Spiritualist healers in Mexico: Successes and failures of alternative Therapeutics.* New York: Bergen and Garvey.

Finucane, R. C. (1977). *Miracles and pilgrims: Popular beliefs in medieval England.* Totowa, NJ: Rowman and Littlefield.

Fiori, K., Brown, E. E., Cortina, K. S., & Antonucci, T. C. (2006). Locus of control as a mediator of the relationship between religiosity and life satisfaction: Age, race, and gender differences. *Mental Health, Religion and Culture, 9,* 239–263.

Flores, A. (1955). Magical realism in Spanish American fiction. *Hispania, 38,* 187–192.

Galanter, M. (1999). *Cults: Faith, healing, and coercion.* New York: Oxford University Press.

Garijo-Guembe, M. M., & Madigan, P. (1994). *Communion of the saints: Foundation, nature, and structure of the church.* Collegeville, MN: Michael Glazier Books.

Gaynor, D. R. (1999). *Changes in cognitive structure associated with experiences of spiritual transformation (transcendente).* Unpublished doctoral dissertation, Institute of Transpersonal Psychology, Palo Alto, CA.

Gebara, I., & Bingemer, M. C. (1987). *Mary, Mother of God, Mother of the Poor.* Maryknoll, NY: Orbis Books.

George, K., & George, C. H. (1955). Roman Catholic sainthood and social status a statistical and analytical study. *Journal of Religion, 35,* 85–98.

Goizueta, R. S. (1996). U.S. Hispanic popular Catholicism as theopoetics. In A. M. Isai-Díaz & F. F. Segovia (Eds.), *Hispanic/Latino theology* (pp. 261–288). Minneapolis: Fortress Press.

Goizueta, R. S. (2004). The symbolic realism of U.S. Latino/a popular Catholicism. *Theological Studies, 65,* 255–274.

Graef, H. (1985). *Mary: A history of doctrine and devotion.* London: Sheed and Ward.

Graziano, F. (2006). Cultures of devotion: Folk saints of Spanish America. *Oxford: Oxford University Press.*

Griffith, J. S. (1992). *Beliefs and holy places.* Tucson: University of Arizona Press.

Griffith, J. S. (2000). *Saints of the Southwest.* Tucson, AZ: Rio Nuevo.

Griffith, J. S. (2003). *Folk saints of the borderlands: victims, bandits and healers.* Tucson, AZ: Rio Nuevo.

Grundler, O. (1922). *Elemente zu einer Religionsphilosophie auf phanomenologischer Grundlage.* Munich: Josef Kosel and Friedrich Pustet.

Gudeman, S. (1976). Saints, symbols, and ceremonies. *American Ethnologist, 3,* 709–729.

Gudeman, S. (1988). The manda and the Mass. *Journal of Latin American Lore, 14,* 17–32.

Haidt, J., & Algoe, S. (2003). Moral amplification and the emotions that attach us to saints and demons. In J. Greenberg, S. L. Koole, & T. Pysczynski (Eds.), *Handbook of experimental existential psychology,* pp. 322–335. New York: Guilford Press.

Hahn, C. (1997). Seeing and believing: The construction of sanctity in early-medieval saints' shrines. *Speculum, 72,* 1079–1106.

Hamington, M. (1995). *Hail Mary? The struggle for ultimate womanhood in Catholicism.* New York: Routledge.

Hardon, J. A. (1954). The concept of miracle from St. Augustine to modern apologetics. *Theological Studies, 15*, 229–257.

Helminiak, D. A. (2001). Treating spiritual issues in secular psychotherapy. *Counseling Values, 45*, 163–189.

Husaini, B. A., Blasi, A. J., & Millar, O. (1999). Does public and private religiosity have a moderating effect on depression? A bi-racial study of elders in the American South. *International Journal of Aging and Human Development, 48*, 63–72.

Jackson, L. E., & Coursey, R. D. (1988). The relationship of God and internal locus of control to intrinsic motivation, coping and purpose of life. *Journal for the Scientific Study of Religion, 27*, 399–410.

Jeske, M. W., Root, M., & Smith, D. R. (2004). *Communio sanctorum: The church as the communion of saints.* Collegeville, MN: Liturgical Press.

Johann, F. G. (2003). *Sarita Colonia: la santa ungida por el pueblo* [Sarita Colonia: The saint annointed by the people]. Peru: Sine Nomine.

Kaptchuk, T. J., & Eisenberg, D. M. (2001). Varieties of healing, 2: Taxonomy of unconventional healing practices. *Annals of International Medicine, 135*, 196–204.

Kearney, M. (1978). Espiritualism as an alternative medical tradition in the borderline area. In B. Velimirovic (Ed.), *Modern medicine and medical anthropology in the United States border population* (pp. 67–73). Washington, DC: Pan American Health Organization.

Kearney, M. (1980). Spiritualist healing in Mexico. In P. Morley & R. Wallis (Eds.), *Culture and curing: Anthropological perspectives on traditional medical beliefs and practices.* (pp. 43–46). Pittsburgh: University of Pittsburgh Press.

Kelly, S., & Rogers, R. (1993). *Saints Preserve Us! Everything you need to know about every saint you'll ever need.* New York: Random House.

Keltner, D., & Haidt, J. (2003). Approaching awe, a moral, spiritual, and aesthetic emotion. *Cognition and Memory, 17*, 297–314.

Kieckhefer, R. (1988). Imitators of Christ: Sainthood in the Christian tradition. In R. Kieckhefer & G. D. Bond (Eds.), *Sainthood. Its manifestations in world religions* (pp. 1–42). Berkeley: University of California Press.

Kieckhefer, R., & Bond, G. D. (1988). *Sainthood: Its manifestations in world religions.* Berkeley: University of California Press.

Klapp, O. E. (1949). The folk hero. *Journal of American Folklore, 62,* 17–25.

Lecuna, Y. (1987). *Bolívar y la historia en la conciencia popular* [Bolívar and history in the popular consciousness]. Caracas, Venezuela: Universidad Simón Bolívar.

Lopez, D. S. (1988). Santification on the Bodhisattva path. In R. Kieckhefer & G. D. Bond (Eds.), *Sainthood: Its manifestations in world religions* (pp. 172–217). Berkeley: University of California Press.

López-Sánchez, S. (1996). Malverde, un bandido generoso [Malverde, a generous bandit]. *Fronteras, 1,* 32–40.

Low, S. M. (1988a). Medical doctor, popular saint: The syncretic symbolism of Ricardo Moreno Cañas and José Gregorio Hernández. *Journal of Latin American Lore, 14,* 49–66.

Low, S. M. (1988b). The medicalization of healing cults in Latin America. *American Ethnologist, 15,* 136–154.

Ludlow, M. (2001). *Universal salvation: Eschatology in the thought of Gregory of Nyssa and Karl Rahner.* New York: Oxford University Press.

Macklin, B. J., & Crumrine, R. (1973). Three north Mexican folk saint movements. *Comparative Studies in Society and History, 15,* 89–105.

Macklin, J. (1974). Belief, ritual and healing: New England spiritualism and Mexican American spiritism compared. In I. I. Zaretsky & M. P. Leone (Eds.), *Religious movements in contemporary America* (pp. 383–417). Princeton, NJ: Princeton University Press.

Macklin, J. (1978). Curanderismo and espiritismo: Complementary approaches to traditional health services. In B. Velimirovic (Ed.), *Modern medicine and medical anthropology in the United States-Mexico border population* (pp. 155–163). Washington, DC: Pan American Health Organization.

Macklin, J. (1988). Two faces of sainthood: The pious and the popular. *Journal of Latin American Lore, 14,* 67–91.

Macklin, J., & Margolies, L. (1988). Saints, near-saints, and society. *Journal of Latin American Lore, 14,* 5–16.

Marceron, J. E. (2002). *Dictionnaire des saints imaginaries et facétieux* [Dictionary of imaginary and humorous saints]. Paris: Seuil.

Margolies, L. (1988). The canonization of a Venezuelan folk saint: The case of José Gregorio Hernández. *Journal of Latin American Lore, 14*, 93–110.

Marsch, M., & Maloney, L. M. (1989). *Healing through the Sacraments.* Collegeville, MN: Liturgical Press.

Martin, J. (2006). *My life with the saints.* Chicago, IL: Loyola Press.

Massolo, M. L. (1995). *Gracias Difunta Correa! Popular devotion and tactics of belonging in Argentina.* Unpublished doctoral disseration, University of California–Berkeley.

Maynard, E. (1988). The Virgin of Solitude: Viability of a Mexican cult. *Journal of Latin American Lore, 14*, 111–121.

Mejido, M. J. (1999). Theoretical prolegomenon to the sociology of U.S. Hispanic popular religion. *Journal of Hispanic/Latino Theology, 7*, 27–55.

Mejido, M. J. (2001). A critique of the "aesthetic turn" in U.S. Hispanic theology: A dialogue with Roberto Goizueta and the Positing of a New Paradigm. *Journal of Hispanic/Latino Theology, 8*, 18–48.

Nájera, F. (1993). *Imán de su silencio: homenaje a nuestro senor Maximón* [Magnet of his silence: Homage to our lord Maximón]. Guatemala City, Guatemala: Ediciones del Caldejo.

Octavec, E. (1995). *Answered prayers. Miracles and milagros along the border.* Tucson: University of Arizona Press.

Orsi, R. A. (1998). *Thank you, St. Jude: Women's devotion to the patron saint of hopeless causes.* New Haven, CT: Yale University Press.

Orsi, R. A. (2005). The cult of the saints and the reimagination of the space and time of sickness in twentieth-century American Catholicism. In L. L. Barnes & S. S. Sered (Eds.), *Religion and Healing in America* (pp. 28-47). Oxford, England: Oxford University Press.

Pater, T. G. (1967). *New Catholic encyclopedia.* New York: McGraw-Hill.

Pédron-Colombani, S. (2004). *Maximón: Guatemalan god, saint, or traitor?* London: Periplus.

Peng, K., & Nisbett, R. E. (2000). Culture, control, and perception of relalationships in the environment. *Journal of Personality and Social Psychology, 78*, 943–955.

Pérez-Pardella, A. (1975). *La difunta Correa.* Buenos Aires: Plus Ultra.

Pieper, J. (2002). *Guatemala's folk saints: Maximon/San Simon, Rey Pascual, Judas, Lucifer and others*. Los Angeles, CA: Author.

Pineda, A. M. (2004). Imagenes de dios en el camino: retablos, ex-votos, milagritos, and murals. *Theological Studies, 65*, 364–379.

Pollak-Eltz, A. (1988). Anima worship in Venezuela. *Journal of Latin American Lore, 14*, 33–48.

Romano, O. I. (1965). Charismatic medicine, folk-healing, and folk-sainthood. *American Anthropologist, 67*, 1151–1173.

Salsean, J. M., Brown, T. L., Brechting, E. H., & Carlson, C. R. (2005). The link between religion and spirituality and psychological adjustment: The mediating role of optimism and social support. *Personality and Social Psychology Bulletin, 31*, 522–535.

Schouppe, F. X. (1983). *Purgatory: Explained by the lives and legends of the saints*. Rockford, IL: Tan Books.

Snyder, C. R. (2002). Hope theory: Rainbows in the mind. *Psychological Inquiry, 13*, 249–275.

Steger, M. F., & Frazier, P. (2005). Meaning of life: One link in the chain from religiousness to well-being. *Journal of Counseling Psychology, 52*, 574–582.

Stevens-Arroyo, A. M. S. (1998). The evolution of Marian devotionalism within Christianity and the Ibero-Mediterranean polity. *Journal for the Scientific Study of Religion, 37*, 50–73.

Talbot, A. M. (2002). Pilgrimage to healing shrines: The evidence of miracle accounts. *Dumbarton Oaks Papers, 56*, 153–173.

Taylor, R. L. (1988). The sage as saint: The Confucian tradition. In R. Kieckhefer & G. D. Bond (Eds.), *Sainthood: Its manifestations in world religions* (pp. 218–242). Berkeley: University of California Press.

Taylor, W. B. (1987). The Virgen of Guadalupe in New Spain: An inquiry into the social history of Marian devotion. *American Ethnologist, 14*, 9–33.

Thompson, J. (1998). Santisima Muerte: On the origin and development of a Mexican occult image. *Journal of the Southwest, 40*(4), 405.

Tilley, M. A. (1991). The ascetic body and the (un) making of the world of the martyr. *Journal of the American Academy of Religion, 59*, 467–479.

Torre, J. L. (1973). *La difunta correa* [The deceased correa]. San Juan, Argentina: Editorial Sanjuanina.

Turner, V., & Turner, E. (1978). *Image and pilgrimage in Christian culture: Anthropological perspectives.* New York: Columbia University Press.

Vanderwood, P. (2001). Juan Soldado: Field notes and reflections. *Journal of the Southwest, 43*(4), 729.

Vanderwood, P. J. (2004). *Juan Soldado: rapist, murderer, martyr, saint.* Durham, NC: Duke University Press.

Village, A. (2005). Dimensions of belief about miraculous healing. *Mental Health, Religion and Culture, 8,* 97–107.

Wald, E. (2001). *Narcocorrido: A journey into the music of drugs, guns and guerrillas.* New York: HarperCollins.

Walliss, J. (2001). Continuing bonds: Relationships between the living and the dead within contemporary spiritualism. *Mortality, 6,* 127–145.

Warnes, C. (2005). Naturalizing the supernatural: Faith, irreverence and magical realism. *Literature Compass, 106,* 1–16.

Watanabe, J. M. (1990). From saints to Shibboleths: Image, structure, and identity in Maya religious syncretism. *American Ethnologist, 17,* 131–150.

Wedig, M. E. (2001). The visual hermeneutics of Hispanic/Latino popular religion and the recovery of the image in Christian praxis. *Journal of Hispanic/Latino Theology, 8,* 6–17.

White, C. S. J. (1988). Indian developments in Hinduism. In R. Kieckhefer & G. D. Bond (Eds.), *Sainthood: Its manifestations in world religions* (pp. 98–139). Berkeley: University of California Press.

White, R. A. (1982). An analysis of ESP phenomena in the saints. *Parapsychology Review, 13,* 15–18.

Wilson, S. (1983). *Saints and their cults: Studies in Religious Sociology, Folklore and History.* Cambridge, England: Cambridge University Press.

Wolf, C. T., & Stevens, P. (2001). Integrating relation and spirituality in marriage and family counseling. *Counseling and Values, 46,* 66–75.

Woodward, K. L. (1990). *Making saints: How the Catholic Church determines who becomes a saint, who doesn't, and why.* New York: Simon and Schuster.

Wulff, D. M. (1977). *Psychology of religion: Classic and contemporary.* New York: Wiley.

Yronwode, C. (1995). Patron saints for various occupations and conditions. Retrieved September 5, 2006 from http://www.luckymojo.com/patronsaints.html

Zavaleta, A. N. (1998). El Niño Fidencio and the Fidencistas [The Child Fidencio and the Fidencistas]. In W. W. Zellner and M. Petrowsky (Eds.), *Sects, cults, and spiritual communities: A sociological analysis* (pp. 95–115). Westport, CT: Greenwood.

Chapter Three

Santería and the Healing Process in Cuba and the United States

BRIAN W. MCNEILL, EILEEN ESQUIVEL, ARLENE
CARRASCO, AND ROSALILIA MENDOZA

The purpose of this chapter is to examine the religious system known as Santería and the implications for the psychological healing process upon the worldviews of its practitioners. While we review the relevant yet sparse literature in relation to the contemporary practice of Santería, much of the information provided herein is based on our own travels to Cuba and the observation of and participation in religious ceremonies, as well as consultations in both Cuba and the United States. In addition, we present qualitative data on the views of psychological health and utilization of resources for psychological issues from the viewpoints of both healers and practitioners. Our intent is to familiarize the reader with the growing practice of Santería in Latina/o communities and facilitate understanding of the psychological healing process that occurs within Santería in which *Babalawos* and *Santeras/os* serve as psychological healers.

LA RELIGIÓN AND ITS MIGRATION: FROM THE CARIBBEAN TO THE UNITED STATES

Cuba has a multitude of faiths, reflecting the island's diverse heritage, ranging from Catholicism, Protestantism, and Judaism to Santería. After the Cuban Revolution, Cuba became officially atheistic and restricted religious practice. Since 1991, restrictions have been eased and the island was even visited by the Roman Catholic Pope John Paul II in 1998. Today, however, given the ancestry and history of the island, its religious practices are marked by syncretisms. Specifically, Cubans combine the elements of the Catholic belief system with other African faiths; this reflects the practice of Santería.

To millions of practitioners and Santeras/os, Santería or Regla de Ocha is known simply as *La Religión* (The Religion). According to González-Whippler (2001), Santería originated in Nigeria along the banks of the Niger River with the Yoruba people, who were brought to the so-called New World by slave traders more than four centuries ago. With the Yoruba came their religion, known in Cuba as *Lucumí*, and in Brazil as *Macumba* and *Candomblé*. The Cuban Lucumís (Yoruba people), however, were deeply influenced by the iconolatry of their Spanish masters, and hid their religious practices for fear of persecution by identifying their deities with Catholic saints. Thus, Santería represents the syncretism or reconciliation between the two different beliefs of the rites of the Yoruba and the traditions of the Catholic Church.

Santería migrated throughout the Caribbean (e.g., from Cuba to Puerto Rico to the Dominican Republic) and to many other Latin American countries, and eventually made its way to the United States. Currently, it thrives in streets and barrios of Chicago, Los Angeles, and New York (Murphy, 1988). The first African American to be initiated into the Santería priesthood was Oba Osejiman Adefunmi I, born Walter King and initiated in Cuba in 1959. He later founded the Yoruba Temple in New York's Harlem neighborhood. Further supporting the integration of the religion in the states, Judith Gleason was one of the earliest Anglo-American priestesses initiated in the United States (Brandon, 1997). The adoption of the religion by other Latina/o groups demonstrates its continuing evolution. For example, Santerismo, a variant of Puerto Rican *Espiritismo*, emerged in the New York City borough of the Bronx in the mid-1960s and like most contemporary spiritist *centros* (centers) serves a multiethnic clientele (Brandon, 1997). Similarly, the "Latinization" of Santería continues with Chicana/o populations in the Los Angeles area (Dianteill, 2002).

The practice of Santería has a substantial historical and contemporary role in the United States within various Latina/o communities. González-Whippler (2001) conservatively estimates that there are more than a hundred million practitioners of the religion in Latin America and the United States.

Today, Latinas/os will vary in their level of belief and practice ranging from rejecting Santería beliefs to occasional visits to botanicas, seeking a *registro/consulta* (reading) when under stress, to formal initiation and full participation as a way of life (Baez & Hernandez, 2001).

THE RELIGION

Santería is a mixture of magic rites of the Yoruba and the traditions of the Catholic Church, where its practitioners identified their gods and goddesses with the saints rooting from the reconciliation of different belief systems between the slaves and the Spaniards (Gonzalez-Wippler, 1987). In Santería, the deities, known as *Orishas,* oversee each person's life and rule over every force of nature and aspect of human life. Specifically, the Orishas interact with the world and humankind as emissaries of God, or Olodumare—a being comprised of three spirits, Olodumare Nzame, Olofin, and Baba Nkwa. Olodumare is the creator; his two companions assisted with the perfection of life, but Olofin is in charge of earth affairs and is humankind's personal god. The spiritual energy that makes up the universe and provides energy to all life and material things is Olorun, the source of *ashé* (power). Driven by energy and ashé, the Orishas are protective guides that aid their followers, providing direction for a better spiritual and material life. Communication between Orishas and humankind occurs through prayer, ritual, divination, song, rhythms, and trance. To show respect and gratitude, offerings for worship include: food, fruits, candies, honey, tobacco, rum, and animal sacrifices—including turtles, ducks, and goats.

The religion includes an array of Orishas to consult for guidance; each Orisha is known for a particular human trait with specific attributes and is associated with a natural component or "force" (Cárdenas, 1997). Each Orisha also has its own colors and ornaments (e.g., specific *collares*, or necklaces, and *pulsos*, or bracelets), annual dates on which they are worshipped and celebrated, specific prayers, foods, songs, drumbeats, and dances. While there are countless deities, the seven African powers most prominent include Obatala (peace and purity); Eleggua (messenger); Orula (divination); Chango (passion and enemies); Oggun (war and employment), Yemaya (maternity), and Ochun (love). Each deity is also known by the forces of nature it rules over and is associated with a Catholic saint. For example, Yemayá lives and rules over the seas, and is syncretized with Our Lady of Regla. (See Holiday, chapter 9, for a table of the most commonly cited and used Orishas).

Santería notes the various stages of spiritual development by granting members various leveled positions. Babalawos are the highest priests (divine spiritual doctors) of the religion, followed by Santeras/os, priests of Santería. In particular, Babalawos are the chosen children of Orula, the owner of the Table of Ifa, a table consulted and used mainly for complicated situations and initiations. Given the divine role of the Table of Ifa, the Babalawo mainly uses *el okuele*, a long metal chain with eight pieces of coconut rinds. Women cannot attain this position in the religion, and only a select few Santeros are selected for this role. Similarly, but with less power and status, Santeras/os are considered consulting experts on human life who use *los caracoles*, or seashells, for their sessions and provide direction by consulting the various saints for guidance.

The first step toward initiation is acquiring protective *elekes* or *collares* (beaded necklaces). The individual (usually a santera/o) who initiates the new member serves as a guide and later becomes known as his or her *madrina* (godmother) or *padrino* (godfather), and the initiate becomes the Santera/o's *ahijado* (godson) or *ahijada* (goddaughter). The relationship between a Santera/o and the godchild is characterized by the godchild's respect, reverence, and obedience to the godparent and the godparent's protection and guidance of the godchild (González-Whippler, 2001). The second step is the making of Eleggua (the god of crossroads, the messenger of the Orishas) and the warriors (which include Oggun, Ochosi, and Osun, who can foretell danger). These gods will fight and protect the initiate, and are placed in their home to ward off dangers and bad occurrences. Many believers stay in this step and simply continue to receive certain deities as they need them for certain life challenges. In the third step, practitioners can aspire to become Santeras/os by "making saint" (i.e., *haciendo santo*). This ceremony costs thousands of dollars and includes numerous ritualistic daily cleansings, sacrifices, consults, and ceremonies that take place over the course of seven days. During this step, blessed by the Babalowo, the practitioner (*iyabo'*) is first crowned only by the santera/o with a guardian angel or protector of life with one of the main Orishas, which is believed to be assigned at birth. It is at this important point that the diviner calls the spiritual parents and requests direct help and protection for the initiate (the godchild, el *ahijado*). Various steps are followed during and after the ceremony leading to the teaching of interpreting the seashells with an *italero* (someone who has made a lifelong study of the *Diloggun*, the seashell divination system). Moreover, during this ceremony, the iyabo´ is given various deities including Obatala, Ochun, Yemaya, and Chango. As noted by Cárdenas (1997) this ceremony carries a "commitment" to Santería and the gods, by which the believer enters the cult of the Orishas.

People consult Santeras/os for a variety of reasons, including physical illness, nervous conditions, and problems in life. The consultation or registro is very similar to a visit with a psychologist or therapist, as the Santera/o listens, attempts to understand the problem, and identifies appropriate solutions. A typical registro may be conducted by the Santera/o through the Diloggun, or reading of the seashells, through which the Orishas speak to the Santera/o to tell them what the problem is and how to remedy it. The solution may be in the form of a ritual cleansing (*despojo*), a Catholic Mass for the dead, or an animal sacrifice (see Holiday, chapter 6, for a description of La Limpia de San Lazaro). In addition, every Santera/o is a competent herbalist who can cure many diseases. The most common herbs include *pasote*, *Álamo*, *yerbabuena*, *mejorana*, *tártago*, and *albaca* for dispelling negative forces and use in despojos (Gonzalez-Whippler, 2001; Pasquali, 1994). As noted by Brandon (1997), it is not surprising that certain Latinas/os of Cuban descent solicit Santeras/os for help. In them, believers find a healer who shares their language, culture, and worldview, and an individual who describes and explains the problems they have, devising a course of action to address them.

MENTAL HEALTH CARE IN CONTEMPORARY CUBA

As Santería holds a substantial role for many Cubans, health care facilities contribute to the overall well-being of the population. In particular, Cuba has been noted for a highly developed system of health care because its constitution makes health care the responsibility of the government and the right of every citizen (Collinson & Turner, 2002). However, this system has been criticized as often limited to treating tourists and foreigners who visit the island. More specifically, the system has been noted for its limited resources and medication in the inner towns of the island. The scope of this chapter is not to cover the debate regarding health care access in Cuba, however; instead, we provide an overview of the system, its structure, and identified services, and psychological practices implemented by practitioners in the island.

In this system of national health care, primary care is provided in *consultorios* (clinics), secondary care in *postclinicos* (specialty clinics), and tertiary care in *hospitales* and *institutos* (hospitals and medical institutes). The *consultorios* address approximately 80% of the health problems, emphasizing health promotion. The family physician and nurse live in the neighborhoods adjacent to their *consultorio*. Patients requiring care beyond the scope of the *consultorio* are referred to the *policlinico*, in which care is provided by interdisciplinary teams offering specialty treatment in a variety of areas including psychiatry and psychology (Dresang, Brebeck, Murray, Shallue, & Sullivan-Vedder, 2005).

According to Kristiansen and Soderstrom (1991), Cuban health psychology builds on the fundamental Marxist-Leninist ideology of Cuban society, as the professional psychologist is obliged to work in the service of the working class. Cubans also apply a biopsychosocial model such that biological, psychological, and social aspects are integrated in each person (Kristiansen & Soderstrom, 1991). Thus, contemporary Cuban health psychology represents a preventive and community-oriented psychology in accordance with the general health philosophy of the country as formulated in 1979 by the Grupo Nacional de Psycologia (National Group of Psychology). Thus, Cuban health psychology encompasses health planning, optimal health promotion, disease prevention, research, education, consultation, psychological treatment, and rehabilitation (Kristiansen & Soderstrom, 1991). Psychologists in Cuba function as generalists performing health education, consultation, therapy, teaching, and research. Priority areas from the Grupo Nacional de Psycologia include education of doctors and nurses in the psychosocial aspects of health, programs for optimal health promotion, reducing unwanted pregnancies, promotion of healthy relations and patterns of communication within family units, and working with educational institutions to promote the physical and psychological well-being of school children.

Collinson and Turner (2002) note that Cuban mental health services address the biomedical aspects of mental health and health promotion while integrating social rehabilitation. Treatment modalities are eclectic, combining rehabilitation, social therapies, occupational therapy, and medication. Our communications with Cuban psychologists have confirmed these impressions; psychologists minimize aspects of the individual personality and individual modalities of intervention, with treatment aimed more toward reintegration of the individual into socialist society.

SANTERÍA AS A SYSTEM OF PSYCHOLOGICAL HEALTH CARE

Sandoval (1979) characterizes Santería as a system of mental health care that addresses matters of the soul, while the orthodox health care system deals with matters of the mind. As noted by Sandoval, there is no conflict between the two systems in the eyes of either Santeras/os and Babalawos, and she argues that the religion's ability to provide for the needs of Cubans has been exported to the Cuban American communities in Florida and other parts of the United States.

Santeras/os as Psychological Healers

As mentioned earlier, registros (or consultations) with a Santera/o are common occurrences for the practitioners of Santería. Specifically, it is common to seek out a Santera through personal contacts and to see her at her place of residence. In a private room filled with sacred objects and symbols, the Santera asks the believer to describe what is disturbing him and listens attentively in attempt to understand. Questions vary regarding family, friends, personal history, personal relationships, work, or deceased relatives. When an individual has a specific question, a Santera/o or Babalawo uses the the caracoles or the okuele for an answer. Certain combinations indicate yes, no, or the answer is indeterminate, and the procedure must be repeated. A "homework" assignment in the form of a task or advice (e.g., visit the shrine of San Lazaro) may be prescribed. At the end, a monetary offering is left; some Santeras/os or Babalawos have a specific fee, while others allow one to give donations.

As noted by Sandoval (1979), a Santera/o may diagnose through the caracoles, but also believe in personal intuition developed through experience. In fact, some Santeras/os even have the power to communicate with *los espiritos* (the spirits) and occasionally combine these practices for guidance. In particular, they ask the spirits and gods what the believer needs in order to improve the situation. Moreover, they provide *consejos* (advice) from their wisdom and insight while the believer attentively takes copious notes on how to proceed with the situation and how to respond to it. Concluding the session, the practitioner has discussed the problem, been provided insight and direction regarding the situation, and typically feels a sense of resolution as a result of the encounter coupled with empowerment and a better sense of well-being.

The palpable presence of Santería in Cuba can cause it to be viewed as a practice that is limited to the island, with a select group still ascribing to it upon emigration to the United States. However, Santería is well documented within the U.S. Cuban American community, and has been noted for its spread across continents and cultures. Hence, it is a practice that encompasses various Cuban American practitioners across generations regardless of their race, age, socioeconomic status, or education.

DATA COLLECTION: INTERVIEWS AND OBSERVATIONS

Given the role of Santeras/os for practitioners in their psychological well-being, we examined the lives of 30 Cubans on the island: their main challenges, social support, religious practices, and perceptions toward psychotherapy. Coupling this data, Santeras'/os' and Babalawos' views of mental or psychological health were examined. In particular, 30 formal, structured interviews were conducted over the course of three months, each taking approximately 30 minutes. More extensively, two qualitative interviews were conducted with Babalawos. All interviews were conducted in Havana, Cuba, during two different trips.

To make a comparison, three Cuban and Cuban American Santeras, one Babalowo, and three Cuban American practitioners were interviewed in the United States regarding their practices and views about psychotherapy. One santera had been "in the religion" for more than 30 years and had been initiated as a santera for 14 years; the other two were initiated as santeras only three to four years prior, but had practiced Santería all their lives (30+ years). The Babalowo was in the religion for more than 20 years, and three practitioners' involvement in *Santería* ranged from two to ten years. Numerous observations were also made of their beliefs and practices with their clients. No comparative data was collected on Cuban Americans, their life challenges, social support, religion, and perspectives toward the practice of psychology.

The 30 interviews in Cuba were divided into three main sections: background information; social struggles and social support; and perceptions toward the practice of psychology. The sample consisted of 19 women and 11 men who were married (10), single (10), divorced (5), separated (2), and widowed (3). Their age ranged from 18 to 80, and they were well distributed by age group: 18–24 (9), 25–35 (3), 36–45 (3), 46–55 (8), 56–65 (3), and 65 and older (3). Similarly, the majority of the group was educated, with eleven having a trade, seven having completed a college education, two in college, six having completed grades 11 or 12, one with a 10th-grade education, and two with less than a 6th-grade education.

The interviews with the Babalowos were prefaced with the questioning of whether they knew about psychological and emotional health and its role on mental health. More importantly, they were asked about their understanding of psychological health and their views of it. The interview protocol consisted of the following five primary questions:

1. What does it mean to you to be mentally healthy?
2. What do you consider to be circumstances (situations) that can negatively affect a person's mental health or well-being?
3. If you found yourself in a difficult situation and were looking for help or a way to feel better (or get back to normal), what would you do? Would there ever be a time when you would go to someone or something other than yourself to feel better? Who or what would that be? Are there other options you would consider?
4. How would doing _____ help you to feel better?
5. As you think about the things that threaten people's well-being, describe what types of things could actually promote good mental health.

In terms of procedures, the interviews were conducted in a nondirective, open-ended fashion that allowed the participants to expand upon their responses. Transcripts were analyzed using consensual qualitative research methodology (Hill, Thompson, & Williams, 1997), which yields themes shared by all interviewees. In particular, the 30 interviews were conducted by a trained student researcher who was provided the questions during an academic trip to Cuba. She was given an interview guide and proper training for the interview process. The Santeras/os and practitioners were interviewed personally by the authors, given the respect of their roles and the honor of their sharing information about the religion. Themes identified in the responses of the participants interviewed with representative comments were identified to highlight the primary findings reported.

Cuban Perspectives and Practices from the Island

The Cuban community identified transportation and the economy as issues of concern in their daily lives. A few indicated that their current living conditions (e.g., housing) were not positive and that they were concerned for their health. Others responded that family separation and the island's current state was a problem, while some participants did not respond to this question, opting instead to remain silent.

A common coping mechanism most often cited by the interviewees was reading; this is not surprising given the educational background of the group. Numerous participants also identified work as an escape through which to forget their challenges. Approximately four people reported smoking as a means to reduce stress, and a few identified watching TV, exercise, and humor as other forms of releasing tension.

The majority of the participants reported not sharing their difficulties with others. In fact, there were individuals who clearly felt everyone has problems, and why burden others with more? One respondent expressed the role of her pillow as an outlet to cry into and let go of her feelings, while others said they enjoyed being independent and their own social support. Although a large majority reported not talking about their problems, the family was identified by more than half of the participants as the support system. In particular, parents, spouses, children, and grandparents were identified as the primary individuals providing emotional support. Not surprising, some indicated feeling understood by their family members, and others did not feel their needs met. No one reported a therapist of counselor as part of a social support system.

Examining the role of religion for the group, seven individuals self-identified as atheists, and seven said they did not have a religion. Five practiced Santería; four were Catholic; two believed in the Christian God; two believed in "everything" but "were nothing," meaning they subscribed to no particular religion; one practiced another African religion;

and two were "spiritual." Those who practiced Santería indicated that they sometimes did what they thought the spirit told them to do. One reported not knowing why she used *cascarilla* (powdered eggshell used in seashell divination and other rites) but recognized that "it works for everything." One participant who practiced the Yoruba religion felt the need to still share a faith in God. Others suggested that their saints helped out in solving problems. Little elaboration was provided about the role of *Santeras/os*.

In relation to psychotherapy, 17 of the 30 participants had not received it. Most important, nine of the participants did not see any benefit to seeing a therapist, and one reported that such practices were only for people who were crazy and really needed help. In total, 12 of the participants had sought and participated in counseling. Three of the twelve had not had a positive experience. One reported the guidance and advice being "absurd," and another mentioned tricking the therapist throughout treatment.

In general, the participants suggested not sharing their challenges with others and primarily identified family as their social support. Almost one-third of the sample (nine) did not view psychotherapy as a promising practice. A small percentage reported a Yoruba religion as their belief system, but two suggested spiritualist tendencies.

Given the limited integration of therapists in the Cuban culture, the perspectives of counseling by many, and the identified role of religion for many Cubans, the following section highlights Santeras'/os' perceptions of mental health, their views on well-being, and practices that promote mental health stability.

The first theme identified by the Santeras/os involved the *meaning of being mentally or psychologically healthy.* To be psychologically healthy, "The person should not be suffering from any psychological problem or mental problem." Intellectual level is not viewed as a guarantee of mental stability—that is, "there are individuals that are very intelligent and hold high positions in their field, yet they are susceptible to a mental breakdown and losing everything." Individuals must also be healthy or stable in both psychological and physiological arenas, although a higher level of distress was identified for mental problems: "Emotional well-being goes hand in hand with one's physical well-being. The root cause of stress is the interaction of these two systems." "We must focus on the mental aspect of each problem in order to treat the physical." "Psychological problems are typically greater than one's physical problems." Treatment of psychological problems was viewed as necessary in order to be mentally healthy, as recognition of one's fears and problems must occur in order to solve them, as well as agreement between one's behaviors and actions: "We help the individual recognize [his] illness and subsequently help [him] work through it." "To be psychologically healthy means to be fully in agreement with your actions or behavior."

The second theme focused on the *circumstances that affect mental health*. Negative circumstances included "Drinking and smoking without moderation" and "Not taking care of oneself or not eating right." The Santeras/os considered personal history and personal relationships important in that "The upbringing of a person is fundamental." While asking "Was their childhood positive or negative?" as well as "the types of friends, the person you grew up with, the Santeras/os focused on "the emotional experiences of the person."

In terms of *help-seeking behaviors*, acknowledgment and self-understanding of the problem is prioritized in that "It is fundamental that you understand the problem or at least convince yourself of its origin. Without either of the two, the problem will remain in your life." A person also has a duty to seek help when needed, as "It is practically an obligation to seek the services of others." Seeking professional help or treatment through a psychologist, physician, or Santera/o is necessary, as the Santeras/os acknowledged that even they would seek outside help for personal issues: "I would seek those in which I trust." "At times, one needs to go to other sources such as the medic or a therapist." "I would... even go see a psychologist." Education and communication with others with whom one is experiencing problems was also viewed as essential: "Listening and reading is the route to knowledge." "If I had a problem with another person, the first thing to do would be to try to communicate with the person."

Perceptions or responses to seeking help include feeling satisfied or fulfilled after communicating with someone about the problem—for example, "It [seeking others] would fill my spiritual hunger. I would feel mentally and spiritually complete." Learning from others and keeping an open mind in receiving help is fundamental, as "Whoever thinks that they know everything is ignorant. I've been a Santero for twenty-seven years and yet I find myself learning from others that have been in this profession for a few months." Sharing similar feelings or perceiving a shared or common situation is also helpful in that "At times, the best person in a given situation is the one that can identify with your own situation."

Finally, the Santeras/os identified various *activities that promote mental health for the person and the community*. For example, "One person might experience happiness hanging out with his friends drinking a bottle of rum and yet another might find the same happiness by listening to music." However, resources must be made available to communities, as barriers result in a lack of opportunities and restrained expression of opinions and beliefs: "When you put limitations on communities, one cannot think the way one would like. I have to swim against the current or else I'll drown." "There are millions of limitations our communities face." "It all depends on the freedoms that are granted to the community." The continuation of therapeutic activities as well as outside activities considered therapeutic were also identified: "By repeating a set of behaviors that are therapeutic, one can attain a certain level of psychological well-being." "By going frequently to a peaceful place, one will benefit from its therapeutic effects."

The themes illustrated in the responses of the Santeras/os indicate that they function in much the same way as a mental health practitioner, of course, within a spiritual context focusing on past behaviors, upbringing, therapeutic actions, and the like. The Santeras/os also expressed their ability to assess and diagnose; one stated, "I could derive from your psychological state if you were suffering from an illness that could lead to a mental breakdown." Spiritualism is not seen as a separate entity, and referral to others with necessary expertise occurs when necessary. It is also apparent that the Santeras'/os' work reflected the common factors (noted in Cervantes, chapter 1 of this volume) responsible for the effectiveness of psychological healing including the therapeutic relationship, a shared worldview, client expectations, and a therapeutic ritual or intervention.

CUBAN AMERICAN PERSPECTIVES AND PRACTICES

Observing the practice of Santería for more than 10 years, the authors can identify a prominent existence of this practice throughout the United States. Within the Cuban American community some individuals believe in the practice and its power, while others critique the practice and shun those who believe it works. Notably, however, there is no socioeconomic factor associated with those who practice. Moreover, some

Cuban Americans who do not practice the religion believe in its power, respect it, and try to avoid negative encounters that can cause *mal de ojo* (the evil eye), *envidia* (envy), and other energy-driven illnesses.

Cuban Americans consult Santeras/os and Babalowos for personal relationships, guidance, mental stability, career changes, and many other personal concerns. The Santeras/os provide guidance to these individuals and identify numerous rituals to perform in order to assist them in the situation. Practitioners who consult Santeras/os report a sense of "feeling more calm" and "at peace and centered" after a consultation. They feel they are guided to solve the problem and have faith that it will be resolved. Occasionally, these individuals will not return for another consultation if things get better. If they need a follow-up or a ceremony, however, their next visit may be shortly after the initial consult.

Through the interviews, the Cuban American practitioners indicated that "energy and the environment influence mental health." One interviewee defined mental health as being "at peace with what you have in life." Others indicated that people can influence one's well-being through "envy, the evil eye, negative interactions, and bad thoughts." Not surprisingly, all three reported having experienced something difficult and challenging that required a consultation, but two of the three reported seeing a psychotherapist in addition to a Santera/o. Although they all were open to the idea of seeking counseling for a problem, the three admitted to consulting their Santeras/os prior to resorting to other support means, given that they have personal relationships with Santeras/os and access to them. Other social support systems included family and friends. Their coping means entailed pursuing activities that would cheer them up, positive thinking, protecting oneself spiritually, performing *un despojo* (a cleansing), and talking with their Santera/o for reassurance and guidance. Negative coping included anxiety, *ataques de nevios* (anxiety attacks), drinking alcohol, and crying.

The Santeras and Babalowo were also asked about their perspectives on mental health and means to improve specific situations when others are having difficulties along their paths. The Babalowo defined mental health as "the ability to live consciously coupled with the task of maintaining balance between your environment and value system." Similarly, the Santeras defined mental health as being "happy," being "content with our decisions," and "the ability to recognize emotional instability, if any, in oneself and to seek out treatment for the problem."

Specific circumstances identified to negatively affect mental health included "stress, imbalance caused by economic, social, and psychological factors," "physical and mental abuse or lack of attention during a person's formative years," "having family issues if you are family oriented," and "negative people." One Santera even admitted to purposely not associating herself with negative people to ensure and protect her well-being.

In difficult situations, they all reported turning to the religion (consulting the oracle), conducting a spiritual ritual mass, or cleansing for coping. One Santera referred to *yerbas*, *colonia 1800* (brand 1800 cologne), and *cascarilla* (eggshell) for protection. Another indicated that Thursdays are the day for spiritual mass given that these are "the day of the holy spirit" and this is when one's soul and body are closest to the divine. On this day, "one should pray to the spirits of the living and those who have passed." The Babalowo very clearly indicated that he would not consult another means (outside Santería) in order to feel better but mentioned that some of his clients meditate and pray.

Finally, they were all asked what people can do to promote well-being. Their responses ranged from "teaching youth the connection between the spiritual and material worlds" to "learning from the lessons that accompany life challenges." Another answer was "going to the ocean, burning incense, and being with people you love."

In general, the observations and interviews confirmed that practitioners, Santeras, and Babalowos recognized the connection between spirit and matter. The practitioners primarily turned to the religion as their practice to address their personal challenges and identify means to feel better about a situation. Simiarly, the Santeras and Babalowos all mentioned a wisdom of life passed down through the guidance of the gods and translated to their clients. They reported that some of their clients occasionally came in distress, seeking life answers during a crisis, while others might seek consultation for improvement of their quality of life. Recognizing this reality, all interviewees identified the religion and its gods as the primary vehicle for assisting individuals in need, and noticed a significant difference in their distress once the problems were attended to spiritually.

CONCLUSIONS

Gonzalez-Whippler (1987) states, in regard to Santería, that "its wisdom is the wisdom of the earth. All that Santería wants to do is embrace nature, but in so doing it embraces the soul of all things" (p. 23). As emphasized by Cárdenas (1997), Santería is "fundamentally associated with affirmation of social and personal identity and with the fostering of community solidarity, often in social circumstances that have made coping with life difficult at best" (p. 493). More specifically, its origins demonstrate a historical impact on its original practitioners (e.g., slaves), individuals who were devoted to their gods for peace of mind and mental stability. Today, migrating across Cuba, the Caribbean, and other cultures, numerous Cubans islanders turn to Santería practices at various levels to live out their current circumstances; political and economic exiles seek consultation to adapt to a new culture; and even non-Cuban rural-to-urban immigrants find refuge in the practice. These believers—those on the island of Cuba, exiles, and immigrants—all share an Orisha religion as a spiritual respite in the stressful circumstances of rapid social change (Cárdenas, 1997). Through the process, the experience of obtaining direction and guidance provides an anchor of security, direction for a hopeful improvement with the circumstance, and a sense of control, given the protection gained through the religion. Hence, Santería is a vigorous force that impacts the lives of Latinas/os across the world. Finally, it is important to note that the influence of the religion spreads beyond those who are seeking positive change for a prosperous future. Believers speak their practices, share their beliefs, and expose other Latinas/os and those from other cultures to their thoughts, perspectives, and practices. This synergy of energy sharing and informal spiritual guidance embedded in daily interactions continues to spread the role of Santería across nations and peoples, emphasizing its influence in daily encounters and its impact on decisions, mental health, and well-being.

REFERENCES

Baez, A. B., & Hernandez, D. V. (2001). Complementary spiritual beliefs in the Latino community: The interface with psychotherapy. *American Journal of Orthopsychiatry, 71*(3), 408–415.

Brandon, G. (1997). *Santería from Africa to the New World.* Indianapolis: Indiana University Press.

Cárdenas, J. S. (1997). *Santería* or Orisha religion: An old religion in a New World. In X. Gossen (Ed.). *South and Meso-American native spirituality: From the cult of the feathered serpent to the theology of liberation* (pp. 474–496). New York: Crossroad.

Collinson, S. R. & Turner, T. H. (2002). Not just salsa and cigars: Mental health care in Cuba. *Psychiatric Bulletin, 26*, 185–188.

Dianteill, E. (2002). Deterritorialization and reterritorialization of the Orisha religion in Africa and the New World (Nigeria, Cuba and the United States). *International Journal of Urban and Regional Research, 26*(1), 121–137.

Dresang, L. T., Brebrick, L., Murray, D., Shallue, A., & Sillivan-Vedder, L. (2005). Family medicine in Cuba: Community-oriented primary care and complementary and alternative medicine. *Journal of the American Board of Family Medicine, 18*, 297–303.

Espin, O. M. (1997). Spiritual power and the mundane world: Hispanic female healers in urban U.S. communities. In *Latina realities: Essays on healing, migration and sexuality* (pp. 157–168). Boulder, CO: Westview Press.

Falicov, C. J. (1998). Belief systems: Religion and health. In *Latino families in therapy: A guide to multicultural practice* (pp. 131–155). New York: Guilford Press.

González-Whippler, M. (2001). *Santeria: The religion*. St. Paul, MN: Llewellyn.

Hill, C. E., Thompson, B. J., & Williams, E. N., (1997). A guide to conducting consensual qualitative research. *Counseling Psychologist, 12*, 517–552.

Kristiansen, S., & Soderstrom, K. (1991). Cuban health psychology: A priority is the primary health care system. In M. A. Jansen & J. Weinman (Eds.), *The international development of health psychology* (pp. 75–82). Philadelphia: Harwood Academic.

Murphy, J. M. (1988). *Santeria: An African religion in America*. Boston: Beacon Press.

Pasquali, E. A. (1994). Santería. *Journal of Holistic Nursing, 12*, 380–390.

Sandoval, M. C. (1979). Santería as a mental health care system: An historical overview. *Social Science and Medicine, 13B*, 137–151.

Part Two

INDIGENOUS AND MESTIZA/O HEALING PRACTICES

Chapter Four

The Use of Psychotropic Herbal and Natural Medicines in Latina/o and Mestiza/o Populations

GERMAN ASCANI AND MICHAEL W. SMITH

INTRODUCTION

Herbal medications have been used for hundreds of years to treat human ailments. In most parts of the world they remain an important treatment—if not the only treatment available—to ease human suffering. The majority of our most valuable drugs today have been isolated from plant and animal sources, exemplifying a most natural evolutionary relationship between humankind and the natural environment. Some of these medications include aspirin, morphine, reserpine (the first antipsychotic), almost all of our antibiotics, digitalis, and such anticancer agents as taxol, vinblastine, and vincristine. During the past decade, traditional systems of medicine have become a topic of global importance. With the advent of modern science, we are now able to better understand the composition of medicinal plants and how they specifically interact with the nervous system. A large and increasing number of patients use medicinal herbs or seek the advice of their physician regarding their use. Interest in medicinal herbs has increased scientific scrutiny of their therapeutic potential and safety, thereby providing physicians with data to help patients make wise decisions about their use.

This chapter is a broad overview of empirical and clinical research currently available in the field of plant medicines. The focus is on psychoactive herbal medicines, and it is not intended to be comprehensive and all-inclusive, but highlights therapeutic applications of herbal medication in relation to psychological illness, its symptomatology, and psychiatric practice. In many cases, the quantity and quality of data are insufficient to make definitive conclusions about a drug's efficacy or safety.

Special consideration is given to ginkgo biloba, *Hypericum perforatum* (Saint-John's-wort), Panax ginseng, and *Valerian officinalis* (Valerian). However, other herbs are mentioned and described because of the specific ethnic and cultural consideration given to mestizo and indigenous healing practices.

The Prevalence of Herbal Medication Use

Currently it is estimated that more than 30% of adults in the United States have utilized at least one form of alternative therapy within the past year (Eisenberg et al., 1993). In subjects evaluated specifically for clinical trials, 59% reported using herbs during their lifetime, and 56% reported using herbs within the past month (Naresh, Emmanuel, Cosby, Crawford, Brawman-Mintzer et al., 1998). Many of these herbal medications have been considered to be relatively free of side effects. They are frequently used for a number of common disorders such as fatigue, insomnia, and the common cold, as well as severe medical problems (Eisenberg et al., 1993).

A study conducted by Eisenberg et al. surprised the field with findings indicating that "alternative" therapeutic approaches, including the use of herbal medicines, were extensively used by Americans. Based on a 1990 nationwide telephone survey of 1,539 adults, they reported that 34% had utilized such services in the past year, which translated to an estimated 427 million such uses nationally, surpassing the total number of visits to all primary care physicians in the U.S. Seven years later, the same group conducted a similarly designed survey with 2,055 adults, and found that more than 40% of Americans used alternative medicine therapies, representing an increase of 25% from the previous study. The total estimated number of visits to alternative medicine practitioners increased by 47% (629 million) in 1997. In comparison, Americans made only 386 million visits to their primary care physicians in the same year. The total expenditures for alternative medicine professional services was estimated at $21.2 billion in 1997, a 45% increase over the 1990 figure (Eisenberg et al., 1998).

The Use of Herbal Medication in Psychiatric Patients

Limited data suggest that the use of alternative therapies may be especially high in specific patient groups. These include 56% among emergency room patients, 57.1% in individuals with physical disabilities (Guilla & Singer, 2000), 51% in patients with inflammatory bowel disease (Rawsthorne et al., 1999) and 7–64% in cancer patients (Lippert, et al., 1999). According to Eisenberg, et al. (1998), a common reason cited for using herbal medication was the treatment of chronic illness such as arthritis, back pain, and lack of energy, which often emerge in the third and fourth decades of life.

Despite the common perception that many of the commonly used herbs are used for psychiatric problems, relatively little information is available regarding the prevalence of their actual use for such. We are aware of only three studies focusing on the use of herbs in psychiatric populations. The first is a survey of 200 outpatients attending an anxiety disorders clinic in Ontario, Canada, in which 55% percent reported a past or current use of herbal preparations (Van Ameringen, Mancini, & Farvolden, 2000). The second surveyed outpatients participating in the Anxiety and Traumatic Stress Program at Duke University Medical Center and a private psychiatric clinic in Raleigh, North Carolina. In this study, 115 out of 213 patients (54%) reported using alternative treatments, 38% of which were herbal medicines (Knaudt et al., 1999), with echinacea and Saint-John's-wort being the most frequently used herbs for physical and psychiatric symptoms, respectively. The third, a pilot study of outpatients attending a university mental health general outpatient clinic (MHC) and a U.S. Veterans Administration (VA) primary care clinic in Albuquerque, New Mexico, was recently conducted. Findings revealed that 56 out of 80 (69%) of the MHC patients versus 16 out of 83 (19%) of the VA patients used herbal medications. Chamomile (*Matricaria recutita, Chamaemelun nobile*), echinacea, ginkgo, ginseng, and Saint-John's-wort were the herbs most commonly reported (Lange et al., 2000).

The Use of Herbal Medicines in Hispanic and Native American Psychiatric Patients in New Mexico

A questionnaire was developed that was specifically designed to assess the use of herbal remedies in psychiatric clinics. The instrument was administered to subjects attending the out-patient psychiatric clinic at the VA Medical Center in Albu-querque, New Mexico. To our knowledge, this is the largest survey of the use of herbal medication in minority psychiatric patient populations. As part of a study examining the barriers to accessing mental health services by minority veterans, data on herbal usage were collected on 538 patients (430 Hispanic Americans and 108 Native Americans). Preliminary data analysis showed that a very high percentage of the patients reported using herbal medicines within the past six months. The use of herbal teas, food supplements, or herbal medica-tions was greater than 55% in both groups, which is much higher than the rates reported by Knaudt, et al. (1999), but is similar to the rate reported in patients attending a Univer-sity of New Mexico Mental Health Clinic (Lange et al., 2000). Although only 10.4% of the Native Americans and 6.4% of the Hispanics reported using herbal medications to treat spe-cific psychiatric conditions, higher rates were reported for the treatment of symptoms associated with psychiatric disorders, such as sadness (6.7% and 14.8%, respectively), anxiety (12.1% and 20.4%), lack of energy (20.5% and 24.3%), and sleep prob-lems (13.5% and 15.7%). Similar to data reported by Eisenberg, et al. (1998), 14% of Mexican American and 18.8% of Native American patients concurrently used herbal and prescription medications. More than 70% of the patients in both groups did not inform their physicians about their herbal medicine usage. In addition, they also reported very low rates of adverse effects associated with herbal treatments for either medical or psychiatric conditions (2% and 5%, respectively).

Although these reports suggest that the use of herbs in psy-chiatric patients is substantial, the generalizability of these data is limited for a number of reasons. For example, they were all conducted in specialty clinics in tertiary care centers. With the exception of the New Mexico study, sample sizes were small and ethnic minority patients were not studied.

The Importance of Herbal Medicine and Indigenous Treatment Methods in Non-Western Societies

There is rich anthropological literature (e.g., Edgerton, 1971, 1980; Fabrega, 1974; Kleinman, 1975a, 1975b, 1980) that clearly indicates that highly developed, sophisticated indigenous heal-ing and patient care systems exist in practically all traditional societies. Numerous herbs have been identified, processed, and utilized for a wide variety of conditions in such contexts. In preliterate societies, such knowledge was typically transmitted orally from generation to generation. In practically all major civilizations, including those of the Arabic (Yunani medicine), Aztecs, Chinese, Egyptians, Greeks, Incas, and Indians (Auryvedic medicine), information regarding the medical use and indications of thousands of botanical products have been carefully codified and annotated throughout the centuries. In most of the non-Western societies (representing more than 75% of the population of the world), the ascendancy of "cosmopolitan" i.e., Western) medicine is a fairly recent phenomenon. Although in most urban areas all over the world Western medicine has gained prominence, its position of dominance is far from complete, and in most non-Western countries it remains in open competition with indigenous practices (Kleinman, 1980). In countries including China (Luo, Shen, & Meng, 1997; Wang, 1998), Korea (Rhi et al., 1995), and Taiwan (Kleinman, 1975a, 1975b, 1980), professional schools for traditional medicine exist and prosper in great numbers, and most hospitals have "specialized" traditional medicine departments and clinics (Lin, 1980). In Japan, where traditional "Oriental medicine" doctors were not allowed to practice after the Meiji Restoration in 1868, Kampo (Han Chinese medicine) is widely available and frequently prescribed by physicians trained in Western medicine (Grierson & Afolayan, 1999; Mizushima & Kamba, 1997), often in combination with conventional Western medication. In the rural Third World, indigenous or traditional practitioners still predominate (Grierson & Afolayan, 1999; Van der Stuyft et al., 1996), and much of the health care of the vast majority of the populace of countries such as India relies on these traditional clinicians. At least partially for the reason of manpower consideration, the World Health Organization has made substantial efforts in promoting the collaboration between Western and traditional (indigenous) practitioners, particularly in terms of the treatment of depression and related conditions in non-Western rural settings.

In the sub-Saharan African region, the ancestral land of the majority of present-day African Americans, the use of botanical products is similarly extensive and sophisticated. As an example, Edgerton (1971) has reported on in-depth observation and interview of an indigenous healer in Tanzania, and found that despite the healer's magicoreligious epistemology he was an astute diagnostician who used a large number of botanical preparations for treating psychiatric patients, some of which are clearly pharmacologically active. (Among his armamentaria is *Rauwolfia serpentina*, which contains reserpine, a prototypical antipsychotic agent extracted from the plant.)

The Role of Herbal Medicine in Mexican and Central and South American Culture

Current popular medical practices in Mexico, Central America, and South American have origins in the ancestors' beliefs that different gods were responsible for health and disease. For example, Mexican folk medicine is based in part on the medical tradition that arose from the worship of the Aztec god of rain, lightning, and agricultural fertility, Tlaloc. Tlaloc was a very important god to all commoners, especially peasants, since he symbolized the need for rain in agriculture. In terms of disease, Tlaloc was associated with diseases caused by water and cold: edema, rheumatism, leprosy, gout. Two particular plants that were associated with Tlaloc were used for divination and curing rites: *Tagetes lucido* (African day flower, also called *yauhtli*) and *Artemisia absinthium* (wormwood; also called *iztauhyatl*). Both yauhtli and iztauhyatl were considered "hot" plants and thus used to treat cold illness. The Aztec also believed that reasoning lay within the heart, and the presence of phlegm in chest (cold illness) could pressure and disturb the heart, causing evil behavior, epilepsy, and madness. Because yauhtli and iztauhyatl were considered "hot" plants they were thus used in treatments for the presence of phlegm (Ortiz de Montellano, 1990). These two plants are reviewed later in this chapter.

In the colonial period, Tlaloc became an even more important figure, and added importance was given to the plants associated with him. These ritual plants were subsequently given Christian names. Therefore, in spite of the Spanish Inquisition, the name changes made it possible to continue old practices and prayers, but under the guise of Christian healing. At that time the Aztecs very likely also adopted rue and rosemary (herbs of European origin) as substitutes for iztauhyatl and yauhtli. Rue and rosemary were also classified as "hot" in the Galenical European system, helping to facilitate the acceptance of these plants by the Aztec. They are used to treat many of the same illnesses iztauhyatl and yauhtli are used to treat, even to this day (Ortiz de Montellano, 1990).

A Mexican national study done by the IMSS-COPLAMAR health program (1983-1985) on the popular uses of traditional medicinal plants for the treatment of central nervous system (CNS) disorders covered 2,242 inquiries obtained from physicians in rural communities (Tortoriello & Romero, 1992). The plants was classified according to their therapeutic uses as anticonvulsants, sedatives (for nervous conditions), or hypnotics (to induce sleep, treat insomnia). A total of 81 different species was named.

Of the three types of therapeutic treatments, plants used as sedatives were the most frequently mentioned (63.7% of the species analyzed), followed by anticonvulsants (51.8%, because in some cases the same species could have more than one use), and hypnotics (27.1%). More than one species of the same genus were often classified in the same group (such as *Artemisia mexicana* and *Artemisia ludoviciana*, both sedatives), probably due to similar chemical composition. Some species could be classified to several groups, such *as Citrus aurantium* (bitter orange, a sedative and hypnotic) and *Ruta chalepensis* (an anticonvulsant and sedative).

The *Tilia* (Linden flower) species is the most often listed plant of the sedatives, but is also listed under anticonvulsants and hypnotics. *Tilia* is widely used as a nervous sedative and is commercialized in almost all Mexican medicinal plant markets. Little scientific information is available on the sedative properties of this plant. *Citrus aurantium* heads the list of hypnotics and is also in both other groups; it is popularly prepared as an infusion of its leaves or flowers, and is said to have sedative and hypnotic properties. While chemical composition and some biological activities of it are well known, its sedative properties are not conclusive. The plants heading the anticonvulsant group include *Ruta chalepensis* and *Chirantodendron pentadactylon* (Flor de la Manita). The former plant is widely used to induce abortion; to stimulate uterine contractions in order to speed childbirth; as an analgesic, anti-inflammatory, and antirheumatic; for mental disorders in Saudi Arabia; and for epilepsy and hysteria in Argentina. It has the pharmacological properties of a CNS depressant, and has proven anti-inflammatory effects. Although *Chirantodendron pentadactylon* has been used as an anticonvulsant since pre-Colombian times, few studies have been conducted to confirm its effects. *Passiflora* (Passiflora Incarnata), which contains alkaloids and flavonoids) and *Valerian* are also mentioned as sedatives and hypnotics.

In Mexico, medicinal plants remain an important part of the indigenous and traditional medical systems (Heinrich et al.,

1998; Taddei-Bringas et al., 1999). At a local family medicine clinic in Mexico, more than 83% of family physicians accept herbal medications' therapeutic value, with more than 75% using it as a therapeutic resource (Taddei-Bringas et al., 1999). At the same clinic, higher rates of acceptance and use were reported by patients and health care workers (92–100% and 90–100%, respectively); Taddei-Bringas, 1999). Similarly high rates (83%) were reported in outpatients attending a rheumatology clinic in Guadalajara, Mexico, with herbal use more frequent among the less educated, in contrast to U.S. reports.

HERBAL MEDICINES USED FOR DEPRESSION

Saint-John's-Wort

General History and Description

Saint-John's-wort (*Hypericum perforatum*) is a perennial herb with round stems and bright yellow flowers with five petals. It was used in Ancient Greece and medieval Europe, where it was believed to ward off evil spirits. Its name derives from *wort*, the Old English word for herb, and the fact that it was harvested in Europe on the eve of St. John's Day, June 24 (Heiligenstein & Guenther, 1998). Traditional uses include treatment of depression, insomnia, enuresis, and anxiety. It has also been topically used for wound healing for centuries. Modern use has focused on its antidepressant effects.

The medicinal properties of Saint-John's-wort were described in the first century. In the European folk medicine tradition it was used as an anti-inflammatory to treat bronchial and urogenital tract inflammations, hemorrhoids, traumas, burns, scalds, and ulcers (Bombardelli & Morazzoni, 1989). In Russia, Saint-John's-wort (or Zveroboi) was used in gastroenteritis, rheumatism, boils, hemorrhoids, coughs, excessive bleeding, wounds, and ulcers (Hutchins, 1991). Native Americans used it to treat fevers and snakebites (Vogel, 1970).

Both the lay public and physicians in Europe perceive Saint-John's-wort to be effective for mild to moderate depression, and to have a benign adverse drug event profile. Saint-John's-wort has been reported to be more effective than placebo, and equally effective as some antidepressants. Although Saint-John's-wort extract is sold in health food stores in the United States, its use as an antidepressant is rarely recommended by U.S. physicians; in fact, few physicians are aware of Saint-John's-wort's antidepressant effects. Yet many patients and physicians would welcome a natural product for the treatment of depression, because some consider psychopharmaceuticals to be toxic chemicals.

Mechanism of Action

The applicable parts of Saint-John's-wort are the dried, above-ground parts. Several active constituents have been isolated. Two constituents that play a significant role are hypericin and hyperforin. Extracts contain at least ten components or groups of components that may contribute to the plant's pharmacological effects. It is not yet possible to correlate all the antidepressive modes of action with specific components, but it is likely that constituents other than hypericin and hyperforin also contribute to the action of Saint-John's-wort preparations. Remaining components in Saint-John's-wort include quinoids (0.6%–0.75%), flavonoids (2.0%–4.0%), xanthone, phenyl propanoid, alicyclic compounds, alkenes, essential oils, and tannin (Snow, 1996).

There are several pharmacological mechanisms possessed by Saint-John's-wort that could account for its reputed antidepressant effect, though much attention has been focused initially on monoamine oxidase (MAO) inhibition. This mechanism is similar to that found in older-generation antidepressant medications, and includes increased monoamine activity through inhibition of degrading enzymes and blocking reuptake, gamma-aminobutyric acid (GABA) receptor activity and blocking reuptake, inhibition of protein kinase C, binding to opioid receptors, and suppression of interleukins. A combined additive or synergisitic effect of the collective actions is feasible (Bennett et al., 1998).

While previous studies report that hypericin inhibits MAO, others have failed to confirm this effect. One possible explanation is that the hypericin used in the study may not be 100% pure and that this could account for the weak enzyme inhibition. In another study it was reported that Saint-John's-wort fractions with the greatest MAO inhibition contain the highest concentration of flavonoid. Complete modeling of *Hypericum* constituents also suggests flavonoids to be the most likely MAO inhibitor fraction, due to a structural similarity to toloxotone and brofaromine, two inhibitors of MAO (Mueller, et al., 1994).

Another investigation focused on the effects of Saint-John's-wort extract on the expression of serotonin receptors. When treated with Saint-John's-wort extract, neuroblastoma cells demonstrated a reduction in the expression of serotonin receptors. The authors suggest that the impaired reuptake of serotonin into the cells may lead to an increased level of neurotransmitters, which may be the mechanism responsible for the antidepressant effect (Holtje et al., 1993), similar to modern-day selective serotonin reuptake inhibitors such as fluoxetine (Prozac), paroxetine (Paxil), sertraline (Zoloft), and others.

Psychological Effects

More than 25 controlled clinical studies of Saint-John's-wort have been published using a variety of commercial alcohol extracts of the plant. These studies have shown Saint-John's-wort's effectiveness in treating mild to moderate depression, as well as its tolerability.

Sixteen studies have compared Saint-John's-wort with placebo, and nine with a reference treatment of imipramine, amitriptyline, maprotiline, desipramine, or diazepam. One multicenter study compared Saint-John's-wort and maprotiline. Effectiveness was determined using the Hamilton Depression Scale (HAMD), the Von Zerssen Depression Scales, and the Clinical Global Impression Scale (CGI). Patients received either 300 mg Saint-John's-wort extract or 25mg maprotiline. Statistical evaluation of the results demonstrated equal efficacy for Saint-John's-wort and maprotilene after four weeks of treatment. Although results were obtained quicker with maprotiline than with Saint-John's-wort, maprotilene treatment resulted in greater number of side effects (e.g., tiredness, mouth dryness, and heart complaints; Harrer et al., 1994).

German researchers published a meta-analysis of 23 randomized trials of Saint-John's-wort with a total of 1,757 outpatients with mild to moderately severe depression. They concluded that the herb was significantly superior to placebo and appeared comparably effective to standard antidepressants (maprotiline, imipramine, and amitriptyline) while producing fewer side effects (Linde et al., 1996). In 13 studies comparing a single Saint-John's-wort preparation with placebo, 55.1% of patients receiving the herb improved, compared with 22.3% given the placebo.

In a double-blind study, 105 patients with neurotic depression or depressive irritation received either 300mg of *Hypericum* extract LI 160 or placebo. Of these, 67% receiving the extract responded to treatment, compared to 28% in the placebo group. Assessments were based on the HAMD scale, which showed significant improvements in easing sadness, hopelessness, uselessness, emotional fear, and difficulty falling asleep. The following items did not improve significantly: "guilt feelings," "disordered sleep maintenance," and "somatic anxiety." There were no notable side effects observed (Harrer et al., 1994). The authors concluded that Saint-John's-wort extract is a low-risk antidepressant for treatment of "mild and moderate depression."

Hubner, Lande, & Podzuweit (1994) conducted a study that focused on the effectiveness of Saint-John's-wort on 39 patients with mild depression and somatic symptoms in a four-week single-center, randomized, placebo-controlled double-blind study. Before treatment had begun, the most common somatic symptoms suffered included lack of drive, fatigue, palpitations, sleep disturbances, and exhaustion. After two weeks, the Saint-John's-wort group showed an obviously lower frequency of such symptoms. Although the placebo group also improved, it was less drastic. After four weeks, the treatment group continued to show improvement while the placebo group either remained static or increased in symptoms. The HAMD scores for the Saint-John's-wort group fell into the normal range after two weeks of treatment while the placebo group improved less. By four weeks, the HAMD scores further improved for the treatment group but actually got worse for the placebo group, consistent with the survey mentioned above. The responder rates for the treatment and placebo groups were, respectively, 70% and 47% (high figures, perhaps because of the mildness of the disease). The authors report that no patients reported any relevant side effects. The authors concluded that the combination of effectiveness and good tolerability, and thus high compliance, *Hypericum* extract LI 160 may be helpful for patients with masked depression.

In a six-week double-blind study conducted by Hansgen, Vesper, and Ploch (1994), 72 depressive patients from 11 physicians' practices were treated with either *Hypericum* extract LI 160 or placebo. Some unique aspects of this study were the authors' efforts to include a broad range of patients (which explains why patients from 11 different practices were included) and the study's duration (to see if improvements in symptoms could be documented with Saint-John's-wort therapy beyond the usual four-week study, which is the length of time recommended in antidepressant drug trial guidelines). For the treatment group, the trial drug was given for the full six weeks; the placebo group received placebo for the first four weeks, then were given trial medication for the final two weeks. All patients were informed that they would receive medication for at least two weeks during the study.

According to the HAMD results, both treatment and placebo groups improved over four weeks, with the treatment group improving more than the placebo group (statistically significant P <.001). For the final two weeks (when all were given medication), the placebo group improved, as did the treatment group. At four weeks, the responder rate for the treatment group was 81%, versus 26% for placebo. According to D-S, the mean scale value for the treatment group fell within the normal range after four weeks and improved further by six weeks. The placebo group failed to reach normal values, although there was significant improvement with subsequent treatment for weeks five and six. The BEB gave similar results. More specifically, the treatment group enjoyed significant improvement for well-being, cardiovascular symptoms, and anxiety/phobia symptoms. The CGI further supports the data. The treatment group was much improved after four weeks, with further improvement by week six. The placebo group improved, but less so, after four weeks, followed by noticeable improvement after taking the medication. Treated patients had greater changes on self-assessment; placebo patients had greater changes on medical assessment. All these data support the efficacy of Saint-John's-wort, which compares favorably with other antidepressants such as imipramine and maprotiline. Saint-John's-wort especially shows good efficacy in responder rate for the HAMD.

Another drug-monitoring study (H. Wolk, 1994) with 3,250 patients composed of 76% women and 24% men assessed the benefits and risks of *Hypericum* extract. The Von Zerssen Depression Scale was used to determine the severity of depression and efficacy of treatment. In this study, 49% of the patients were mildly depressed, 46% intermediately depressed, and 3% severely depressed. Patients received *Hypericum* extract for a period of four weeks. After treatment, 79% and 82% assessed by patients and physicians, respectively, demonstrated improvement (44).

Side Effects and Toxicity

Ingestion of Saint-John's-wort can cause sickness and death in grazing animals. It has been noted to cause phototoxicity in cell cultures, dermatitis, and inflammation of nasal mucosa in animals that consume the plant (Wolk et al., 1994). Hypericin is thought to be the phototoxic constituent in Saint-John's-wort. It is absorbed from the digestive tract into the bloodstream and distributed to the vessels in the skin. When the skin of the animal is exposed to sunlight, an allergic reaction takes place, causing blistering and burning.

The only recorded research cases of phototoxicity in humans were with patients receiving high doses of intravenous hypericin (McAuliffe et al., 1993). A research study to investigate the phytotoxicity of hypericum was conducted with human keratinocytes. The data from the study indicated that the usual therapeutic doses of *Hypericum* extracts are about 30 to 50 times below the level of phytotoxicity (Seigeris, 1993).

In an open study with 3,250 subjects, the most common side effects reported by Wolk et al. (1994) were gastrointestinal irritation (0.6%), allergic reactions (0.5%), fatigue (0.4%), and restlessness (0.3%). A review of case reports, clinical trials, postmarketing surveillance, and drug monitoring studies concurrently showed that the most common side effects were gastrointestinal problems, dizziness/confusion, and sedation (Ernst, Rand, Barnes, & Stevinson, 1998). These side effects were comparable to placebo levels in the study.

A meta-analysis (Linde, 1996) found greater incidence of side effects reported by patients taking pharmaceutical antidepressants (52.8%) than those taking *Hypericum* (19.8%).

Contraindications and Interactions with Other Drugs

Practitioners recommend that due to the possible MAO inhibition of hypericin, those under therapy should avoid foods high in tyramine (cheese, beer, wine, yeast) and medications that interact negatively with MAO inhibiting drugs (tryptophan, amphetamines).

The risk of consuming these products when taking an MAO-inhibiting substance is an acute extreme rise in blood pressure (hypertensive crisis), with the risk of stroke. However, these recommendations are based on the interactions of pharmaceutical MAO inhibitors (MAOIs), which have a much stronger MAO inhibiting effect when compared with Saint-John's-wort. Fair-skinned people are advised to stay out of strong sunlight due to the possible photosensitivity action of Saint-John's-wort. *Hypericum* preparations are not advised for the treatment of severe depression.

Evidence suggests that Saint-John's-wort induces the cyto-chrome oxidase enzyme isoform CYP3A4 (Ernst, 1999). This raises the potential for pharmacokinetic interactions with drugs metabolized by the same enzyme. Interactions have been reported with warfarin, digoxin, carbamazepine, nor-triptyline, and cyclosporine.

Furthermore, concomitant use of Saint-John's-wort with antidepressants can lead to increased adverse effects and increase risk of serotonergic side effects, including serotonin syndrome. This effect has been reported with nefazodone (Ser-zone), paroxetine (Paxil), and sertraline (Zoloft) by Jellin et al. (2002). As with any other medication, interactions should be considered when taking a combination of drugs.

Yerba Mate

General History and Description

Yerba mate (*Ilex paraguarensis*) is a tree that originates from Paraguay but is also grown extensively in northern Argen-tina. Yerba mate is a tealike beverage brewed from the dried leaves and stemlets of yerba mate and consumed mainly in Argentina, southern Brazil, Paraguay, and Uruguay. The word *mate* is derived from the Quichua word *matí*, which names the hollowed-out gourd (*Lagenaria vulgaris*) that is traditionally used for drinking the infusion. Approximately 300,000 tons of yerba mate are produced each year. (Vasquez & Molina, 1986).

The flavor of yerba mate is somewhat sweet, bitter, and alfalfalike, similar to that obtained from tea (Camellia sinen-sis). Of the 196 volatile chemical compounds found in yerba mate, 144 are also found in tea. The infusions of *Ilex paragua-rensis* are less astringent than those of tea.

Native Guarani use yerba mate to boost immunity, cleanse and detoxify the blood, tone the nervous system, restore youthful hair color, retard aging, combat fatigue, stimulate the mind, control the appetite, reduce the effects of debilitating disease, reduce stress, and eliminate insomnia. It is used in popular medicine and employed in commercial herbal prepa-rations as a diuretic, antirheumatic, and stimulant to the cen-tral nervous system.

Mechanism of Action

Yerba mate contains xanthines, including caffeine, theophyl-line, and theobromine, well-known stimulants also found in coffee and chocolate. It also contains vitamins, minerals, amino acids, antioxidants, and chlorophyll, all of which may contribute to the "good" energy most people associate with mate. Yerba mate also contains caffeoyl derivatives (caffeic acid, chlorogenic acid, 3,4-dicaffeoylquinic acid, 3,5-dicaffeoylquinic acid and 4,5-dicaffeoylquinic acid) and flavonoids (quercetin, rutin, and kaempferol).

Physiological effects include a subjective feeling of wakefulness, focus, and alertness reminiscent of most stimulants, but often without the negative effects typically created by other beverages containing caffeine, such as anxiety, diarrhea, jitteriness, and heart palpitations.

Ilex paraguariensis extract inhibits the formation of advanced glycation end products more efficiently than does green tea (Lunceford & Gugliucci, 2005). Advanced glycation end products are implicated in the development of diabetic complications.

Ilex paraguariensis extract also attenuates the myocardial dysfunction provoked by ischemia and reperfusion, and this cardioprotection involves a diminution of oxidative damage through a nitric oxide-dependent mechanism (Schinella, Fantinelli, & Mosca, 2005).

Psychological Effects

Yerba mate is reported to produce mental stimulation, fatigue reduction, stress reduction, insomnia elimination, appetite control, body immunization, blood detoxification, nervous system toning, and restoration of hair color and preservation of youth. A person who drinks yerba mate is said to be mateado, which translates to happy, awake, and energized. These effects would be useful in treating depressive symptoms.

Side Effects and Toxicity

Side effects similar to caffeine toxicity are possible from drinking too much yerba mate tea or taking too high a dose of yerba mate supplements.

Contraindications and Interactions with Other Drugs

Although the exact mechanism of carcinogenesis of maté is unknown, available information suggests that yerba mate drinking is a risk factor for upper airway cancer (Goldenberg, Golz, & Joachims, 2003).

HERBAL MEDICINES USED FOR ANXIETY AND INSOMNIA

Chamomile

General History and Description

Chamomile (*Matricaria recutita*, *Chamaemelun nobile*) has been used throughout history, including in ancient Egyptian, Greek, and Roman cultures. The two species look very much like tiny daisies, with white petals and a yellow central disc. They are both native to Europe, Africa, and Asia, and have been naturalized in North America. The most common form of ingestion is to dry the flower tops and brew them as tea. Although there are many reported uses of this plant, it is best known for its antispasmodic, anti-inflammatory, and mild calming effect (Gruenwald, Brendler, & Jaenicke, 1998).

Mechanism of Action

The sedative and anxiolytic effects of chamomile are likely mediated by the ability of apigenin, a flavanoid, to bind to benzodiazepine receptors (Viola et al., 1995).

Psychological Effects

The plant is said to have a calming, soothing (anxiolytic) effect. It is a common ingredient in herbal hypnotic teas.

Side Effects and toxicity

It appears that chamomile has very few toxic effects. It has been listed as "generally regarded as safe" by the U.S. Food and Drug Administration (FDA). Adverse reactions may include allergic reactions to the pollen in the flowers (Kowalchik & Hylton, 1987).

Contraindications and Interactions with Other Drugs

There are no known interactions. The anti-inflammatory activity of chamomile can be seriously inhibited by phenobarbital, as well as by certain other sedatives and hypnotics, such as chloral hydrate and meprobamate.

Although the coumarin content of chamomile is not high at normal usage levels, it is important to note that coumarins can affect the action of almost any drug. It should also be noted that the presence of azulenes in chamomile may interfere with the actions of bradykinin, histamine, acetylcholine, and serotonin. To the extent that chamomile's action depends on the presence of cholinergic substances, its action will be affected by the decrease in cholinergic receptor stimulation produced by anticholinergics. In the absence of other hard data, it may still be assumed that observable interactions may occur between the many central nervous system drugs and the psychoactive principles in chamomile.

Hops
General History and Description

Hops (*Humulus lupulus*) are a climbing perennial vine that vigorously grows 20–35 feet each year. *Humulus lupulus* is a member of the hemp family, which has grown wild since ancient times in Europe, Asia, and North America. The female flowers mature in late summer and are used to add bitterness, favor, and aroma to beer. In ancient times the young shoots were eaten as a vegetable and the dried flowers were used for their slight narcotic effect and sedative action in the treatment of mania, toothache, earache, and neuralgia (Haas, 1995). Modern herbal medicine practitioners continue to use hops as a sedative and mild hypnotic, as well as for its endocrine, free radical scavenging, and antitumor properties.

Mechanism of Action

The majority of hops' medicinal actions have been attributed to its flavonoid constituents. Flavonoids are composed of different chemical classes such as flavones, isoflavones, flavonols, flavanols, flavanones, and chalcones (Stevens, Ivancic, Hsu, & Deinzer, 1997).

The endocrine properties of hops are due to the high estrogenic activity of the prenylated flavonoid 8-prenylnaringenin. (Milligan et al., 2000) Other prenylated flavonoids, including isoxanthohumol and xanthohumol, have exhibited high chemopreventive, antiproliferative, and cytotoxic effects in human cancer cell lines (Henderson et al., 2000; Miranda et al., 1999). Humulon, one of the bitter hop acids essential for brewing, has been used as an antibiotic and antifungal agent. The antimicrobial activity of humulon is used primarily for preserving beer (Simpson & Smith, 1992).

A study on mice has revealed that the chemopreventive activity of hops flavonoids appears to be due to induction of quinone reductase (a hepatic phase II detoxifying enzyme) and reduced expression of CYP1A1 (a phase I enzyme that activates chemical carcinogens; Miranda et al., 2000). Prenylated flavonoids from hops decrease growth and destroy human breast, colon, and ovarian cancer cells in vitro (Miranda et al., 1999). Hops flavonoids have also exhibited the ability to scavenge reactive nitrogen and oxygen species (Stevens et al., 2002) The sedative and sleep-inducing activity of hops is poorly understood.

Evaluation of the estrogenic activity of hops has shown significant competitive binding to estrogen receptors (ER-alpha and ER-beta), induction of alkaline phosphatase activity, up-regulation of progesterone receptor mRNA in cultured endometrial cells, and up-regulation of preselin-2, another estrogen-inducible gene (Liu et al., 2001).

Psychological Effects

Hops are often used as a mild sedative for anxiety, nervousness, and insomnia. Much of this use is based on the observation of sleepiness in European hops pickers. Blumenthal (1998) lists hops as an approved herb for mood disturbances such as restlessness, anxiety, and sleep disturbances. Although there have been no meaningful clinical studies to support hops as a sedative, several European studies have demonstrated formulas combining hops with other sedative herbs that are effective for insomnia. A pilot study using a preparation containing 500mg of valerian extract combined with 120mg of hops extract at bedtime for 30 patients with mild-to-moderate, nonorganic insomnia resulted in a decline in sleep latency and wake time. Insomnia was diagnosed using a polysomnographic standard examination, and a positive treatment effect was based on two weeks of treatment with reexamination (Fussel, Wolf, & Brattstrom, 2000). Additionally, a similar hops-valerian preparation demonstrated efficacy and tolerability equivalent to benzodiazepine for the treatment of nonchronic and nonpsychiatric sleep disorders (Schmitz & Jacket, 1998). Combinations of hops with valerian and passionflower (*Passiflora incarnata*) or lemon balm (*Melissa officinalis*) are also approved by the German Commission E as sedative and sleep-promoting formulas. Further studies are needed to determine if hops act as a mild sedative independently, as a synergist, or are absent of sedative action.

There is evidence supporting the use of hops for female endocrine disturbances. Common menstrual disturbances among female hops pickers suggest a potential endocrine effect of the hops plant. In Germany, hops baths were used to treat gynecologic disorders and hops extracts have been reported to reduce hot flashes in menopausal women (Goetz, 1990).

Results from in vitro assays for estrogen activity suggest potential use for hops as a dietary supplement in the treatment of menopausal symptoms, although animal and human studies are currently lacking. In vitro investigation of active constituents showed that 8-prenylnaringenin alone competed the strongest against 17[beta]-estradiol for binding to both alpha- and beta-estrogen receptors (Milligan et al., 2000). It also has been suggested that 8-prenylnaringenin has activity equal to or greater than other established plant estrogen (Milligan et al., 1999). Isoflavonoid phytoestrogens have been associated with a reduction in incidence of breast and prostate cancer, cardiovascular disease, and menopausal symptoms (Cassidy & Milligan, 1998; Knight & Eden, 1996).

Cancer Prevention

Three flavonoids (xanthohumol, dehydrocycloxanthohumol, and isoxanthohumol) from hops cause a dose-dependent decrease in growth of human breast, colon, and ovarian cancer cells in vitro. (Miranda et al., 1999; Prochaska & Santamaria, 1988; Prochaska & Talalay, 1988). Induction of QR in mouse hepatoma cells is used to assess the potential anticarcinogenic activity of components of the human diet. Additionally, topical application of humulon, one of the bitter agents in hops, markedly suppressed the promotion of skin tumors in mice (Yasukawa, Takeuchi, & Takido, 1995).

Side Effects and Toxicity

Humulus lupulus is believed to be nontoxic. However, as with all plants, it may cause allergic reactions in sensitive individuals. Hops are known to cause a contact dermatitis in hops pickers, attributed to myrecene in fresh hop oil. Additionally, a mechanical dermatosis has been attributed to the rough hairs on the stem and secretions of the yellow glandular hairs on hops (Estrada, Gozalo, Cecchini, & Casquete, 2002). No clinical cases of allergy or anaphylaxis resulting from therapeutic use of hops have been published.

Contraindications with Other Drugs

Limited evidence from one animal study suggests that hops may potentiate the effects of sedative drugs (Lee, Jung, & Song, 1993). The phytoestrogenic effects of 8-prenylnaringenin theoretically could have an impact on hormonal therapies, although no studies have been conducted to confirm this.

Kava

General History and Description

Kava (*Piper methysticum*) is a plant native to the South Pacific islands, including Fiji, Hawaii, the Marshall Islands, New Guinea, New Zealand, Samoa, the Solomon Islands, Tahiti, and Tonaga. Kava is a bush that grows 6–10 feet in height, with large heart-shaped leaves (Gruenwald, Brendler, & Jaenicke, 1998). The large rhizome is the part of the plant used medicinally.

Kava was discovered by Captain James Cook, who named the plant "intoxicating pepper." In the South Pacific, kava is a popular social drink, similar to alcohol in Western societies. Kava is also prepared in a defined ritual manner and used for ceremonial purposes. Commercially, it is available as kava extract and prepared from the dried root of *Piper methysticum*.

It is known traditionally for producing relaxation. In contrast to many other sedative herbs and pharmaceutical drugs that commonly cause sleepiness, kava is reputed to produce an alert, relaxed mental state.

Mechanism of Action

Kava's anxiolytic effects may be due to effects on ion channels in the CNS, similar to effects observed with mood stabilizers like lamotrigine (Grunze, Langosch, & Schirmacher, 2001), as well as interactions with $GABA_A$, dopamine D2, and opioid (mu and delta) and histamine (H1 and H2) receptors (Dinh, Simmen, & Bueter, 2001). The active constituents are thought to be several compounds (kawain, dihydrokawain, methysticin, dihydromethysticin) known as kavalactones. Kava in its raw state typically contains 3.5% of these kavalactones; however, the kava extracts that were utilized in clinical studies, contained 30–70% kava lactones (Pittler & Ernst, 2000). The majority of kava products sold in the United States utilize the 30% kava lactone preparation. Of the above mechanisms, GABA facilitation and the blockading of voltage-gated cation channels would best account for the sedative properties of kava.

Psychological Effects

In a systematic review of 14 double-blind randomized clinical trials of kava extract as a symptomatic treatment for anxiety, seven studies were identified as suitable for meta-analysis (Pittler & Ernst, 2000). Although seven of the studies were excluded due to duplication, use of kava or use in combination with a benzodiazepine, meta-analysis of the remaining seven did suggest that kava extract was superior to placebo. The studies employed standardized doses of kavalactones ranging from 60 to 240mg per day, and were four to twenty-four weeks in duration (Pittler & Ernst, 2000). Subjects presented with anxiety symptoms that were diagnosed with criteria from the American Psychiatric Association's *Diagnostic and Statistical Manual of Mental Disorders* (third edition, revised) and/or several psychometric measures of anxiety (e.g., the Hamilton Anxiety Scale and Adjective Check List, the Anxiety Status Inventory, and Zung's Self-Rating Anxiety Scale). Some studies found kava to be effective using only two acute doses, while others found benefit after chronic doses.

Side Effects and Toxicity

In a large study (N = 4,049) of Kava safety, a very low rate of side effects was reported (Schulz, Hansel & Tyler, 1998). Side effects reported with kava include allergic dermatitis, dizziness, headache, gastrointestinal upset, and disturbances of oculomotor equilibrium and accommodation. Although two studies reported no impairment of cognitive function (Munthe et al., 1993; Heinze et al., 1994), kava may impair the ability to drive or operate machinery, as evidenced by several reportedly kava-related citations for "driving under the influence" (Lickteig, 2000; Stannard, 2000; Swensen, 1996).

A new and more serious concern has recently come to light as case reports (presently about 30) have associated the consumption of kava extract products with liver damage (Escher et al., 2001; Russmann, Lauterberg, & Hebling, 2001; Shaver, 2001; Strahl, Ehret, & Damn, 1998). Although liver toxicity is associated with prolonged use (Singh & Blumenthal, 1997), several cases of death or need for liver transplant were observed after only one to three months of use (Escher et al., 2001; Russmann, Lauterberg, & Hebling, 2001; Strahl et al., 1998). In one case, liver toxicity occurred after only three weeks of use and a single episode of alcohol consumption (Shaver, 2001). Symptoms reported have included jaundice, fatigue, and dark urine (Escher et al., 2001; Russmann, Lauterberg, & Hebling, 2001). Liver function tests can be elevated after three to eight weeks of use, possibly followed by hepatomegaly and the onset of encephalopathy (Escher et al., 2001). These reports have resulted in the suspension of the sale of all kava products in France, Great Britain, and Switzerland

(limited to the acetone extract of kava) until further evalua-
tions are completed (Shaver, 2001), and the U.S. Food and Drug
Administration has asked all physicians to review charts of
patients with liver disease to assess whether they have a history of kava ingestion.

Chronic use of kava has also been associated with puffy
face, hematuria, decreased platelets, and lymphocytes (Singh &
Blumenthal, 1997), generalized abnormal movements (Spillane,
Fisher, & Currie, 1997), as well as a pellagra-like dermopathy
with symptoms of dry flaky skin and yellow discoloration of
the skin, nails, and hair (Mathews et al., 1988; Schulz, Hansel, &
Tyler, 1998). This syndrome is unresponsive to treatment with
niacinamide and resolves only with lowering or discontinuing
kava consumption (Norton & Ruze, 1994). Although the mechanism of this skin disorder is unknown, it may be due to interfer-
ence with cholesterol metabolism (Norton & Ruze, 1994).

Contraindications and Interactions with Other Drugs

There is one case study of an individual who was hospital-
ized due to lethargy and disorientation when kava was used
concomitantly with alprazolam, a sedative hypnotic. There is
a theoretical risk of drowsiness and motor reflex depression
when kava is used with CNS depressants such as alcohol, barbiturates, and benzodiazepines.

There are concerns that kava can adversely affect the liver,
and concomitant use with other potentially hepatotoxic drugs
might increase the risk of developing liver damage. Some of
these drugs include acarbose, amiodarone, atorvastatin, carbamazepine, diclofenac, gemfibrozil, isoniazid, ketoconazole, lovastatin, nitrofurantoin, pravastatin, rifampin, ritonavir, simvastatin,
tacrine, tomoxifen, and valproic acid (Jellin et al., 2002).

Bitter Orange

General History and Description

Bitter orange (*Citrus aurantium*) is used for a number of ailments, including colds, fevers, liver disorders, gall bladder
problems, rheumatism, internal and external bruising, skin
blemishes, digestive problems, epilepsy, emotional shock,
insomnia, and anxiety (Facciola, 1998; Molina, 1999).

Mechanism of Action

Bitter orange has a high flavonoid content (limonene, hes-
peridin, naringin, neohesperidin and tangaretin), as well as

furanocoumarins (Bisset & Wichtl, 1994). Active components found in bitter orange fruit include synephrine and octopamine, which are similar to epinephrine and norepinephrine (Airriess, 1997), both of which are important neurotransmitters involved in endogenous depression.

The dried peel of the unripe or ripe fruit is used to stimulate appetite and gastric secretions and is a common ingredient in remedies for gastrointestinal disorders (Bisset & Wichtl, 1994). The flowers are used by the indigenous people of Mexico and Puerto Rico for their sedative properties (known there as *azahares de naranja*), and often combined with other herbs such as valerian, linden flowers (*Tilia cordata, Tilia Europea, Tilia platypus*) and white zapote (*Casimiroa edulus,* Hernandez et al., 1984; Martinez, 1991). More recently, with the FDA ban on the use of ephedra, bitter orange has been increasingly used as a component in natural weight-loss products, theoretically due in large part to the synephrine content of the fruit. However, there is only one study of a combination of Saint-Johns-wort, caffeine, and bitter orange for weight loss, and it found no difference from the use of a placebo (Colker, Kalman, Torina, Perlis, & Street, 1999).

Psychological Effects
Bitter orange is commonly used to overcome sleep disturbances and nervousness.

Side Effects and Toxicity
Synephrine's effects on blood pressure would be expected to increase the risk of cardiovascular events, especially in those with preexisting cardiovascular disease (Hofstetter, Kreuder, & Von Bernuth, 1985).

Contraindications and Interactions with Other Drugs
Bitter orange juice is a potent inhibitor of liver enzyme CYP3A4, and has been reported to increase the blood level of several drugs metablolized by this enzyme (Di Marco, Edwards, Wainer, & Ducharme, 2002; Malhotra, Bailey, Paine, & Watkins, 2001; Penzak et al., 2002). These include a wide array of antipsychotic, antidepressant, and mood stabilizer medications as well as cardiac and antibiotic medications.

Passionflower
General History and Description
Passionflower (*Passiflora incarnata*) is a colorful flowering plant with five white or lavender petals, a purple or pink

corona, and five brightly colored stamens. The parts of the plants use for medicinal effect are the whole plant or aerial parts. It is native to the mid- to southeastern United States. It has a history with Native Americans as a poultice to treat bruises, and as a tea for sedative/anxiolytic effects (Kowalchik & Hylton, 1987).

In 1569, Spanish explorers discovered passionflower in Peru. They believed that the flowers symbolized Christ's passion and indicated his approval of their explorations. Passionflower was utilized in the United States in combination with herbal sedative products until it was banned in 1978 by the FDA due to a lack of proven effectiveness (Gruenwald, Brendler, & Jaenicke, 2000).

Passionflower is used for nervous restlessness, mild insomnia, and nervous gastrointestinal complaints (Schulz, Hansel, & Tyler, 1998). As a member of a six-ingredient combination product, it was effective in relieving symptoms in a double-blind, placebo-controlled trial of adjustment disorder with anxious mood, as scored on the Hamilton Anxiety Rating Scale (Bourin et al., 1997).

Mechanism of Action

Possible mechanisms of passionflower's anxiolytic effects include reports of its constituent chrysin/apigenin binding to central benzodiazepine receptors (Wolfman, Viola, Paladini, Dajas, & Medina, 1994). Despite neuropharmacological and animal data to support sedative and anxiolytic effects of passionflower, there have not been any such controlled studies in humans. Two studies have been published that examined the effects of combined herbal extracts—including passionflower—on anxiety (Akhondzadeh, 2001). Although there were significant effects, a combined herbal treatment confounds the ability to selectively identify the effects of passionflower.

Psychological Effects

Although passionflower is used by herbalists for the treatment of anxiety disorders, insomnia, anxiety associated with heroin withdrawal, and attention deficit hyperactivity disorder (ADHD), few rigorous studies have been conducted (Akhondzadeh, 2001). In a double-blind study of passionflower extract, 45 drops per day of an extract of passionflower taken for four weeks was as effective as 30mg per day of oxazepam (Serax), a medication used for anxiety (Speroni & Minghetti, 1988). A small study utilizing passionflower in 36 subjects with generalized anxiety disorder has reported some benefit after a month. Studies utilizing combination products, however, have reported mixed findings (Bourin, Bougerol, Guitton, & Broutin, 1997).

Side Effects and Toxicity

Adverse reactions reported with passionflower use include vasculitis, altered consciousness, severe nausea, vomiting, drowsiness, prolonged QT interval, and episodes of nonsustained ventricular tachycardia (Bourin, Bougerol, Guitton, & Broutin, 1997). A case report of a 34-year-old woman who developed severe nausea, vomiting, drowsiness, and heart symptoms was attributed to self-administration of passionflower (Fisher, Purcell, & Le Couteur, 2006). A single case report of an "idiosyncratic hypersensitivity reaction" to passionflower extract causing urticaria and cutaneous vasculitis in a 77-year-old man has also been reported (Speroni & Minghetti, 1988); the man developed pruritic erythematous rashes over the anterior and posterior aspects of his chest while taking an herbal tablet (Naturest), which contained passionflower extract, for his insomnia.

Use during pregnancy is not advised due to one of the indole alkaloid constituents, which may have uterine stimulating effects.

Contraindications and Interactions with Other Drugs

Theoretically, passionflower can potentiate MAOI activity and concomitant use can potentiate the effects of sedative drugs, including antihistamines and barbiturates. There have yet to be any such reports of such an interaction, however.

Linden

General History and Description

Flowers from several linden species (*Tilia cordata*, *Tilia Europea*, *Tilia platypus*), known also as lime blossoms or *flor de tila*, are found in Europe and North America. The flowers are gathered immediately after flowering in the midsummer. They are dried carefully in the shade and prepared as tea.

Linden flowers are utilized for the relief of nervous conditions such as anxiety and insomnia, and as a prophylactic against the development of arteriosclerosis and hypertension (Barreiro Arcos et al., 2006). Tea prepared from the flowers may be given to allay irritability and restlessness, and to promote sleep. The diaphoresis produced by the hot infusion is employed to check diarrhea from cold, and for colds and upper respiratory infection, and also—either hot or cold—may be used for restlessness, nervous headaches, painful and difficult digestion, and mild hysteria. It is commonly combined with passionflower, valerian, bitter orange, and white zapote.

Mechanism of Action

The dried linden flower has antispasmodic, diaphoretic, diuretic, sedative, and mild astringent properties. Active ingredients include flavonoids, volatile oil, and mucilage components (Coleta, Campos, Cotrin, & Proenca de Cunha, 2001; Toker, Asian, Yesilada, Memisoglu, & Ito, 2001). In vitro, its antispasmodic activity is attributed to p-coumaric acid and the flavonoid constituents (Jellin et al., 2002). Antinociceptive and anti-inflammatory activities are purported to be due to the two main flavonoid glycosides: kaempferol-3, 7-O-alpha-dirhamnoside and quercetin-3, 7-O-alpha-dirhamnoside isolated from the leaves (Toker, Kupeli, Memisoglu, & Yesilada, 2004).

One study has found that a complex mixture of compounds, primarily flavonoids, reduced anxiety in mice through interactions with benzodiazepine receptors (Viola et al., 1994).

Psychological Effects

The flowers are used to make tea for the treatment of anxiety and insomnia.

Side Effects and Toxicity

No interactions are known to occur, and there is no known reason to expect a clinically significant interaction with dried linden flowers. Orally, frequent use of linden flower tea is associated with cardiac damage, but this is rare (Jellin et al., 2002).

Valerian

General History and Description

Valerian is native to Europe and Asia, but now grows in most parts of the world. *Valeriana officianalis* is the species most commonly known and studied, but approximately 200 species are known. The plant grows 1–3 feet in height, with an erect stem with pinnate leaves and numerous small pink-white flowers at the top. The parts of the plant used medicinally are the roots and rhizomes (Kowalchik & Hylton, 1987).

Valerian has been used medicinally for thousands of years. Its reported uses are broad (digestive aid, muscle relaxant, antipyretic, anti-epileptic, etc.), but it is commonly known for the treatment of insomnia and anxiety (Gruenwald, Brendler, & Jaenicke, 1998; Kowalchik & Hylton, 1987). It is widely used and approved in Europe as a mild hypnotic to induce sleep and relieve anxiety. Traditionally, valerian is used for hysterical states, excitability, hypochondria, and migraine headaches (Jellin et al., 2002).

Mechanism of Action

Although the mechanism of action responsible for the sedative properties is unknown, it most likely involves inhibition of the GABA reuptake transporter and stimulation of GABA release from synaptosomes (Santos et al., 1994). The valerian constituents valerenic acid and valepotriates demonstrate GABA-enhancing effects and/or sedate the central nervous system (Houghton, 1999). Some binding of valerian extract occurs at $GABA_A$ receptor; this has been attributed to the amino acid content of the extract and deemed insufficient by itself to explain valerian's CNS depressant effects.

Collectively, valerian extracts show a variety of GABAergic mechanisms. The predominant mechanism has yet to be determined, but an additive or synergisitic interaction among the several mechanisms is possible.

Psychological Effects

Several behavioral effects of valerian have been noted in animals. These include suppression of the orienting response in an open-field paradigm, and decreasing spontaneous and caffeine-induced motor activity (Dunaev, Trzhetsinskii, Tishkin, Fursa, & Lineko, 1987). Valerian extracts show sedative and anxiolytic effects. Whereas passionflower and chamomile have relatively specific anxiolytic effects, valerian shows more general sedative effects, but all effects occur in a dose-dependent manner (Leuschner, Muller, & Rudmann, 1993). The sedative effects of valerian extract are moderate when compared to diazepam and the neuroleptic chlorpromazine (Leuschner, Muller, & Rudmann, 1993).

Sleep-promoting effects have been reported in several controlled studies (Leathwood et al., 1982; Lindahl & Lindwall, 1989) and have shown consistent benefit in reducing the time to sleep onset (sleep latency) and subjective improvement in sleep quality in patients.

Side Effects and Toxicity

Valerian can cause headache, excitability, uneasiness, cardiac disturbances, and insomnia (Schinella, Fantinelli, & Mosca, 2005). Occasionally, valerian causes morning drowsiness (Kuhlmann et al., 1999). Although most reports describe a lack of residual morning effects on alertness and concentration, a few reports suggest that impairment in alertness and information processing does occur (Kuhlmann et al., 1999). Impairment is dose dependent and peaks within the first few hours after an oral valerian dose (Kuhlmann et al., 1999). One case report of a 23,500mg overdose reportedly resulted in fatigue, abdominal cramps, chest tightness, lightheadedness, and foot and hand tremor (Willey et al., 1995). No residual effects were observed 24 hours later.

Although it has been used for many years, very little is known about valerian's potential for side effects, including impaired vigilance. In a placebo-controlled study of two plant-based sleep remedies (one containing valerian, and the other a valerian and hops combination) with flunitrazepam, no hangover effect was noted for the herbal preparations (Gerhard, Linnenbrink, Georghiadou, & Hobi, 1996). However, the valerian or valerian-hops mixture did produce some slight impairment of performance during the first few hours after ingestion.

Contraindications and Interactions with Other Drugs

Theoretically, valerian can potentiate the sedative effects of alcohol, barbiturates, benzodiazepines, and other sedating medications. There is preliminary evidence that valerian can inhibit the cytochrome p450 (CYP450) 3A4 enzyme, and increase levels of drugs metabolized by that enzyme. However, this interaction has not been reported in humans. Drugs metabolized by CYP3A4 include chemotherapeutic agents (etoposide, paclitaxel, vinblastine, vincristine, vindesine), fozofenadine, itraconazole, ketoconazole, lovastatin, triazolam, and numerous others (Jellin et al., 2002).

White Zapote

General History and Description

The common white sapote, called *zapote blanco* by Spanish-speaking people, *abché* or *ahache* by Guatemalan Indians, and Mexican apple in South Africa, is widely identified as *Casimiroa edulis*. The genus *Casimiroa* derives its name from

Cardinal Casimiro Gomez de Ortega, a Spanish botanist of the 18th century. The woolly-leaved white sapote was known to the Maya as *yuy* and in Guatemala as *matasano de mico*. The ancient Nahuatl name for the fruits, *cochiztzapotl*, is translated as "sleepy sapote" or "sleep-producing sapote," and it is widely claimed in Mexico and Central America that consumption of the fruit relieves the pains of arthritis and rheumatism. Extracts from the leaves, bark, and especially the seeds have been employed in Mexico as sedatives, soporifics, and tranquilizers. Mexican traditional medicine uses it to treat hypertension and insomnia and to facilitate dreaming. Derivatives of white sapote were among the herbal medicinal products displayed at the St. Louis, Missouri, World's Fair (Louisiana Purchase Exposition) in 1904 and described in the *Materia medica Mexicana*. The seed extracts, in liquid, capsule, or tablet form, continue in use in Mexico, one product bearing the trade name Rutelina.

Mechanism of Action

Several active ingredients, including three alkaloidal glycosides—casimirin, casimiroine and casimiroedine—have been isolated. N-benzoyltyramine has also been isolated and may display physiological effects similar to tyramine, one of the active ingredients found in ergot (*genus Claviceps*) and mistletoe. The main alkaloid of the seeds is casimiroedine, representing 0.143% (Panzica & Townsend, 1973).

Hydroalcoholic extract of white zapote demonstrates potential anxiolytic and antidepressant properties in vitro (Molina-Hernandez, Tellez-Alcantara, Garcia, Lopez, & Jaramillo, 2004; Mora et al., 2005), while aqueous extracts resulted in anticonvulsant (Garzon-de la Mora et al., 1999) and vasodilating effect (Baisch, Urban, & Ruiz, 2004).

Two firmly established antiepileptic drugs in human therapy, phenytoin (PHT) and phenobarbital (PB) abolished 90% of MES-induced seizures, whereas an 80% and 100% absence of clonic seizures was attained in an METsc test, correspondingly. The seizure abolition observed in white zapote and VDA–treated rats was comparable with the anticonvulsive pattern exhibited by PHT and PB. These results suggest that potentially antiepileptic compounds are present in *Casimiroa edulis* extracts that deserve the study of their identity and mechanism of action (Navarro Ruiz, Bastidas Ramirez, Garcia Estrada, Garcia Lopez, & Garzon, 1995).

Psychological Effects

For many years, extracts from the leaves, bark, and especially the seeds of white zapote have been employed in Mexico as sedatives, soporifics, and tranquilizers.

Side Effects and Toxicity

Safety profiles have not been established. White zapote should not be combined with other hypotensive medications as their effects may be increased. The seeds of white zapote have a narcotic effect and are potentially toxic; tinctures or preparations made from the seeds should be avoided in patients with cardiovascular disorders (Gruenwald, Brendler & Jaenicke, 1998).

Contraindications and Interactions with Other Drugs

The following statement (translated from Spanish) is made in a communication received from the Sección Administrativa, Dirección de Control de Medicamentos, Secretaria de Salubridad y Asistencia in Mexico City (1961): "In Mexico, the white zapote is not used other than in folk medicine and not in any way by pharmacists nor doctors; neither is it an official drug in the Pharmacopoeia."

HERBS USED AS ADAPTOGENS OR NOOTROPICS

Ginseng
General History and Description

Ginseng (*Panax ginseng*) has been used for medicinal purposes for more than 2,000 years and across several cultures (Hobbs, 1996). The name *ginseng* is used traditionally to refer to several related species of plants. Most ginsengs belong to the genus *Panax*. Chinese or Korean ginseng refers to "true ginger" and is the most studied form of ginseng in the scientific research literature. *Panax ginseng* is indigenous to China, but also cultivated in Japan, Korea, and Russia (Gruenwald, Brendler & Jaenicke, 1998), as well as the United States. *Panax* is a Latin term derived from the Greek words *pan* ("all") and *akos* ("cure"). As the name implies, it has been used in traditional herbal medicine to treat a wide variety of ailments. Orally, ginseng is used as a so-called adaptogen for increasing resistance to environmental stress and as a general tonic for improving well-being. It is also used for stimulating immune function; improving physical and athletic stamina; and improving cognitive function, concentration, memory, and work efficiency. It has also been used orally for depression and anxiety, and as a diuretic.

The contents of commercial preparations labeled as containing *Panax ginseng* can very greatly. Ginger can be referred to as red or white ginseng, which distinguishes how some ginseng roots are prepared. This distinction has potential pharmacological implications because different chemicals are produced in the process. Heat treatment of ginseng at a temperature and pressure higher than what is conventionally used to prepare red ginseng has been found to cause increased production of ginsenosides, the active ingredients. *Panax ginseng* is a perennial plant with a round stem and terminal whorls of five to eight palmate leaves (Gruenwald, Brendler & Jaenicke, 1998). The rhizome is the principal part for medicinal interest.

While studies on ginseng, particularly *Panax ginseng* (Chinese/Korean ginseng) and *Panax quinquefolius* (American ginseng) are plentiful, few actually focus on the psychiatric aspects of ginseng despite its use for such purposes. Ginseng has traditionally been given as a remedy in China to alleviate chronic psychotic patients who need to *wenyang bushen*—that is, to correct imbalances that require "warming" the *yang* (the positive functions of body), and to recruit the functions of the kidney (Liu, 1981). Most existing modern studies, however, focus on ginseng's effects on memory and have already drawn clear clinical pictures of ginseng's memory-enhancing effects (Benishin, Lee, Wang, & Liu, 1991).

Mechanism of Action

The major active constituents are the ginsenosides. There are many identified ginsenosides and a system of nomenclature consisting of a capital R followed by a lowercase letter and/or number. For example, ginsenoside Rb_1 was shown to increase the amount of acetylcholine release (Benishin, 1992). Another ginsenoside, Rg_2, has an effect on the amino acid GABA, and the ginsenosides Rb and Rg_1 on monoamine turnover (Itoh, Zang, Muri, & Saito, 1989). Additionally, ginseng affects neurotropins and blocks Ca channels and is a vasodilator through nitric oxide mechanisms. There is an extensive literature that deals with the effects of ginseng on CNS function, but effects are also seen in neuroendocrine function, carbohydrate and lipid metabolism, the immune system, and cardiovascular function.

Psychological Effects

The ginsenosides have been found to affect long-term potentiation (Abe, Cho, & Saito, 1994). Decreased c-fos mRNA and fos protein are observed in the hippocampus during aging, and ginsenoside Rg_1 increases the expression of mRNA, a protein in both young and aged rats (Liu & Zhang, 1996). Also increased are levels of cAMP in the hippocampus. Thus, ginsenoside Rg_1 may improve cognitive function by altering c-fos and cAMP in cerebral structures.

One of the symptoms of aging includes memory loss; extracts of numerous plants have been used in hopes of reversing or lessening it. In senile dementia of the Alzheimer type (SDAT), the disease involves the degeneration of the cholinergic nerve tracts projecting from the medial forebrain complex to cortical and hippocampal regions. Various studies have reported alterations in the cholinergic parameters in SDAT brains, such as choline uptake sites, choline acetyltransferase, acetylcholinesterase (AChE), and muscarinic and nicotinic receptors.

Ginseng may have benefits for learning and memory, as well as promoting nerve growth. A study was designed to examine the mechanism of action of the ginsenoside Rb_1 and its beneficial action on preventing memory deficits induced by scopolamine in rats (Benishin, 1992). Anticholinergics such as scopolamine cause memory impairment, which mimics dementia. The rats were tested for memory in a passive avoidance learning framework by being exposed to an electrical shock by a prod, the aversive stimulus. Scopolamine shortened the latency to retouch the prod due to amnesia. Administration of either Rb_1 or saline (control) would demonstrate whether the rat showed decreased learning deficit if the latency period to retouching prod increased. Rb_1 did partly reduce the scopolamine-induced amnesia. No sedative properties were found to affect data. Scopolamine, which bound to muscarinic receptors, was not displaced by Rb_1, which doesn't interact with synaptosomal muscarinic receptors. Neither does Rb_1 inhibit AChE, whose inhibition will increase available ACh and increase activity. It is thought that Rb_1 increases the quantity of ACh released during depolarization. It does so by a "dose-dependent increase in the high-affinity uptake of the precursor, choline, which is specific for cholinergic nerves, and is consistent with an increase in ACh turnover." Benishin calls this a "new undefined mechanism." This ginsenoside seems to be extremely beneficial to improving central cholinergic function. There are also suggestions that ginsenosides, especially Rb_1, are able to potentiate the effects of nerve growth factor.

Side Effects and Toxicity

There have been reported incidences of adverse reactions supposedly attributed to ginseng (DeSmet, Keller, Hansel, & Chandler, 1992). However, overall, ginseng has been shown to be well tolerated, with few side effects. Authors are critical of the literature, which documents adverse effects of ginseng because most of the reports provide incomplete data, such as the type of ginseng product, dose, and duration of ingestion. Also, the literature on adverse ginseng effects come from Australia, Great Britain, and North America, where ginseng is classified as a "health food" that does not require high government drug standards. Indeed, these ginseng "health foods" often contain no ginseng, replacing it with less-related plants, adulterations of ginseng, or mixtures of other toxic plants and chemicals. Some "ginseng products" contained no ginsenosides (DeSmet, Keller, Hansel, & Chandler, 1992).

Ginsenosides show low toxicity in pharmacological studies (Chen, Sawchuk, & Staba, 1980). A "ginseng abuse syndrome" was reported as consisting of hypertension, irritability, nervousness, and sleeplessness (Siegel, 1979). The people in this study were also taking very high doses, such as 15g per day, whereas conventional doses are 1g to 2g per day (Gruenwald, Brendler, & Jaenicke, 1998).

Contraindications and Interactions with Other Drugs

There is some evidence from one case that ginseng can decrease the effectiveness of warfarin (Coumadin). Theoretically, concomitant use of ginseng and antiplatelet agents might increase risk of bleeding, but this effect has not been reported in humans. Additionally, concurrent use might interfere with immunosuppressive therapy, since ginseng might have immune-system-stimulating properties (Jellin et al., 2002).

There is some evidence that ginseng can inhibit the cytochrome p450 2D6 (CYP2D6) enzyme by 6%. Although this effect is unlikely to produce clinically significant interactions, it might cause elevated levels of drugs metabolized by the CYP2D6 enzyme. Some of these drugs include amitriptyline, clozpine, desipramine, donepezil, fentanyl, fluoxetine, methadone, olanzapine, tramadol, and trazodone (Jellin et al., 2002).

Ginkgo
General History and Description
Ginkgo (*Ginkgo biloba*), also known as the kew or maidenhair tree, is a species of gymnosperm that has been in existence for 200 million years; it is the oldest living tree species in the world. It is a seed-bearing tree that typically grows to a height of 35–80 feet. It has green leaves that are fan shaped and produce an acid that is resistant to insects. The seeds (referred to as fruit) are round, fleshy, and have a yellow or green color (Gruenwald, Brendler, & Jaenicke, 1998).

Ginkgo use for asthma and bronchitis was described in the first pharmacopoeia, *Chen Noung Pen T'sao*, dating to 2600 B.C.E. (Diamond et al., 2000). The ginkgo tree was not brought to Europe and North America until the 18th century, and common use of ginkgo in the West did not occur until the 1960s. Today, ginkgo extracts are marketed under a variety of registered trade names. Ginkgo is among the most commonly prescribed drugs in France and Germany, making up 1% and 4% of their prescriptions, respectively (Field & Vadnal, 1998).

Preparations include dried leaf, tincture, and several extracts (Field & Vadnal, 1998). Different extracts of ginkgo are used in research, and the relative composition of its chemical constituents varies depending on preparation type.

Mechanism of Action
Ginkgo's active chemical constituents are classified into flavonoid glycosides, biflavones, and terpene lactones. Ginkgo has effects on several neurotransmitter and physiological systems. Additionally, ginkgo has vasodilating effects through platelet-activating factor (PAF) and nitric oxide (NO) systems (See Table 4.1).

Ginkgo enhances the release of acetylcholine and alters cholinergic receptors. Both direct in-vitro application and long-term oral administration increases presynaptic uptake of choline in hippocampal synaptosomes (Kristofikova, Benesova, & Tejkalova, 1992). The increase in choline uptake is due to an increase in the number of choline uptake transporters and/or rate of transport. The nootropic drugs tacrine and donepezil, used in treatment of Alzheimer's disease, similarly enhance cholinergic transmission by preventing breakdown of acetylcholine. Although not the only effect of ginkgo, cholinergic mechanisms could well account for its cognitive effects.

Table 4.1

	Effects
Cholinergic	Increased uptake of choline and release of acetylcholine
	Increased number of muscarininc receptors
Monoamine	Increased uptake of 5-HT
	Inhibition of MAOa and MAOb
	Prevent of desensitization and age-related reduction of 5-HT1a
	Altered norepinephrine turnover
	Reduced b-adrenergic binding and activity
	Reversal of age-related decline in alpha2 adrenergic receptors
GABA	Elevation of GABA levels
	Increased glutamic acid decarboxylase activity
Vasoactive	PAF inhibition
	NO-dependent vasodilation

Psychological Effects

A number of studies have shown cognitive benefits from ginkgo extracts. Many studies have been done in subjects with some form of dementia (Alzheimer's disease, vascular dementia, age-associated decline, etc.) and focus primarily on clinical and functional ratings of memory and information processing. Meta-analysis indicates a modest but consistent benefit from ginkgo in controlled studies. Cognitive improvement is not found in all measures administered, and results may depend on several methodological factors.

A meta-analysis of studies using rigorous methodological inclusion criteria was carried out (Oken, Storzbach, & Kaye, 1998). Collectively, the studies supported a real effect on ginkgo extracts on cognition in people with Alzheimer's disease. A small effect size was found, but it is substantial when compared to the prescription nootropic donepezil (Oken, Storzbach, & Kaye, 1998).

Recent publications have provided ample clinical support for ginkgo's role as a cognition and memory enhancer. Ginkgo extract (GE), considered a nootropic (memory-enhancing drug), has been demonstrated to increase reaction time to learned tasks in elderly subjects with mild to moderate memory impairment, indicating more rapid information processing (Rai, Shovlin, & Wesner, 1991). It has also been shown to dramatically improve attention in humans (Deberdt, 1994) and to increase the memory of rats in conditioned-reflex experiments (Petkov et al., 1993). Its effectiveness as a nootropic drug on persons with mental insufficiencies may be further enhanced through active memory training and therapy (Deberdt, 1994). Hypotheses suggest that ginkgo's actions lies in its ability to improve cerebral blood circulation, since old age, decreased cerebrovascular function, and memory appear to correlate (Petkov et al., 1993). Differences in electroencephalograph (EEG) readings have also been found between GE-treated patients and placebo-treated patients (Rai, Shovlin, & Wesnes, 1991).

Improved cognitive function was noted in a double-blind, placebo-controlled parallel group study of ginkgo in elderly patients with mild to moderate memory impairment (Rai, Shovlin, & Wesnes, 1991). Assessments included the Folstein Mini-Mental State Examination (MMSE), the Kendrick Battery for detection of dementia in the elderly, the digital recall task (computer version), the classification task (computer version), latency of auditory event related potential, and EEG. GE-treated patients scored significantly better than placebo patients on the Kendrick Battery at both week 12 and week 24, and in median reaction time of the classification task at week 24. There were no significant changes for either group on the MMSE. Mixed results were found for the digit recall task at week 24, as the GE-treated group showed worsening of performance in "number correct before an error is made" at week 24. The GE-treated group showed improvement of performance in "magnitude of error." These results show that GE has a beneficial effect on mental efficiency in mild to moderately mentally impaired elderly patients. The other results are inconclusive due to inconclusive data and the short period of study.

Other studies tested the effect of GE on performance of a dual-g previous studies have shown that GE administered acutely to elderly subjects facilitated dual coding and rate of memory information processing. Coding rate is important because it determines other memory processes. The authors concluded that ginkgo was beneficial for memory (Allain, Pascale, Lieury, LeCoz, & Gandon, 1993).

Side Effects and Toxicity

No serious side effects are reported in large clinical studies of ginkgo (Field & Vadnal, 1998). Mild gastrointestinal symptoms or allergic skin reactions may occur. Other side effects are headaches, dizziness, and heart palpitations.

The side effect of most concern probably relates to ginkgo's hematologic effects. Because it potently inhibits PAF, those at risk of bleeding disorders should be closely monitored.

Contraindications with Other Drugs

Concomitant use of other medications that affect platelet aggregation could theoretically increase the risk of bleeding in some people. Some of those drugs include aspirin, enoxaparin (Lovenox), heparin, indomethacin (Indocin), and warfarin (Coumadin).

MISCELLANEOUS HERBAL MEDICINES

Marigold

General History and Description

Native to Mexico and Central America, marigolds have been used for more than 2,000 years for ornamental, medicinal, and ritual purposes. Considered to have magical powers by the Aztec people, they were an integral part of rituals honoring dead ancestors. The first recorded use of marigolds is in the *Códice de la Cruz Badiano* of 1552. This herbal records the use of marigolds for treatment of hiccups, being struck by lightening, or "for one who wishes to cross a river or water safely." The last use confirms the magical properties ascribed to marigolds. They are still utilized on the Day of the Dead in Mexico and South America, where marigolds are used to decorate the graves of the dead.

Though native to the Americas, marigold species are known by many different names, such as Aztec marigold and African marigold (*Tagetes erecta*), French marigold (*Tagetes patula*; such misnomers as these latter two can be attributed to the plant's travels from the Americas to Africa and Europe and back again). In the southwestern United States, Mexico, and Central and South America, the herb has long been used in medicinal teas and beverages, and in Chile and Argentina as a condiment for stew and rice dishes. The Zapotecs use the marigold as a primary herb in purification rituals. The plant is popular with the Tarahumara Indians of Chihuahua, and is smoked by the modern Huichol Indians in their religious (peyote) rituals to enhance closed-eye visions.

The flower head and foliage of the marigold have been taken orally as an anthelmintic, a menstrual flow stimulant, and for treating colic. African marigolds are also used orally in treating whooping cough, cough, colds, mastitis, and sore eyes. It is used orally for improving digestion, stimulating appetite, a sedative in gastric pain, an antiflatulent, a bile flow stimulant, and antiabortifacient.

Mechanism of Action

The applicable parts of the marigold are those that grow above ground. Some evidence suggests that *Tagetes* oil might have tranquilizing, hypotensive, bronchodilatory, spasmolytic, and anti-inflammatory properties. The constituent ocimenone demonstrates insecticidal activity against mosquito larva and nematodes (Petkov et al., 1993).

Psychological Effects

Indigenous peoples consider it a "hot plant," and it is used to induce sweating; its root is used to heal *frio en la matriz* ("cold in the womb"; Gregory, 2005).

Side Effects and Toxicity

Topically, Tagetes can cause contact dermatitis. It can also cause an allergic reaction in individuals sensitive to the Asteraceae (Compositae) family, which includes chrysanthemums, daisies, marigolds, and ragweed, among other plants.

Contraindications and Interactions with Other Drugs

No interactions are known to occur, and there is no known reason to expect a clinically significant interaction with marigolds (Petkov et al., 1993).

Ginger

General History and Description

Ginger (*Zingiber officianale*) is a rhizome, or underground stem. It is a tropical perennial that grows 6- to 12- inch stalks with dense, conelike flowers. Ginger's use was well known among the ancient Greeks and Romans, and was a common import from Asia during the 11th and 13th centuries C.E. (Kowalchik & Hylton, 1987). It was known in China as early as the 14th century B.C.E. It is mentioned in the Koran as part of a divine drink. The Spanish had been using it as early as the 16th century, and introduced it to Jamaica and the West Indies, where it is now widely cultivated. Ginger is used for therapeutic effects on digestion and gastrointestinal function, and is widely known as a cooking spice.

Mechanisms of Action

Four main mechanisms have been cited to explain the diverse physiological mechanisms of ginger. These are (1) eicosanoid inhibition; (2) serotonin antagonism; (3) substance P release; (4) Ca/ATPase activity.

If ginger alone exerts anxiolytic effects, one potential mechanism is by serotonin antagonism. Another potential mechanism is the eicosanoid inhibition. Apart from direct neuronal effects of eicosanoids, arachidonic acid and its metabolites inhibit GABAa transmission. The interactions between eicosanoid and GABA are complex, but arachidonic acid levels increase along with increases in intracellular Ca and GABA efflux, suggesting that it may be acting as an intrinsic feedback modulator in GABAergic neurons (Asakura & Matsuda, 1984).

The antithromboxane effect of ginger is of potential significance in stress and depression. Hypercortisolism is found in approximately 50% of patients with major depression. Plasma thromboxane B level has been correlated in a group of depressed patients with high levels of cortisol, but not depressed individuals with low cortisol or with normal controls (Piccirillo et al., 1994).

Psychological Effects

Two studies have been done to date that address ginger's anxiolytic effects in an animal model. Unfortunately, both of these used a combined treatment of ginger and ginkgo, so they do not allow for differentiation of effects. The combination had diazepamlike effects in an animal model of anxiety (Hasenohrl et al., 1998). Unlike diazepam, the ginger/ginkgo combination did not have memory-impairing effects on spatial navigation memory (in a water maze test) or inhibitory avoidance learning. A standard preparation with a ratio of ginger to ginkgo of 2.5:1 had anxiolytic efficacy, whereas other ratios (1:1 or 1:2.5) were ineffective across all doses tested.

Side Effects and Toxicity

There is little known toxicity in ginger. It is listed by the FDA as "generally regarded as safe" (Petkov et al., 1993). Some patients taking ginger can have some abdominal discomfort, heartburn, diarrhea, and a pepper-like irritant effect in the mouth and throat.

Contraindications and Interactions with Other Drugs

Concominant use of herbs that have coumarin constituents or affect platelet aggregation could theoretically increase the risk of bleeding in some people. Due to claims that ginger rhizomes increase stomach acid, they might interfere with antacids, H-2 antagonists, or proton pump inhibitors. It may also interfere with cardiac drugs due to inotropic effects.

Lobelia

General History and Description

The species Lobelia also includes the species *Lobelia cardinalis*, *Lobelia chinensis*, and *Lobelia inflata*, and *Lobelia siphilitica*, all of which are used as herbal medicines. (The genus name *Lobelia* honors the Flemish botanist Mathias L'Obel.) The most common medicinal lobelia is Indian tobacco (*Lobelia inflata*; also known by the names asthma weed, emetic weed, and pukeweed, among others), a branching annual that grows to three feet in height with leaves that are 1–3 inches in length; it produces small, violet-pinkish-white flowers situated in axils of alternate leaves, the bottom of which greatly inflate in the fruiting stage. The parts of the plant typically used include the leaves, flowers, and seeds. Lobelia is an indigenous North American annual or biennial plant found in pastures, meadows, and cultivated fields of the eastern United States, and as far west as Arkansas and Nebraska. The roots of lobelia plants were used by the Iroquois to treat syphilis; hence the species name *Lobelia siphilitica*. Lobellia was also placed in the bed of quarreling couples years ago to help them rekindle their love. It was also both chewed and smoked by Native Americans.

Mechanism of Action

The primary known constituents of lobelia include piperidine alkaloids (lobeline, isolobeline), lobelic acid, chelidonic acid, glycoside (lobelacrin), essential oils, resins, and fats. Lobeline, an extract from *Lobelia inflata*, is used in antitobacco therapy. It is also used as a stimulant, antiasthmatic, and expectorant in cases of bronchitis (Fetrow et al., 1999).

Lobelia is one of the most useful systemic botanical relaxants available. Its primary historic use has been in its application to bronchitic asthma and bronchitis. An analysis of the action of the alkaloids present in this herb reveals apparently paradoxical effects. Lobeline is a powerful respiratory stimulant, while isolobelanine is an emetic and respiratory relaxant that will stimulate catarrhal secretion and expectoration while relaxing the muscles of the respiratory system. The overall action is a truly holistic combination of stimulation and relaxation.

Lobelia has a general depressant action on the central and autonomic nervous systems, and also on neuromuscular action. It may be used in many conditions in combination with other herbs to further their effectiveness if relaxation is needed. The piperidine alkaloids (e.g., lobeline) are thought responsible for its activity. Animal and in-vitro studies show that lobeline crosses the blood-brain barrier, has similar activity to nicotine, and stimulates the release of dopamine and norepinephrine (Santha et al., 2000). At low doses lobelia has stimulant effects, but higher doses result in CNS depression.

Lobeline has high lipophilicity and distributes widely throughout the body. Additional pharmacokinetic data is not available (Damaj et al., 1997).

In the past, Lobelia has been used particularly for its antispasmodic qualities to treat asthma and whooping cough, and also in large amounts to induce vomiting. Externally, this herb can be made into a poultice for bruises, felons (inflammations of the fingers or toes), insect bites, poison ivy irritation, ringworm, and sprains.

Psychological Effects

Animal studies report that lobeline has anxiolytic and cardiovascular effects and increases cognitive performance. Lobelia causes CNS stimulant activity, dilates bronchioles, and increases respiration rate at low doses, but higher doses cause CNS and respiratory depression (Terry et al., 1998). In rat and mouse models, Lobeline increases dopamine release from striatal synaptosomes, increases norepinephrine release from the hippocampus (Santha et al., 2000), and binds extensively to nicotinic receptors both centrally and peripherally (Damaj et al., 1997). In vitro, lobeline redistributes dopamine pools in presynaptic vesicles and antagonizes their release following amphetamine stimulation. Lobeline can have both antagonistic and synergistic effects when combined with nicotine, and does not induce receptor up-regulation as seen with nicotine (Terry et al., 1998). Intravenous administration of approximately 12mcg/kg lobeline to healthy human subjects resulted in cough, apnea, prolonged inspiration, and expiratory pause, the feeling of choking, and pressure in the throat and chest (Raj et al., 1995). Animal studies suggest that beta-amyrin palmitate, another derivative of *Lobelia inflata*, stimulates the release of norepinephrine in the brain, possibly leading to an antidepressant effect (Subarnas et al., 1993).

Although 16 studies have been performed evaluating lobelia for smoking cessation, none met inclusion criteria set by Stead and Hughes (2002). Trials evaluated only short-term efficacy (up to 14 days) of lobelia use with no long-term follow-up performed. Reduction in number of cigarettes used—not abstinence—was the primary outcome for a majority of the studies reviewed. No evidence supports the hypothesis that lobelia is effective for smoking cessation (Stead and Hughes, 2002).

Side Effects and Toxicity

Lobelia is known to cross into breast milk and should not be consumed by pregnant or nursing mothers. Some adverse reactions have been reported including bradycardia, cough, depression (in high doses), dizziness, hypertension, nausea, respiratory stimulation (in low doses), seizures, sweating, and vomiting. Significant toxicity has occurred following use, including arrhythmia, bundle branch block, cardiovascular collapse, coma, seizures, and vomiting (Fetrow et al., 1999).

Contraindications and Interactions with Other Drugs

Lobelia may have additive toxicity when combined with nicotine. Clinical studies evaluating lobelia for smoking cessation do not support its use (Stead & Hughes, 2002); patients should be warned not to use this supplement.

Wormwood

General History and Description

Wormwood *(Artemisia absinthium)* is the principal flavor ingredient in absinthe, a 136-proof alcoholic beverage popular at the turn of the century. From European origin, this plant today grows extensively in Mexico. In the central part of the country it is known as *hierba maestro*.

It is often taken as tea in combination with other herbs. Absinthe is historically associated with addiction, acts of violence, damage to the nervous system, and mental deterioration. Vincent van Gogh's self-amputation of his left ear is attributed to absinthe addiction. Absinthe was banned in many countries by 1915, including the United States; it has recently made a comeback, however, among European and U.S. youths (Gambelunghe & Melai, 2002; Holstege, Baylor, & Rusyniak,

2002). The flowers, leaves, and stems of wormwood plants are used as flavoring in alcoholic bitters and vermouth (Jellin et al., 2002), and medicinally (taken orally) they are used to treat loss of appetite, anxiety, indigestion, biliary dyskinesia, and gastrointestinal complaints such as gastritis. They can also be used topically as an aide to healing wounds and insect bites.

Mechanism of Action

Wormwood contains bitter principles (absinthe and anabsinthin) and volatile oil composed of up to 70% thujone. Thujone is the primary constituent of essential oils derived from a variety of plants including wormwood (*Artemisia absinthium*), mugwort (*Artemisia vulgaris*), sage (*Salvia officinalis*), clary sage (*Salvia sclarea*), tansy (*Tanacetum vulgare*), and yellow cedar (*Thuja occidentalis*; see Albert-Puleo, 1978). Essential oils containing thujone have been used in traditional medicine as an anthelmintic. Some researchers think thujone has a mind-altering effect similar to tetrahydrocannabinol, THC, the active ingredient in marijuana (Jellin et al., 2002).

In small doses, wormwood acts as an aromatic bitter. As the amount ingested increases, the toxic effects of thujone become more pronounced, leading to increased salivation and increased blood flow to mucous membranes and pelvic viscera. Chronic thujone poisoning leads to seizures, delirium, and hallucinations.

The convulsant effect of alpha-thujone, the psychotropic component of absinthe, is attributed to noncompetitive blockading of the GABA-gated chloride channel and possibly the 5-HT3 receptor Deiml (Hold, Sirisoma, & Casida, 2001, Jellin et al., 2002). Although a recent study questions the role of theorem in the development of absinthism due to the low levels found in absinthe (Lachenmeier, Emmert, Kuballa, & Sartor, 2006), studies in rats reveal that low-dose intraperitoneal injections of thujone (0.2ml/kg) can induce electrocortical seizures associated with myoclonic activity (Millet et al., 1981).

Psychological Effects

In a study to determine if the impacts of absinthe on attention performance and mood were different from those experienced with alcohol alone (Dettling et al., 2004), a total of 25 healthy subjects consumed three drinks with an identical amount of alcohol but with different amounts of thujone and then completed an attention test and mood questionnaires. Simultaneous administration of alcohol containing a high

Table 4.2

Botanical Name	Common Names	Psychiatric Symptoms Treated
Artemisia absinthum	Wormwood; also *Artemisia Mexicana* (Sp.)	Anxiety
Citrus aurantium	Bitter orange; also *naranja agria* (Sp.)	Insomnia
Humulus lupulus	Hops; also *cebada* (Sp.), common hops, European hops.	Insomnia
Hypericum perforatum	Saint John's-Wort; also fuga daemonum, demon chaser, goatweed	Depression
Illex paraguayensis	Yerba maté; also Jesuit's Brazil tea, Paraguay tea, St. Bartholemew's tea.	Depression, fatigue, poor concentration
Lobelia inflata	Indian tobacco; also asthma weed, emetic weed, pukeweed	Smoking cessation, anxiety, depression
Chamomilla recutita, Matricaria recutita	Chamomille; also amerale, babunnej, bayboon, German chamomile, kami-ture, *manzanilla* (Sp.), papatya	Insomnia, anxiety
Panax ginseng	Ginseng	Memory, concentration
Passiflora incarnata	Passionflower; also apricot vine, *Corona de Cristo* (Sp.), *Madre Selva* (Sp.), maypop, *passiflora* (Sp.), passionblume, water lemon	Anxiety
Piper methysticum	Kava	Anxiety
Tegetes erecta		
Tegetes patula	Marigold; also African day flower; African marigold; Aztec marigold, *Chinchilla enana* (Sp.), Mexican marigold	Anxiety
Tilia europea, Tilia cordata, Tilia platypus	Linden; also *flor de tila* (Sp.), small-leaved lime	Anxiety
Valeriana officianalis	Valerian; also *amantilla* (Sp.), baldrian, garden Indian valerian, Mexican valerian, *valeriana* (Sp.)	Insomnia, anxiety
Zingiber officianale	Ginger; also *jenjibre* (Sp.)	Anxiety, insomnia

concentration of thujone had a negative effect on attention performance, with effects being most prominent at the time of the first measurement. This is contrary to what was observed for alcohol alone, or for alcohol containing a low thujone concentration. Mood state assessment has revealed high thujone concentration temporarily counteracted the anxiolytic effect of alcohol. The authors speculated that this was due to the antagonistic effect of thujone on GABA receptors.

Side Effects and Toxicity

When taken in excess, thujone produces giddiness and attacks of epileptiform convulsions. Reports of poisonings in France after victims had taken large doses of thujone-containing oils were characterized by tonic-clonic or solely clonic seizures (Millet et al., 1981). A case report of agitation and incoherence several hours after consumption of 10ml of essential oil of wormwood was noted. Although the subject showed improvement with treatment he later developed acute renal failure (Dettling et al., 2004).

Contraindications and Interactions with Other Drugs

Theoretically, due to claims that wormwood increases stomach acid, it might interfere with antacids, sucralfate, H-2 antagonists, or proton pump inhibitors. It may also interfere with the effectiveness of anticonvulsant drugs due to wormwood's potential to cause seizures (Jellin et al., 2002).

REFERENCES

Albert-Puleo, M. (1978). Mythobotany, pharmacology, and chemistry of thujone-containing plants and derivatives. *Econ. Bot., 32*(1), 65–74.

Barreiro Arcos, M. L., Cremaschi, G., Werner, S., Coussio, J., Ferraro, G., & Anesini, C. (2006). *Tilia cordata, mill.*: Extracts and scopoletin (isolated compound): Differential cell growth effects on lymphocytes. *Phytother Res, 20*(1), 34–40.

Damaj, M. I., et al. (1997). Pharmacology of lobeline, a nicotinic receptor ligand. *J Pharmacol Exp Ther, 282*, 410–419.

Dettling, A., Grass, H., Schuff, A., Skopp, G., Strohbeck-Kuehner, P., & Haffner, H. T. (2004). Absinthe: Attention performance and mood under the influence of thujone. *J Stud Alcohol, 65*(5), 573–581.

Diamond, B. J., Shiflett, S. C., Feiwel, N., et al. (2000). Ginko biloba extract: Mechanisms and clinical indications. *Arch Phys Med Rehabil,* (81), 668–678.

Di Marco, M. P., Edwards, D. J., Wainer, I. W., & Ducharme, M. P. (2002). The effect of grapefruit juice and Seville orange juice on the pharmacokinetics of dextromethorphan: The role of gut CYP3A and P-glycoprotein. *Life Sci, 71,* 1149–1160.

Dunaev, V. V., Trzhetsinskii, S. D., Tishkin, V. S., Fursa, N. S., & Lineko, V. I. (1987). [Biological activity of the sum of the valepotriates isolated from *Valeriana alliarifolia*]. *Farmakol Tokskol, 50*(6), 33–37.

Edgerton, R. B. (1971). A traditional African psychiatrist. *Southwestern Journal of Anthropology, 27,* 259–278.

Edgerton, R. B. (1980). Traditional treatment for mental illness in Africa: A review. *Culture, Medicine and Psychiatry, 4,* 167–189.

Eisenberg, D. M., Kessler, R. C., Foster, C., et al. (1993). Unconventional medicine in the United States: Prevalence, costs, and patterns of use. *New England Journal of Medicine, 328,* 246–252.

Eisenberg, D. M., Davis, R. B., Ettner, S. L., et al. (1998). Trends in alternative medicine use in the United States, 1990–1997: Results of a follow-up national survey. *JAMA, 280,* 1569–1575.

Ernst, E. (1999). Second thoughts about safety of St. John's wort. *Lancet, 354*(9195), 2014–2016.

Ernst, E., Rand, J. I., Barnes, J., & Stevinson, C. (1998). Adverse effects profile of the herbal antidepressant St. John's Wort (*Hypericum perforatum L.*). *Eur J Clin Pharmacol, 54*(8): 589–594.

Escher, M., Desmeules, J., Giostra, E., et al. (2001). Drug points: Hepatitis associated with kava, an herbal remedy for anxiety. *BMJ, 322,* 139.

Estrada, J. L., Gozalo, F., Cecchini, C., & Casquete, E. (2002). Contact urticaria from hops (*Humulus lupulus*) in a patient with previous urticaria-angioedema from peanut, chestnut, and banana. *Contact Dermatitis, 46,* 127.

Fabrega, H., Jr. (1974). Problems implicit in the cultural and social study of depression. *Psychosomatic Medicine, 36*, 377–398.

Facciola, S. (1998). *Cornucopia II: A source book of edible plants*. Vista, CA: Kampong.

Fetrow, C. W., et al. (1999). Professional's handbook of complementary and alternative medicines. Philadelphia: Springhouse.

Field, B., & Vadnal, R. (1998). Ginkgo biloba and memory: An overview. *Nutr Neurosci, 1*, 2565–2567.

Fisher, A. A., Purcell, P. le. & Couteur, D.G. (2000). Toxicity of *Passiflora incarnata L. J Toxicol Clin Toxicol, 38*, 63–66.

Gambelunghe, C., & Melai, P. (2002). Absinthe: Enjoying a new popularity among young people? *Forensic Sci Int, 130*(2–3), 183–186.

Garzon-de la Mora, P., Garcia-Lopez, P. M., Garcia-Estrada, J., Navarro-Ruiz, A., Villanueva-Michel, T., Villarreal-de Puga, L. M., et al. (1999). Casimiroa edulis seed extracts show anticonvulsive properties in rats. *J Ethnopharmacol, 68*(1–3), 275–282.

Gerhard, U., Linnenbrink, N., Georghiadou, C., & Hobi, V. (1996). [Vigilance decreasing effects of 2 plant-derived sedatives]. *Schweiz Rundsch Med Prax, 85*(15), 473–481.

Goetz, P. (1990). [Treatment of hot flashes due to ovarian insufficiency using a hops extract (*Humulus lupulus*)]. *Rev Phytotherapie Pratique, 4*, 13–15.

Goldenberg, D., Golz, A., & Joachims, H. Z. (2003). The beverage mate: A risk factor for cancer of the head and neck. *Head Neck, 25*(7), 595–601.

Gregory, J. (2005). Cross-Cultural Medicine. *Am Fam Physician, 72*, 2267–2274.

Grierson, D. S., Afolayan, A. J. (1999). An ethnobotanical study of plants used for the treatment of wounds in the Eastern Cape. *South African Journal of Ethnopharmacology, 67*, 327–332.

Gruenwald, J., Brendler, T., & Jaenicke, C. (1998). *PDR for Herbal Medicines*. Montvale, NJ: Medical Economics.

Gruenwald, J., Brendler, T., & Jaenicke, C. (Eds.). (2000). *PDR for Herbal Medicines* (2nd ed.). Montvale, NJ: Medical Economics.

Grunze, H., Langosch, J., Schirrmacher, K., et al. (2001). Kava pyrones exert effects on neuronal transmission and transmembraneous cation currents similar to established mood stabilizers: A review. *Prog Neuropsychopharmacol Biol Psychiatry, 25,* 1555–1570.

Gulla, J., & Singer, A. J. (2000). Use of alternative therapies among emergency department patients. *Annals of Emergency Medicine, 35,* 226–228.

Haas, L. F. (1995). Neurological stamp: *Humulus lupulus* (hop). *J Neurol Neurosurg Psychiatry, 58,* 152.

Hansgen, K. D., Vesper, J., & Ploch, M. (1994). Multi-center double-blind study examining the antidepressant effectiveness of the hypericum extract LI 160. *Journal of Geriatric Psychiatry and Neurology, 7*(1), S15–18.

Harrer, G., et al. (1994). Effectiveness and tolerance of the hypericum extract LI 160 compared to maprotiline: A multi-center double blind study. *Journal of Geriatric Psychiatry and Neurology, 7,* 24–28.

Harrer, G., et al. (1994). Treatment of mild/moderate depressions with hypericum. *Phytomedicine, 1,* 3-8.

Hasenohrl, R. U., Topic, B., Frisch, C., Hacker, R., Mattern, C. M., & Huston, J. P. (1998). Dissociation between anxiolytic and hypomnestic effects for combined extracts of zingiber officinale and ginkgo biloba, as opposed to diazepam. *Pharmacol Biochem Behav, 59*(2), 527–535.

Heiligenstein, E., & Guenther, G. (1998). Over the counter psychotropic: A review of melatonin, St. John's wort, valerian, and kava-kava. *J Am Coll Health, 46*(6), 271–276.

Heinrich, M., Ankli, A., Frei, B., et al. (1998). Medicinal plants in Mexico: Healers' consensus and cultural importance. *Social Science Medicine, 47,* 1859–1871.

Heinze, H. J., Munthe, T. F., Steitz, J., et al. (1994). Pharmacopsychological effects of oxazepam and kava-extract in a visual search paradigm assessed with event-related potentials. *Pharmacopsychiatry, 27,* 224–230.

Henderson, M. C., Miranda, C. L., Stevens, J. F., et al. (2000). In vitro inhibition of human P450 enzymes by prenylated flavonoids from hops, Humulus lupulus. *Xenobiotica, 30,* 235-251.

Hernandez, L., Munoz, R.A., Miro, G., et al. (1984). Use of medicinal plants by ambulatory patients in Puerto Rico. *Am J Hosp Pharm, 41,* 2060–2064.

Hobbs, C. (1996). Ginseng: *The energy herb.* Loveland, CO: Botanica Press.

Hofstetter, R., Kreuder, J., Bernuth, G. von (1985). [The effect of oxedrine on the left ventricle and peripheral vascular resistance]. *Arzneimittelforschung, 35*, 1844–1846.

Hold, K. M., Sirisoma, N. S., & Casida, J. E. (2001). Detoxification of alpha- and beta-thujones (the active ingredients of absinthe): Site specificity and species differences in cytochrome P450 oxidation in vitro and in vivo. *Chem Res Toxicol, 14*(5), 589–595.

Holstege, C. P., Baylor, M. R., & Rusyniak, D. E. (2002). Absinthe: Return of the green fairy. *Semin Neurol, 22*(1), 89–93.

Holtje, H. D. et al. (1993). Molecular modeling of the antidepressive mechanism of hypericum ingredients. *Nervenheilkunde, 12*, 339–340.

Houghton, P. J., (1999). The scientific basis for the reputed activity of Valerian. *J Pharm Pharmacol, 51*, 505–512.

Hubner, W. D., Lande, S., & Podzuweit, H. (1994). Hypericum treatment of mild depressions with somatic symptoms. *Journal of Geriatric Psychiatry and Neurology, 7*(1), S12–14.

Hutchins, A. R. (1991). *Indian herbology of North America.* Boston: Shambhala.

Itoh, T., Zang, Y. F., Murai, S., & Saito, H. (1989). Effects of Panax ginseng root on the vertical and horizontal motor activities and on brain monoamine-related substances in mice. *Planta Medica, 55*(5), 429–433.

Jellin, J. M., Gregory, P. J., Batz, F., Hitchens, K., et al. (2002). Pharmacists' letter/prescriber's letter natural medicines comprehensive database (4th ed.). Stockton, CA: Therapeutic Research Faculty.

Kanba, S., Yamada, K., Mizushima, H., et al. (1998). Use of herbal medicine for treating psychiatric disorders in Japan. *Psychiatry Clinical Neuroscience, 52*, S331–S333.

Kleinman, A. M. (1975a). Medical and psychiatric anthropology and the study of traditional forms of medicine in modern Chinese culture. *Bulletin of the Institute of Ethnology, 39*, 107–123.

Kleinman, A.M. (1975b). The symbolic context of Chinese medicine: A comparative approach to the study of traditional medical and psychiatric forms of care in Chinese culture. *American Journal of Chinese Medicine, 3*, 103–124.

Kleinman, A. M. (1980). *Patients and healers in the context of culture.* Berkeley: University of California Press.

Knaudt, P. R., Connor, K. M., Weisler, R. H., et al. (1999). Alternative therapy use by psychiatric outpatients. *Journal of Nervous and Mental Disease, 187,* 692–695.

Knight, D. C., & Eden, J. A. (1996). A review of the clinical effects of phytoestrogens. *Obstet Gynecol, 87,* 897–904.

Kowalchik, C., & Hylton, W. H., (Eds), (1987). *Rodale's illustrated encyclopedia of herbs.* Emmaus, PA: Rodale Press.

Krauss, H. H., Godfrey, C., Kirk, J., et al. (1998). Alternative health care: Its use by individuals with physical disabilities. *Archives of Physical Medicine and Rehabilitation, 79,* 1440–1447.

Kristofikova, Z., Benesova, O., & Tejkalova, H. (1992). Changes in high-affinity choline uptake in the hippocampus of old rats after long-term administration of two nootropic drugs (tacrine and Ginkgo biloba extract). *Dementia, 3,* 304–307.

Kuhlmann, J., Berger, W., Podzuweit, H., et al. (1999). The influence of valerian treatment on reaction time, alertness and concentration in volunteers. *Pharmacopsychiatry, 32,* 235–241.

Lachenmeier, D. W., Emmert, J., Kuballa, T., & Sartor, G. (2006). Thujone: Cause of absinthism? *Forensic Sci Int, 158*(1), 1–8.

Lange, C. W., Yager, J., Etsitty, V., et al. (2000). *Herbal remedy use by psychiatric patients.* Paper presented to the American Psychiatric Association Annual Conference.

Leathwood, P. D., Chauffard, F., Heck, E., et al. (1982). Aqueous extract of valerian root (*Valeriana officinalis L.*) improves sleep quality in man. *Pharmacol Biochem Behav, 17,* 65–71.

Lee, K. M., Jung, J. S., Song, D. K., et al. (1993). Effects of *Humulus lupulus* extract on the central nervous system in mice. *Planta Medica, 59,* A691.

Leslie, C. (1976). *Asian medical systems: A comparative study.* Berkeley: University of California Press.

Leuschner, J., Muller, J., & Rudmann, M. (1993). Characterisation of the central nervous depressant activity of a commercially available valerian root extract. *Arzneimittelforschung, 43*(6), 638–641.

Lickteig, M. A. DUI charge for drinking tea. Retrieved May 4, 2000, from http://09.207.168.170/local/Wnews/03kavadui_ a3empirea.html.

Lin, K. M. (1980). Traditional Chinese medical beliefs and their relevance for mental illness and psychiatry, in normal and abnormal behavior in Chinese culture. In A. Kleinman & T. Y. Lin (Eds.), (pp. 95–111).

Lindahl, O., & Lindwall, L. (1989). Double-blind study of a valerian preparation. *Pharmacology Biochemistry and Behavior, 32*, 1065–1066.

Linde, K., et al. (1996). St. Johns wort for depression: An overview and meta-analysis of randomized clinical trials. *BMJ, 313*, 253–258.

Lippert, M. C., McClain, R., Boyd, J. C., et al. (1999). Alternative medicine use in patients with localized prostate carcinoma treated with curative intent. *Cancer, 86*, 2642–2648.

Liu, J., Burdette, J. E., Xu, H., et al. (2001). Evaluation of estrogenic activity of plant extracts for the potential treatment of menopausal symptoms. *J Agric Food Chem, 49*, 2472–2479.

Liu, M., & Zhang, J. T. (1996). Effects of ginsenoside Rg_1 on c-fos gene expression and cAMP levels in rat hippocampus. *Chung Kuo Yao Hsueh Pao, 17*(2), 171–174.

Liu, X. (1981). Psychiatry in traditional Chinese medicine. *British Journal of Psychiatry, 138*, 429–433.

Lunceford, N., & Gugliucci, A. (2005). *Ilex paraguariensis* extracts inhibit AGE formation more efficiently than green tea. *Fitoterapia, 76*(5), 419–427.

Luo, H. C., Shen, Y. C., & Meng, F. Q. (1997). Therapeutic effect of shuxuening combining neuroleptics for the treatment of chronic schizophrenia: A double-blind study. *Chung Kuo Chung Hsi I. Chieh Ho Tsa Chih, 17*, 139–142.

Malhotra, S., Bailey, D. G., Paine, M. F., & Watkins, P. B. (2001). Seville orange juice–felodipine interaction: Comparison with dilute grapefruit juice and involvement of furocoumarins. *Clin Pharmacol Ther, 69*, 14–23.

Martinez, M. (1991). *Las plantas medicinales de Mexico.* Mexico City: Libreria y Ediciones Botas.

Mathews, J. D., Riley, M. D., Fejo, L., et al. (1988). Effects of heavy usage of kava on physical health: Summary of a pilot survey in an aboriginal community. *Med J Aust, 148*, 548–555.

McAuliffe, V. et al. (1993). *Phase one dose escalation study of synthetic hypericin in HIV infected patients.* Paper presented at the National Conference on Human Retrovirus Related Infections.

Millet, Y., Jouglard, J., Steinmetz, M. D., Tognetti, P., Joanny, P. & Arditti, J. (1981) Toxicity of some essential plant oils: Clinical and experimental study. *Clin Toxicol, 18*(12), 1485–1498.

Milligan, S. R., Kalita, J. C., Heyerick, A., et al. (1999). Identification of a potent phytoestrogen in hops (*Humulus lupulus* L.) and beer. *J Clin Endocrinol Metab, 84*, 2249–2252.

Milligan, S. R., Kalita, J. C., Pocock, V., et al. (2000). The endocrine activities of 8-prenylnaringenin and related hop (*Humulus lupulus* L.) flavonoids. *J Clin Endocrinol Metab, 85*, 4912–4915.

Miranda, C. L., Aponso, G. L., Stevens, J. F., et al. (2000). Prenylated chalcones and flavanones as inducers of quinone reductase in mouse Hepa 1c1c7 cells. *Cancer Lett, 149*, 21–29.

Miranda, C. L., Stevens, J. E., Helmrich, A., et al. (1999). Antiproliferative and cytotoxic effects of prenylated flavonoids from hops (*Humulus lupulus*) in human cancer cell lines. *Food Chem Toxicol, 37*, 271–285.

Mizobuchi, S., & Sato, Y. (1985). Antifungal activities of hop bitter resins and related compounds. *Agric Biol Chem, 49*, 399–403.

Mizushima, H., & Kanba, S. (1997). Use of Kampo medicine for the treatment of psychiatric disorders in Japan. *Indian Journal of Pharmacology, 29*, 344–346.

Molina, G. V. (1999). Plantas medicinales en el pais Vasco [Medicinal plants in the state of Vasco]. San Sebastian, Spain: Editorial Txertoa.

Molina-Hernandez, M., Tellez-Alcantara, N. P., Garcia, J. P., Lopez, J. I., & Jaramillo, M. T. (2004). Anxiolytic-like actions of leaves of *Casimiroa edulis (Rutaceae)* in male Wistar rats. *J Ethnopharmacol, 93*(1), 93–98.

Mora, S., Diaz-Veliz, G., Lungenstrass, H., Garcia-Gonzalez, M., Coto-Morales, T., Poletti, C., et al. (2005). Central nervous system activity of the hydroalcoholic extract of *Casimiroa edulis* in rats and mice. *J Ethnopharmacol, 97*(2), 191–197.

Muller, W. E. G. et al. (1994). Effects of hypericum extract on the expression of serotonin receptors. *Journal of Geriatric Psychiatry and Neurology, 7*, 63–64.

Munthe, T. F., Heinze, H. J., Matzke, M., et al. (1993). Effects of oxazepam and an extract of kava roots (*Piper methysticum*) on event-related potentials in a word recognition task. *Neuropsychobiology, 2*(7), 46–53.

Naresh, P., Emmanuel, N. P., Cosby, C. C., Crawford, M., Brawman-Mintzer, O., Book, S. W., et al. (1998). *Herb Use in Subjects Assessed for Clinical Trials.* Paper presented at the Annual Meeting of the American Psychiatric Association, Toronto, Ontario, Canada.

Navarro Ruiz, A, Bastidas Ramirez, B. E., Garcia Estrada, J., Garcia Lopez, P., & Garzon, P. (1995). Anticonvulsant activity of *Casimiroa edulis* in comparison to phenytoin and phenobarbital. *J Ethnopharmacol, 45*(3), 199–206.

Norton, S. A., & Ruze, P. (1994). Kava dermopathy. *J Am Acad Dermatol, 31*, 89–97.

Oken, B. S., Storzbach, D. M., & Kaye, J. A. (1998). The efficacy of ginkgo biloba on cognitive function in Alzheimer disease. *Arch Neurol, 55*(11), 1409–1415.

Panzica, R. P., & Townsend, L. B. (1973). The total synthesis of the alkaloid casimiroedine, an imidazole nucleoside. *Am Chem Soc, 95*(26), 8737–8740.

Penzak, S. R., Acosta, E. P., Turner, M., Edwards, D. J., Hon, Y.Y., Desai, H. D., et al. (2002). Effect of Seville orange juice and grapefruit juice on indinavir pharmacokinetics. *J Clin Pharmacol, 42*, 1165–1170.

Petkov, V. D., Kehayov, R., Belcheva, S., Konstantinova, E., Petkov, V. V., Getova, D., et al. (1993). Memory effects of standardized extracts of Panax ginseng (G115), ginkgo biloba (GK501), and their combination, Gincosan (PHL-00701) *Planta Medica, 59*(2), 106–114.

Piccirillo, G., Fimognari, F. L., Infantino, V., Monteleone, G., Fimognari, G. B., Falletti, D., et al. (1994). High plasma concentrations of cortisol and thromboxane B2 in patients with depression. *Am J Med Sci, 307*(3), 228–232.

Pittler, M. H., & Ernst, E. (1999). Efficacy of kava extract for treating anxiety: Systematic review and meta-analysis. *Journal of Clinical Psychopharmacology*, 20, 84–89.

Pittler, M. H., & Ernst, E. (2000). Efficacy of kava extract for treating anxiety: Systematic review and meta-analysis. *J Clin Psychopharmacol,* (1), 84–89.

Prochaska, H. J., & Santamaria, A. B. (1998). Direct measurement of NAD (P) H: Quinone reductase from cells cultured in microtiter wells: A screening assay for anticarcinogenic enzyme inducers. *Anal Biochem, 169*, 328–336.

Prochaska, H. J., & Talalay, R. (1988). Regulatory mechanisms of monofunctional and bifunctional anticarcinogenic enzyme inducers in murine liver. *Cancer Res, 48*, 4776–4782.

Rai, G. S., Shovlin, C., Wesnes, K. A. (1991). A double-blind, placebo controlled study of Ginkgo biloba extract ("Tanakan") in elderly outpatients with mild to moderate memory impairment. *Current Medical Research and Opinion, 12*, 350–355.

Raj, H., et al. (1995). Sensory origin of lobeline-induced sensations: A correlative study in man and cat. *J Physiol, 482*, 235–246.

Rawsthorne, P., Shanahan, F., Cronin, N. C., et al. (1999). An international survey of the use and attitudes regarding alternative medicine by patients with inflammatory bowel disease. *American Journal of Gastroenterology 94*, 1298–1303.

Rhi, B. Y., Ha, K. S., Kim, Y. S., et al. (1995). The health care seeking behavior of schizophrenic patients in 6 East Asian areas. *International Journal of Social Psychiatry, 41*, 190–209.

Russmann, S., Lauterberg, B. H., & Hebling, A. (2001). Kava hepatotoxicity. *Ann Intern Med, 135*, 68.

Santha, E., et al. (2000). Multiple cellular mechanisms mediate the effect of lobeline on the release of norepinephrine. *J Pharmacol Exp Ther, 294*, 302–307.

Santos, M.S., Ferreira, F., Cunha, A.P., et al. (1994). Synaptosomal GABA release as influenced by valerian root extract--involvement of the GABA carrier. *Archives Internationales de Pharmacodynamie et de Therapie, 327*, 220–231.

Schinella, G., Fantinelli, J. C., & Mosca, S. M., (2005). Cardioprotective effects of Ilex paraguariensis extract: Evidence for a nitric oxide-dependent mechanism. *Clin Nutr, 24*(3), 360–366.

Schmitz, M., & Jackel, M. (1998). [Comparative study for assessing quality of life of patients with exogenous sleep disorders (temporary sleep onset and sleep interruption disorders) treated with a hops-valarian preparation and a benzodiazepine drug]. *Wien Med Wochenschr, 148*, 291–298.

Schulz, V., Hansel, R., & Tyler, V. E. (1998). *Rational phytotherapy: A physician's guide to herbal medicine.* Berlin, Germany: Springer.

Seigeris, C. P., et al. (1993). Phototoxicity caused by hypericum. *Nerveaheilkund, 12*, 320–322.

Shaver, K. (2001). Liver toxicity with kava. *Pharmacist's Letter/ Prescriber's Letter, 18*, 180115.

Siegel, R. K. (1979). Ginseng abuse syndrome: Problems with the panacea. *JAMA, 24*(15), 1612–1615.

Simpson, W. J., & Smith, A. R. (1992). Factors affecting antibacterial activity of hop compounds and their derivatives. *J Appl Bacteriol 72*, 327–334.

Singh, Y. N., & Blumenthal, M. (1997). Kava: An overview. *HerbalGram, 39*, 33–44, 46–55.

Smith, G. W., Chalmers, T. M., & Nuki, G. (1993). Vasculitis associated with herbal preparation containing Passiflora extract. *Br J Rheumatol, 32*(1), 87–88.

Snow, J. M. Hypericum Perforatum, L. *Protocol Journal of Botanical Medicine, 2*(1), 16–21.

Sonnenborn, U., & Hansel, R. (1992). Panax ginseng. In P. A. G. M. DeSmet, K. Keller, R. Hansel, & R. F. Chandler (Eds.), *Adverse Effects of Herbal Drugs* (vol. 1, pp. 179–192). Berlin: Springer-Verlag.

Chapter Five

Brazil's Ultimate Healing Resource
The Power of Spirit

SANDRA NUÑEZ

INTRODUCTION

Brazil is not typically associated with Latin American culture because of a language difference with its neighbors. Having been colonized by Portugal, Brazil's official language is Portuguese. With the exception of language, however, Brazil and Spanish Latin America share other historical and cultural similarities: European colonization, a native indigenous culture, a history of slavery, African ancestry, and an important spiritual legacy. Brazil, considered by its people to be the heart and soul of the world, believes it will lead the world in its healing and spiritual evolution.

Contained in this chapter is a presentation of the unique combination of scientific and supernatural knowledge utilized in Brazilian spiritual healing and psychic surgical practices within the context of the world's spiritual and scientific evolution. This unique Brazilian medical repertoire provides patients with a practical path toward self-discovery, personal transformation, and self-responsibility in the healing process. Spiritual healing intervenes on the conscious plane and provides appropriate behavioral guidelines that are capable of freeing the patient's soul from obstructions that could otherwise lead to disease and/or suffering. It is the moral teachings contained in the Christian Gospel that constitute principles concerning behavior in all instances of private and public life, having a direct impact on the individual's health. In their spiritual quest to lead the world in the humanization of medicine, Brazilians have come to be great educators who are working on the construction of an effective integrative model of health. Brazilian spirituality (spiritism), and its major concepts, teachings, history, and how Brazilians have utilized it for healing will be the highlight of this chapter's multidisciplinary effort.

Included herein is a description of the spiritual diagnostic and treatment protocols, the spiritual surgical procedures, and an explanation of how these actively promote healing. A presentation of the scientific, philosophical, and moral aspects of Brazilian spiritual healing will be followed by a practical discussion (based on a medical and humanistic perspective) of the need for cooperation between science and religion. Professional as well as individual patient experiences involving Brazilian spiritual healing, along with other medical and spiritual knowledge found in ancient traditions, can—when analyzed critically and in depth—offer a greater understanding of what makes a health care delivery system more effective and efficient; provide genuine integral health; and focus on prevention (as opposed to maintenance-oriented care) while also curtailing costs and maintaining an integrity that does not sacrifice quality or treatment outcomes.

Although this form of unorthodox healing may initially not "digest well," this information will definitely challenge some established common-sense assumptions of the world—in particular as these apply to biomedicine and what most perceive as the only "real knowledge." Even when empirical observation and facts are presented, such information may still be difficult to accept because comprehending it contradicts individual secular teachings and/or religious upbringing. The goal of this chapter is to present valuable information objectively in order to analyze it in its most critical form without directly or indirectly discrediting any related educational, scientific, medical, or religious institution or individual. The objective of this work is to provide insight to some of the many misconceptions about spiritual/psychic healing and surgical practices within the larger context of medical science, philosophy, and morality. Bringing forth the ideological foundations found in these three disciplines is essential; they are the integral components behind a collaborative global working relationship between humanity's spiritual and healing traditions and biomedicine.

Spiritual healing has a deep connection to the human soul. Its diagnosis and treatment cannot be dealt with through classic medicine alone, as it does not yet have the required knowledge, preparation, or training to adequately understand, formulate, and implement a required transcendental model of health. Principles that have been validated by facts and observations derived from all academic disciplines, and collected in different parts of the world, warrant consideration. In acknowledging and humbling itself to other important aspects of the human experience and incorporating these into the current medical paradigm, biomedicine—as well as humanity in general—will finally have met a most important evolutionary objective.

A BRIEF HISTORY OF THE ORIGINS OF BRAZILIAN SPIRITUAL HEALING

The idea of spirits influencing thoughts, actions, health, and illness was not born of the spiritist doctrine, nor was it born in Brazil. It has existed since the time of early human life on earth. All religions preach in a direct or indirect way about the existence of a spiritual world; none completely deny these spiritual interventions. Throughout time, many religious institutions have created dogmas and ceremonial rituals related to this universal belief of the spirit world, and today it is not uncommon to find the faithful praying in fellowship with spirit entities (such as angels, saints, or benevolent spirits), asking them to take their prayer petitions before their creator. Nor is it unusual in today's modern times for exorcisms (a practice done before and after Apostolic times, to expel evil spirits from a possessed person) to take place. Only from a historical perspective can Brazil's mediumistic medicine be completely assessed and appreciated.

The native Amerindians of Brazil, the Tupinamba, had certainly suffered illness prior to the arrival of the Europeans; they counted, however, on the village shaman to intercede for their good fortune and health. Gifted with specialized universal, esoteric, and empirical knowledge and being aware of universal cosmic rules concerning calendrical matters, agriculture, weather, horticulture, astronomy, and cosmology, shamans were allowed to harness the forces of nature in order to meet the health and survival needs of their people. It is evident that European medicine did nothing for the native population. For the village shaman who succumbed to the

European priests' conversion efforts, the harmony and future of his community was altered.

Concerned with the successful conversion of pagans, the church and its priests saw in these supernaturally powerful men a significant threat to their conversion efforts and decided they would have to strip them of their power. In their efforts to convert "heathens" to "people of reason," European friars reduced the shamanic healing tradition to one that was disreputable, ignorant, and incompetent. This left the sole power in the hands of the priest, now the principal intermediary between the physical and the superior spiritual spheres—most notably, the latter. The friars did not hesitate to learn from the indigenous advanced ethnobotanical knowledge, which exerted great influence on the developing European pharmacopoeia.

By 1530, African slaves arrived in Bahia in northeast Brazil, bringing their own healing medicine and magic. African healers, their knowledge, and a belief system strongly influenced by stories of *orixás* (spirits) soon adapted to the indigenous and European healing traditions. But once baptized as Christians—as the indigenous peoples had been before the slaves' arrival—African slaves creatively adopted the Christian spirits and combined them with their own orixás. "Olorun, god of creation, was thought of as God the Father, or Jehova. Obatala, god of the heavens and purity, merged with Jesus Christ. His daughter, Yemanja, merged with the Virgin Mary" and her children with various other Christian saints, notes Krippner (1987, pp. 274-275). He adds,

> There was no direct counterpart for Satan in Yoruba mythology. The closest that could be derived were the *ifas* and the *exus,* messengers of the gods and guardians of the temples who were quite mischievous, sometimes mixing up people's prayers and granting them someone else's request. (p. 275)

Spirits were considered to be very important in healing ceremonies.

African-based medicine was received with a higher level of contempt than was that of the indigenous peoples of Brazil. The African worldview as seen by Portuguese and Spanish colonists was one that was more deeply submerged in idolatry, superstition, and allegiance to supernatural powers than was its indigenous counterpart. Africans' dominion over supernatural powers extended into prevention and removal of spells, as well as white magic (Voecks, 1997, p. 47). In Brazil this idea of African magic and medicine came to be known as a type of deviant science, and the resultant backlash was to go as far as to prohibit African slaves the use of plants for medicine or surgery; consulting a slave on any medical issue was banned.

While the precolonial Portuguese worldview undoubtedly included the existence of mystical forces, the church, as far as it was concerned, considered these mundane activities to be neither good nor bad, but morally neutral. Supernatural activities, such as love potions, amulets, and divination, were used for specific ends; they were not negatively viewed nor considered dangerous. It was only in the centuries that followed colonization that Christianity redefined magic and supernatural powers as the handiwork of Satan (Voecks, 1997). African slaves, realizing their inferior position in the New World, perceived European magic as far more powerful than their own; that they were slaves and the Europeans were masters was enough proof that Europeans, too, had control of supernatural forces. Rather than relinquish their practices, slaves adopted the European repertoire. This syncretism gave the Afro-Brazilian practitioner a new position of considerable status and power among his people, as well as among the ruling class. The role of folk healer, herbalist, diviner, and shaman, as well as that of magician and sorcerer—which had long been vacated by the demise of the Tupinamba—would come to be occupied by *pais* and *maes-de-santo*, Afro-Brazilian priests and priestesses of the Yoruba religion known as Candomblé, the religion of the orixás.

This syncretism among the indigenous, African, and Catholic religions occurred effortlessly as they all had great similarities and parallel orientations toward finding resolution of practical problems. Notes Voecks (1987):

> The cosmologies of both religions are essentially pantheistic; both recognize a high god, distant and largely inaccessible to mortals, as well as a pantheon of lesser divinities, to whom direct appeal can be made during periods of adversity. Like the Yoruba gods and goddesses, who are viewed as deified heroes of African antiquity, the Catholic saints once were mortal beings, whose exceptional deeds are immortalized in myth. And, like their West African counterparts, the saints took on certain

qualities: dominion over nature, control of fertility, and influence over health. (Pp. 59–60)

The Yoruba belief that transcendental communication is a means to an end continued on with Candomblé in the state of Bahia and is found in many other religious ceremonies and rituals.

From the fertile grounds of the Candomblé spirit tradition, a new influence came almost three centuries later with Kardec's *The Spirits' Book* (2003). Making its debut in Brazil in 1875, this book, published in France in 1857, was channeled from spirit and helped establish important principles of communication between the physical and spiritual worlds. Kardec's work stresses the need for inner transformation and self-knowledge as avenues to fulfillment and personal realization on earth. It is considered a classic of spiritual literature and has been translated (thus far) into 45 languages. Kardec's other books—among them *The Gospel According to Spiritism*—helped redefine concepts of human suffering, imperfection, and disease for many Brazilians. *Kardecismo* offered a new therapeutic regimen. A new life based on a systematic study of illuminating spiritual and scientific texts offered a promising evolutionary path to a greater self. By the end of the 19th century in Brazil, spiritism (Kardecism) and the now deep-seated homeopathic movement brought from Germany would prove to be the impetus to the next Brazilian phenomena, the spiritist healing movement.

The humanization of medicine in Brazil was accomplished through the selfless works of Dr. Adolfo Bezerra de Menezes. After studying philosophy and the spiritist doctrine, Bezerra de Menezes immediately identified with the spiritual knowledge of Kardec's books, becoming a devout defender of the Gospel teachings of Christ. He was a most influential figure in the spiritist healing movement as well as other social movements of the time. Known as the Doctor of the Poor and the Brazilian Kardec, Bezerra de Memezes spent his entire lifetime fighting for many human causes, including human rights for the poor and the rights and freedom of both slaves and spiritists. As Brazil's most consciously active and vocal figure of the 19th century, he erected a multitude of spiritist centers and communities throughout Brazil, and in 1888 he became the president of the Brazilian Spiritist Federation. He served poor patients without ever expecting or receiving any form of payment. Even after his passing he has remained a type of folk saint among Brazilians of all classes. Many believe his benevolent spirit continues to work from the spirit realm through mediumistic healers, such as João de Deus at the Casa de Dom Inacio in Abadiania, Brazil.

By the turn of the 20th century (1904), another spiritist group, Umbanda, was founded, which emphasized the importance of spirit incorporation in healing ceremonies, venerating Jesus Christ, and using Christian, rather than African, names. While all three major spiritist groups differ in the ceremonial and ritualistic aspect (Kardecism is ritual-free), they hold several beliefs in common. These three major syncretic groupings—Candomblé, Kardecism, and Umbanda—helped shape an integral part of the Brazilian worldview as we know it today. While these three spiritist groups are responsible for much of Brazilian ideology, there have been many other important figures in the history of Brazilian spiritism who have also collaborated to Brazil's humanization and transcendental efforts.

Brazilian healing phenomenon João de Deus of Abadiania and world-renown medium from Uberaba, Francisco (Chico) Candido Xavier, have been pivotal figures in the history of Brazilian spirituality. Xavier, a preeminent world figure, authored via "channeling" more than 412 books, following the illuminating messages of Kardec and Bezerra de Menezes, and the books have been translated into dozens of languages. Xavier donated all proceeds from his divine gift to the poor; he never profited from royalties. His most noteworthy achievement was his ability to reconcile the Kardecist-spiritist doctrine with traditional Catholicism, a monumental challenge when considering the geographical size, multicultural diversity, and large Catholic population of Brazil (including more than 2.5 million spiritists, a majority of whom are also practicing Catholics, which indicates that many have identified with Xavier's honest purpose). By achieving this, Xavier creatively elaborated a new form of Brazilian popular Catholicism. Brazilians, in order to transcend to Kardec's spiritism, had to replace long-established antagonistic systems characterized by traditional, institutional, and dogmatic order with a more humane order. In 1981 Xavier was nominated for the Nobel Peace Prize, and until his death in July 2002, he remained a most humble and loving expression of the teachings of Christ.

Brazil, in its immortal expression of spirit life, has come to represent for the entire world the foundation of a new way of thinking. With the instrumental help of Kardec, Bezerra de

Menezes, Xavier, João de Deus, and other genuine mediums, Brazil promises to be a country that will lead humanity to its greater self. Professional classes have already organized themselves to study and extend spiritist doctrine paradigms in all professional areas, as can be seen in the National Congress of Spiritist Medical Doctors and the national (as well as international) Medical Spiritist Association. The latter organization, whose mission is to contribute to the scientific studies and research of medicine and spiritism, aims to educate health professionals about the importance of respecting and tolerating patients' beliefs and religions in practicing spiritual medicine; to promote the medical spiritist paradigm through courses and communication means, books, and other publications; to contribute with the implantation of this new medical paradigm throughout the world; and to assist with the goal of creating more humanistic medical professionals and facilities.

SPIRIT HEALING WITHIN THE CONTEXT OF OTHER HEALING SYSTEMS AND BIOMEDICINE

Medical anthropology, the exciting field that looks at the way individuals throughout the world have approached issues of health, illness, and healing, has found that many ancient healing traditions still exist even though the civilizations that once practiced them have been nonexistent for centuries. In the advent of a growing popularity for alternative or complementary methods of healing, many of these old traditions are making a comeback. In comparing modern medicine to ancient methods of healing, some similarities are found, with the most significant difference being the missing spiritual element from the current medical paradigm.

The classification of diseases of supernatural etiology has been completely disregarded by classic medicine. It is important to keep in mind that the exclusion of a spiritual classification of disease in the current classic model does not mean that it does not exist, but simply that we choose not to include it in the current classification. We need only to recall cosmology (the science that deals with the systematic origin and structure of the universe) in its earlier years of development, based solely on metaphysical examination. Eventually, after much rigorous study, cosmology gained acceptance to the physical sciences.

It is likely only a matter of time before spiritual/psychic healing becomes an accepted field in classic scientific medicine.

The wealth of medical knowledge that is available to us from many of the ancient world healing systems validates important cosmological and theological principles that are missing from today's modern medicine. Common among these ancient traditions are: (1) the importance of a harmonious balance (inner and external) in achieving health; (2) working with human energy fields; (3) modification of lifestyle, diet, and exercise; (4) the existence of spirits in disease and the supernatural dimension of healing (faith and prayer); and (5) the ideologies of true knowledge, purity, harmony, and goodness. Important aspects of health are prevention (through diet, exercise, relaxation/meditation/ritual), detoxification, and regulating the humors to achieve physical, emotional, and mental balance. At the root of all these ancient healing traditions is the ultimate goal of the spirit liberating itself. We find the same element in Brazilian spiritual healing.

The spiritual life Portuguese Latin Americans have come to know surpasses the religious sense. Brazilians, when compared to their Spanish Latin American counterparts, have taken on a stronger spiritual (vs. religious) character. While mediumistic healing has definitely had a place in Spanish Latin American culture and healing traditions, it has existed covertly behind the larger traditional dogmatic teachings of institutionalized religion, which in Latin America has been predominantly represented by the Catholic Church. For spiritist Brazilians it is only a matter of time before the truth is revealed about the current secular world; they understand that with the changing and manipulating of the truths of the universe, the natural forces of nature have been antagonized, reflecting on the entire social, economic, and political spectrum. Living in a secular world that is primarily focused on the acquisition of things, and too often characterized by selfishness, has caused humanity to not only lose many valuable aspects of the human experience but to disguise them with other truths. This is a serious problem, particularly as these common misconceptions affect all aspects of the human experience. This has been the case for Dr. Stanley Krippner, Note the following observation he made during an interview with Jeffrey Mishlove, Ph.D., regarding spiritual healing as a phenomenon that tends to be disguised with a mystical cult or sorcery: You know, the worst black magic is the black magic we commit against ourselves. It is the sorcery that hurts ourselves when we think negative thoughts, or we hold onto a destructive self concept [*sic*], or when we allow ourself [*sic*] to say negative, hostile things about ourselves and the people around us, and those sentences go over and over in our mind. It is no wonder, then, that people get stomach aches and backaches and headaches with those negative thought images going around." And yes, to me that sounds like something's that sorcery, and if that can be exorcised, so much the better. If you want to call this a malevolent spirit, fine. If you want to call it negative thinking, fine. But either the spiritist or the psychotherapist, or both of them, really have to approach that negativity and get rid of it if the person's going to recover (Krippner, 1998, n.p.).

Undeniably, grasping the sacredness of spirit healing (with the assistance of benevolent spirits), cannot be experienced equally by all, particularly if the sacredness of life is not equally perceived by everyone. Discernment, the spirit of truth, takes on new meaning here.

An example is demonstrated in the *Aquarian Gospel*, when Jesus speaks to people at the temple about his messiahship:

> You cannot hear the voice of God, because your ears are closed. You cannot comprehend the works of God, because your hearts are full of self. And you are busybodies, mischief-makers, hypocrites. You take these men whom God has given me into your haunts and try to poison them with sophistries and lies, and think that you will snatch them from the fold of God. (Dowling, 1979, p. 214)

Some have attempted to stone Jesus, but he stops them and asks them for which of his good works he is being stoned—healing the sick, or expelling evil spirits?

Through modernization, secularization, and technological advances, the spirit of truth has undeniably been distorted, directly affecting all value systems and the sacredness of life. From a technicist standpoint, most conventional medical schools have taught illness as a series of technical problems that are to be approached with an application of specific technical solutions. As a result, society has professional medical performance that is excellent in technical terms but poor in humanistic terms, as can be observed in our health care system's evolutionary path. How both folk medicine and biomedicine differ from this essential reference point is significant in understanding why the two work, and why they produce strikingly different outcomes.

In underlining the difference between conventional medicine and folk medicine traditions Finkler notes, "Spiritualism is embedded in a sacred world while biomedicine is sanctioned by secular science" (1994, p. 179). Both folk medicine and biomedical models have different physical settings, etiological beliefs, diagnosis and treatment repertoires, and reasons for practicing, and of most importance is the difference in the practitioner-patient relationship as it relates to each method's particular focus. In biomedicine the focus of a patient's healing is on the *physician*—his persona, knowledge, and reputation. The patient who follows the doctor's treatment plan, and gets the desired results or even an undesired outcome, attributes those results to the physician. He gets better (or worse) because of the doctor's ability (or inability) to cure him. In this model the patient looks to the doctor for the alleviation of his suffering. The patient, even after diet modification and following the doctor's plan of treatment rigidly, waits for the healing to occur. Here the doctor only treats the *effect* of the disease.

In contrast, the focus of folk/spiritual healing is on the *patient*. In this case the healer identifies the *cause* of the disease and guides the patient so *she herself* discovers what needs to be done to effectively resolve it. In spiritual healing the patient improves because of what the patient changes *in herself* to resolve the cause of the problem—not simply because she followed someone else's orders. The patient ultimately is the only one who can change what is causing her problem (even with the assistance of a spirit being). Here the patient looks to herself for the alleviation of her own suffering (Finkler, 1994). This is the fundamental difference between spiritual healing and biomedicine.

Although similar to the spiritual component found in universal holistic and homeopathic health models, Brazil's spiritual concept differs slightly—specifically in its use of mediumistic healing techniques. Working with the help of benevolent spirits may initially sound bizarre and almost impossible for many to conceptualize; it is not until the present work is read in its entirety, and is followed with additional personal and independent study, that the individual can make a sound assessment. Having said this, I propose the reader step aside and try to see Brazilian spiritual healing not from his particular worldview but rather from the unique Brazilian (spiritist) mind set.

THE SPIRITIST HEALING MODEL
OF HEALTH: AN OVERVIEW

For Brazilian spiritists, educating the soul with fundamental moral concepts of the laws of nature is believed to create the personal transformation that is required for complete healing. Much of this spiritual knowledge is gained through knowledge of the Christian Gospel and an extension of it, the spiritist doctrine (*Kardecismo*)—a scientific, philosophical, and moral way of life that promotes preventative care and a more complete diagnostic and treatment regimen for many known and unknown medical conditions. Unlike the classic model of medicine, the relationship between soul and body is inextricably linked to a person's health. Without adequate diagnosis (many having origins in the soul) and inappropriate treatment, higher levels of consciousness cannot be achieved, personal transformation is inevitably hindered, and healing will not truly take effect. From a health perspective the spiritist doctrine provides a clear and ample connection between a person's moral condition (the soul's condition), the balance or imbalance of her energetic organism, and her current health condition—in other words, a strong interrelationship among soul, perispirit, and body, respectively.

A central tenet of spiritual healing is that everything, including health and illness, occurs around the theory of relativity found in quantum physics and the spiritual law of reciprocity. When the *soul* is in equilibrium with the *perispirit* (the semimaterial, spiritual and physical, human envelope) and the *physical body*, the individual enjoys good health; but when disequilibrium occurs, disease sets in.

THE SCIENTIFIC, PHILOSOPHICAL, AND MORAL/
RELIGIOUS ASPECTS OF BRAZILIAN HEALING

Brazilian doctors trained in modern medicine who practice the spiritist way of life, as well as other non-Brazilian physicians who are rediscovering a renewed sense of sacredness in scientific medicine, now acknowledge the great need to study beyond the physical-chemical phenomena related to the person's biological metabolism. They believe that classic medicine has reduced studies to only the organic body and has completely ignored the multidimensional aspect of the human organism. The current Western psychiatric model, too, follows a purely organic etiology in mental functioning as it has been structured within the complexities of the neuroen-docrine metabolism (Costa, 2001).

The soul as it relates to healing, from a purely scientific standpoint, has been most commonly rejected; it is thought to exist only outside the empirical arena, thus not fitting into the standard observation, measurement, and experimentation of research investigation. The soul, not having received the attention it deserves, lacks scientific explanation. This has made the soul nonverifiable, nonexistent, and therefore difficult to explain or comprehend in scientific terms. However, for Brazilians who believe it is their natural legacy to develop this area of scientific inquiry, spiritual healing is not about presenting information that has no basis or validity. The public is not expected to accept information crudely; rather, spiritual healing in Brazil is a legitimate field of inquiry that has been and continues to be approached critically at the scientific, philosophical, and moral levels. Unlike what many people think, spiritual healing is not explained by myth, but instead by such validating disciplines as biology, cosmology, medical anthropology, medicine, philosophy, physiology, parapsychology, quantum physics, religion, theistic psychology, and theology.

Increasing scientific discoveries—in particular, discoveries related to transpersonal psychology—have recently opened new horizons for the study and interpretation of many psychic phenomenon, recognizing established concepts of consciousness, subconsciousness, and superconsciousness. Growing interest and study of the faculty of mediumship—in particular, *healing mediumship* (psychic healing)—now permits us to classify it scientifically as a psychobiological predisposition inherent to those who under certain conditions are allowed to capture the thoughts of discarnate spirits, can experience the astral plane, and can also establish contact with the spirit world. Brazilians, studying the organic and psychic phenomena of mediumship for more than a century, are leading the world in establishing an essential understanding of mediumistic healing principles.

Modern-day investigations of spiritual healing demonstrate healers possess energetic fields with unique properties that allow an actual exchange of energy between healer and patient. Researchers such as Sister Justa Smith, a biochemist, have found spiritual healing not to be the result of psychosomatic effects, as has been a common misconception for centuries. Smith's research suggests that healers have the ability to selectively affect different enzyme systems in a direction toward greater organization and energy balance. By speeding up different enzymatic reactions, healers assist the body to heal itself (something Western physicians are not trained to do). Healers therefore provide the patient with the needed energetic boost to push the patient's total energetic system back into homeostasis. A healing boost of this magnitude has special negatively entropic, self-organizational properties that assist the cells in creating order from disorder along selectively defined routes of cellular expression. This as well as other recent discoveries involving plants and animals are scientific examples of a healer's effect on the healing process of biological organisms. It is important to note that the biological organisms that are mentioned here were all nonhuman. The animal (mouse), plant, and enzyme systems were utilized instead of a human being to remove the suggestion or belief on the part of the test subject. Such studies demonstrate the validity of the existence of a concretely observed and measured therapeutic energy exchange between healers and biological systems (Smith, 1973). These research studies direct us to further investigate the energetic body. The future of medical advances may well be in our ability to control such energy, and in helping people in ways we have not as yet been able to do. Research studies such as these have left some scientists with a firm conviction that magnetic fields play an important role in the body's healing and immunological processes.

The field of parapsychology has been supported by the work contributed by Michael Persinger, head of the Neuroscience Research Group (Psychophysiology Laboratory) at Laurentian University in Sudbury, Ontario, Canada. His hypotheses—that extremely low frequency (ELF) Shumann waves may serve as carrier for psi information (psychic phenomena involving the sixth sense; i.e., automatic writing, channeling, clairsentience, clairvoyance, clairaudience, distant healing, mental telepathy, etc.)—resulted positive, finding fewer psi experiences reported during periods of geomagnetic disturbance, thus impairing the propagation of ELF waves. Most interesting however, is his observation of the variation in the earth's electromagnetic field. The area having the lowest magnetic intensity on the planet (25 gauss) is in Brazil, near Rio de Janeiro. This geographical advantage in terms of the growing psychic phenomenon and spirituality in Brazil could explain certain Brazilians' ability to communicate with the spirit world and to lead the world in its spiritual evolution.

While scientific research on the health benefits of prayer is still in its infancy, and while some of the studies done on the effect of prayer on the therapeutic process have shown it has no effect on the therapeutic process, there is still a small and growing body of evidence of the positive effect prayer has on overall health and well being. In the *Handbook of Religion and Health* (2001), Koenig, McCullough and Larson acknowledge intercessory prayer to be good for both one's mental and physical health. In their review of 1200 research studies and 400 reviews, they found religious involvement to have a direct correlation with many aspects of healthy living (e.g. well being, happiness, fulfillment, greater hope and optimism, less anxiety and greater purpose and meaning of life).

In yet another source supporting these findings, *The Relaxation Response* (2000), Dr. Herbert Benson, a Harvard behavioral medicine specialist has studied the effect of meditation and prayer on health for more than thirty years. In his book, he shows that patients can successfully overcome many stress-related ailments by repeating a word, a sound, or a prayer. At his Institute for Mind Body Medicine, his effective and essential self-care modalities are growing in acceptance to potentially become a third modality in health care, next to surgical interventions and pharmaceuticals.

Larson, Milano, and Lu (1988), researchers who also investigated the effect of prayer on healing, also regard as positive the effect spirituality has on the therapeutic process and added it is a research area that has definite benefits for humanity and thus requires further investigation. Despite the published studies, which have demonstrated religion's ameliorating effect on a patient's suffering, and lowering self-destructive behaviors to aid in the promotion of a healthy lifestyle, the empirical evidence has not received the proper attention nor have these issues received the appropriate research focus.

Unlike classic medicine, spiritual healing reestablishes the connection between the patient and the greater cosmic principles of her existence—those of karma (cause and effect) and reincarnation, which in the treatment protocols help identify a true etiology for a patient's ailment. Spiritual healing offers, above all, philosophical depth, promoting a revolution of ideas and critical thinking about the individual and her world, particularly where social, political, economic, health, and moral conditions are irrational.

Since the exploration of emotions, feelings, thoughts and ideas cannot be expressed in material or physical terms alone

(because human consciousness, the soul, requires it be studied from the less explored, spiritual realm of knowledge), a
broader understanding will occur when investigators reach
beyond the human (physical) senses. Transcendental knowledge that goes beyond the realm of sense is found in the teachings of Christ. In the *Aquarian Gospel*, Jesus enlightens Greek
philosophers about the seen and unseen realities:

> I come not here to speak of science, of philosophy, or
> art: of these you are the world's best masters now. But
> all your high accomplishments are but stepping stones to
> worlds beyond the realm of sense; are but illusive shad-
> ows flitting on the walls of time. But I will tell you of a
> life beyond, within; a real life that cannot pass away....
> Unaided by the Spirit-breath, the work of intellection
> tends to solve the problems of the things we see, and
> nothing more. The senses were ordained to bring into the
> mind mere pictures of the things that pass away; they do
> not deal with real things; they do not comprehend eter-
> nal law. But man has something in his soul, a something
> that will tear the veil apart that he may see the world
> of real things. We call this something, spirit conscious-
> ness; it sleeps in every soul, and cannot be awakened till
> the Holy Breath becomes a welcome guest.... There is no
> power in intellect to turn the key; philosophy and sci-
> ence both have toiled to get a glimpse behind the veil; but
> they have failed. The secret spring that throws ajar the
> door of soul is touched by nothing else than purity in life,
> by prayer and holy thought. (Dowling, 1979, p. 84)

It is a revealing message—that neither science nor philosophy alone have all the answers, and that they will gain the
ability to find true meaning in everything only when together
with morality they develop a keen sense of discrimination and
discernment. Humankind, through inborn powers and knowledge of the kingdom of the soul, is naturally led to the higher
self. *Genuine* healers (medium and psychic) possess advanced
understanding and a critical extrasensory perception of the
spirit realm.

Finally, spiritual healing as Brazilians know it requires a
moral understanding of essential human aptitudes: universal
love and a sense of justice, respect, and tolerance of others (fraternal solidarity), as these are essential natural instruments
that allow the individual to live in perfect harmony with his

surroundings, thus allowing him to live his existence in a more complete sense.

THE HUMAN SOUL

For Brazilians the soul and spirit are, in fact, two aspects of a single entity. The soul is that which lives in the biological body and participates in the constitution of the human body. As soul, the spirit takes on a biologically evolutionary form in order to purify and become more lucid through the earthly knowledge and experiences it acquires. All souls are created *equal*: simple and ignorant. Through successive rebirths in different physical bodies (reincarnation), the soul acquires through its own effort conditions that allow higher levels of consciousness. Reincarnation in accordance with the law of immortality of the soul contends that the soul survives physical death and makes available the opportunity to participate in a new existence (a new biological form) in order that it may reach its highest level of evolution and maintain its individuality throughout the successive incarnations (Kardec, 2003).

Reincarnation allows a faulty soul from a previous incarnation the opportunity to be born again to repay previous debts and make amends for previous errors. For spirits who have no debts to repay, reincarnation allows the soul to gain the greatest level of spiritual evolution. According to the spiritist doctrine, there are not *many* lives, but *one* eternal life with various phases of evolution in different physical incarnations. The reincarnated soul is not newly born to this planet, as it brings with it a predisposition directly related to its previous lives—influences, knowledge, and experiences that remain imprinted on the soul. This fundamental concept of reincarnation, a central pillar of spiritism, is intricately related to the concepts of human imperfection, disease, and suffering. Disease, in the context of human suffering, is seen as the purifying agent necessary for the soul to evolve.

After physical death, this entity is no longer soul and instead is transformed to spirit outside the physical body, as it now exists freely in the spirit realm. It is at this point that the spirit entity is no longer considered part of living physical matter. The soul, when not united with a body, is a spirit. It is spirit entities from the higher order who no longer need to reincarnate to the physical plane that assist mediumistic healers. These spirits continue to elevate in the spirit plane by the extent of their benevolence. It is the natural law of cause and effect that becomes manifest in this or future phases of the evolutionary path. According to this rigorous law, each person receives according to what deeds she has practiced (good, bad, productive or unproductive, etc.)—particularly as practiced for the common good. This natural law is the highlight of Christ's parable of the sower: reap what you sow.

Karmic law is the natural "equalizer" that allows individuals to see their hardships, difficulties, and sufferings as the past actions or inactions they must now tend to and repair in order to harmonize the cosmic imbalance they originally created. Expiation and reparation are therefore the best therapeutic modalities in eliminating the spiritual, psychological/emotional, and physical ill effects brought about by past errors. Forgiveness alone, while being a divine grace, is not enough to delete human error; expiation and reparation are also necessary to restore individual, societal, and cosmic balance. Understanding that a great deal of infractions (individual and collective) are committed in the presence of laws that regulate human behavior has helped patients understand their suffering as the result of their own free will.

THE SOUL-MIND-BODY CONCEPT

It is within a comprehensive understanding of the soul and perispirit that mediumistic healers diagnose physical disease. Diagnosing illness within the spiritual paradigm requires that healing mediums understand that the many health problems patients have spring from emotional, mental, and spiritual imbalances, and that for healing to occur *all* of these imbalances must be identified, adequately addressed, and carefully and individually treated. "Medicine considering only the material (physical) aspect, is deprived of an incessant cause of action. Knowledge of the *peri-spirit* is the key to a crowd of medical problems hitherto inexplicable," notes Estrich-Pellegrino (1997, p. 79). The perispirit (formed of subtle wrappings of atoms) is the semimaterial envelope that links the soul and the body during biological life; it is the means by which the soul (spirit) acts upon matter, and matter acts upon soul (spirit). Spiritual influence has biological repercussions, and psychorganic behaviors have influence upon spirit. The mind, in housing feelings and emotions, turns out to be a more powerful agent in generating disease and disharmony than are known bacterias and viruses. The physical body within the spiritual paradigm therefore serves as the impurity filter of the soul and provides the means for its spiritual evolution.

With spiritual beings living a physical experience (as opposed to physical beings having a spiritual experience) there is a reciprocal force between soul and body, a merging of responsibility that takes place in the human mind. According to Brolio (1999), the differences in human behaviors are fundamentally related to the soul, since their thought, intellect, will, and free choice—as well as other psychic manifestations that characterize the way a person thinks and acts—are shaped by the soul's predisposition. The soul (conscience), containing the totality of knowledge acquired throughout its entire existence, contains organic, psychic, and spiritual aspects of the human being, which is formed by the conscience, subconscience, and superconscience (Brolio, 1999; Schubert, 2004). These three areas of the human brain ("rooms of the mental house") balance and restore the forces of the physical organism.

Brazilian health care professionals, understanding how thought comes before form (emotional, physiological, and/or biological forms) and consciousness exists before matter, can approach all morbid processes as essentially being mentally commanded by the soul. Brazilian spiritist-psychologist Schubert, in her book *Os Poderes da Mente* [*Powers of the Mind*] (2004) emphasizes the mind's capabilities as being totally dependent on the soul. The soul's attributes produce a chain of thoughts that are sorted and directed in the mental house composed of the primary brain, the cortex motor, and the frontal lobes. The primary brain (our nervous system) houses habitual and automatic impulses, archives our immortal life, and represents the subconscious (our past lives). The second part, the cortex motor (the intermediary zone), is the motor to our human energy system, where effort and freewill reside. This is the conscious part of our being (our present life), where our present noble qualities (which we are currently edifying) are being stored. Finally, the frontal lobes, the areas of the brain that are least known by science and researchers, house superior notions (ideals and superior goals) and the materials of our sublime order that are gradually conquered by our efforts for spiritual ascension—the superconscious, the future; the area that allows the human mind to preview the future. The human mind responsible for translating the contents of the soul, with all its baggage from past lives and its perspective of the future, helps in the construction of the individual's present reality, signaling thought, emotional, and physiological processes as a total expression of the soul's evolutionary condition, and thus establishes a direct spiritual dimension to a patient's health and well-being. (Costa, 2001; Schubert, 2004). According to this model, thought, feelings, and emotions imprinted on the soul have definite and direct influence on health and illness. Pain and suffering of the physical body is only transitory; it is moral suffering that serves as a catalyst of spiritual evolution—an etiological agent rarely considered by classic medicine.

THE HUMAN ENERGY SYSTEM AND THE ROLE OF EMOTIONS IN HEALTH

To understand the transferring of energies used by healing mediums (through the incorporation of benevolent spirit entities) a complex understanding of the perispirit and the human energy fields that protect the human body and give it essential life force is required.

Modern physics has demonstrated that matter is a form of energy. In philosophical terms, form without matter is energy. God being immaterial (form without matter) is also energy. Humans composed of energy contain a sophisticated human electromagnetic field, which provides essential life force that is in the early beginnings of scientific development. These are important revelations for the field of science and medicine; many Brazilians believe further studies of electromagnetic energy will lead physicists to the source of human electromagnetic energy. Physicists knowing that electromagnetic energy requires a source in order for it to function are helping science better understand the human energy system and its role in biological function.

Many healing and spiritual world traditions include principles of the human energy system in their medical repertoires. Brazilians, too, have come to utilize similar principles. As a system of inner and external light energy, many believe that the human energy field comprises an aura: the fluctuating egg-shaped energy field that externally surrounds the body, and seven chakras: the spinning wheels of lights in the human body that function as vortices of energy. Think of the chakras as the human system of inner light; the aura and the chakras work systematically via a network of fine energy channels in the body called *meridians*. Essential life energy flows through the human being via these centers; when blockages occur in the channels it cause illness. Both information and light energy flows from the cosmos through the aura, into the charkas, filtered through the meridians. This is how the spirit world inspires us, and how light reaches the body cells, giving them potential life-sustaining energy. Each of the energy fields has a particular function and influences various emotional, mental, and physical (physiological) processes.

As disease begins in the outer layers, energy fields lose their vibrancy. The physical body being the one with the lowest frequency reflects the disharmony that has formed into dense energy in the physical body. If alcohol and/or drug abuse or other unclean living has occurred, the energy fields become weakened, can be attacked, and can attract undesirable (spirit) attachments. A more lucid explanation of "attachments" is given by Schwimmer in Robert Estrich-Pellegrino's book, *The Miracle Man*:

> Look on an attached spirit as we would bacterium. When we are healthy, our immune system takes care of even deadly bacterium. When our immune system is weakened or damaged, then bacteria or viruses enter to create havoc. The same can be said for spirit attachment. If one's energy field is healthy and strong, spirits will not be able to enter. (1997, p. 87)

Negative perceptions and emotions such as anger, bitterness, envy, fear, greed, hate, hypocrisy, intolerance, pride, rage, resentment, sadness, vanity, and even fanatic religiosity, being definite forms of energy, play a fundamental role in the creation of blocked energies (Souza, 2001). It is believed that a curse, or a bad action, emotion, feeling, thought, or word is poison to the individual soul, poisoning its every atom. Poisonous thoughts and emotions produce discordant tones and inharmony. Brazilian spiritists believe negative feelings that consequently consume a great deal of vital energy in the process of energetic metabolism create larger amounts of unhealthy, wasted energy. When the production of these negative energies exceeds the capacity of distribution and elimination, it accumulates in a corresponding organ or chakra, thus clogging vital energy in important energy terminals, creating fertile ground for the beginning of the physical disease process. Ignoring the fact that individuals absorb and emit energy at all times through their actions, thoughts, and words has not allowed traditional medicine to consider the symbiotic aspect of human emotions, energy, and thoughts in the pathological disease process. By dismissing the soul's influence over individual behavior, traditional medicine's effort (to modify human temperament and ill emotions) has yet to be supported before the moral dispositions of the spirit, resisting any therapeutic intervention. This may explain why efforts by traditional medicine to modify human temperament are yet to be successful.

THE SACRED MISSION OF HEALING MEDIUMS

Brazilian spiritists believe therapy for the soul requires soul doctors, soul clinics, the assistance of benevolent and highly evolved spirits from the spirit world, and a key treatment modality: soul knowledge. The individuals whom have been entrusted with care of the human soul are healing mediums. A sensorial perception function, *mediumship* is a condition by which relations between men and spirits is established. It is a natural human faculty, inherent to all human beings, at different levels and types. It is the attunement between an incarnate (living) and disincarnate (nonliving) being that allows an adequate channel for perception of thoughts, will, and sentiments. This faculty may appear in any person regardless of the religious doctrine he embraces. History has revealed great mediums of all creeds and in all epochs, going back to the most ancient civilizations, including many that are mentioned in the Bible. It is through mediumship that humankind has been able to be conscious of immortal spiritual responsibilities (Kardec, 2003).

Christ, acknowledging the reality of a spirit world, taught humanity about secret doctrines. In the *Aquarian Gospel* we read,

> Forbid not any man to do the works of God. There is no man who can pronounce the sacred Word, and in the name of Christ restore the sick and cast the unclean spirits out, who is not a child of God.... The man of who you speak is one with us. Whoever gathers in the grain of heaven is one of us. (Dowling, 1979, p. 190)

Mediums fulfill a sacred mission. They are specialists in the sacred and masters of spirit. Healing mediums are not supposed to promise a cure, nor give false hope. Their mission is to put the patient back on track with her spirituality, reconnecting her with the spirit world. If needed, they can help identify a patient's obsessor, attempt disobsession procedures, minister passes, and provide fluidic magnetized water (energized with the healer's energy), ultimately activating the patient's own cure. Mediumistic healing practices, as unorthodox and controversial as they may initially appear, have never contradicted the Gospel teachings of Christ, nor have they opposed working collaboratively with allopathic medicine.

The following insightful selection from the *Aquarian Gospel* explains healing mediumship as an influential treatment modality. It is from the lesson of Udraka, among the sudras and visyas, the life and works of Jesus in India during an 18-year period when Christ is said to have traveled, learning from the masters, seers, and wise men in the temples and schools of Tibet, Egypt, India, Persia, and Greece:

> The healer is the man who can inspire faith. The tongue may speak to human ears, but souls are reached by souls that speak to souls. He is the forceful man whose soul is large, and who can enter into souls, inspiring hope in those who have no hope, and faith in those who have no faith in God, in nature, nor in man. A thousand things produce inharmony and make men sick; a thousand things may tune the harpsichord, and make men well. That which is medicine for one is poison for another one; so one is healed by what would kill another one. The virtue from the hand or breath may heal a thousand more; but love is queen. Thought, reinforced by love, is God's greatest sovereign balm. But many of the broken chords in life, and discords that so vex the soul, are caused by evil spirits of the air that men see not; that lead men on through ignorance to break the laws of nature and of God. These powers act like demons, and they speak; they rend the man; they drive him to despair. But he who is healer, true, is master of the soul, and can, by force or will, control these evil ones. Some spirits of the air are master spirits and are strong, too strong for human power alone; but man has helpers in the higher realms that may be importuned, and they will help to drive the demons out. Of what this great physician said, this is the sum. And Jesus bowed his head in recognition of the wisdom of this master soul, and went his way." (Dowling, 1979, pp. 58–59)

Mediumship is a vocation and a God-given gift that requires that it be practiced in a sacred and devout manner. The healing medium in relaying healing energies, through good spirits channeling divine energy, can never charge for his service. As Jesus told his disciples, "'Heal the sick, raise the dead, cleanse those who have leprosy, drive out demons. Freely you have received, freely give'" (Matthew 10:8, quoted in Kardec, 1978, p. 247). "God gave these gifts to them in order to ease others' suffering and to spread the faith," notes Kardec. "So Jesus told His disciples not to commercialize their gifts, i.e., to use them to earn profits or make a living" (1978, p. 251). Where there is no profit to be made, deceit is unlikely; and misuse is subject to divine accountability; Kardec posits that "those endowed with this gift will have to account for the use to which they have put it, since they only received it in order to do good to their fellow human beings" (1978, p. 276). Cultivating mediumship therefore requires a sincere disposition to serve.

João de Deus, deemed by many to be among the most powerful mediumistic healers existing at the present time, has worked as a healing, physical, and unconscious medium for more than four decades at the Casa de Dom Inacio in the small town of Abadiania in central Brazil. This healing phenomena fulfills João de Deus's sacred mission of serving humanity in humanizing medicine by setting a living example and providing a new model of medicine for the rest of the world "I do not heal anyone—God alone is the healer," he continuously answers to the never-ending expressions of gratitude from the multitudes he has treated while "in entity" (Estrich-Pellegrino, 1997, pp. 1–6).

João de Deus has dedicated his life to humanity, and his is a twofold purpose in life: to heal the sick, and to make people aware that we are here on the earth to improve our level on the "other side"—to elevate and better the position of our souls in the hereafter by what we do in this physical life (Estrich-Pellegrino, 1997). At the young age of sixteen, João de Deus "accepted the responsibility of devoting his life to spirit incorporation for the purpose of healing the sick. He accepted a lifelong task that would demand much of him and frequently repay him with abuse, personal deprivation, persecution, and unlawful incarceration" (Estrich-Pellegrino, p. 6). He is a humble and devout God-loving man, and accepts and treats all without prejudice or religious bias. João de Deus has been endowed with faith, goodwill, and an understanding of the spirit's predominance over the physical (material) world. Most important, he and other genuine healing mediums teach their patients to act on internal direction and to learn to discriminate between thoughts motivated by strength (faith) and those motivated by fear and illusion (which characterize human weakness).

At the Casa de Dom Inácio, the entities that João de Deus incorporates are benevolent spirits of deceased doctors, surgeons, healers, psychologists, and theologians who cite God as the only healing source. Through João de Deus as the medium or vessel, the discarnate entities (spirits) assist him with the diagnosis and treatment of those who are ill and have made the long journey to the small town. At this healing sanctuary, conventional medical physicians and Brazilian allopathic-trained spiritist doctors (*medico-espiritas*), assist healing-medium João de Deus while learning from the greater realms of medicine. These partnerships (healers, spirits, and doctors) are seen throughout the many healing sanctuaries (*casas* or *centros espiritas*) in Brazil. Serving as both sanctuaries and health care facilities, casas and centros provide patients with comprehensive medical care. Patients report the attention to be more personal, compassionate, effective, and efficient.

The casas' simple and unbureaucratic nature saves the patient a tremendous amount of the unneeded frustration and aggravation that is typical of the complex organization found in most conventional settings. They also serve as a teaching institution for health care professionals as well as individuals for whom the casas provide education and training that was excluded from conventional medical school curriculums. Casas and centros also serve as important research centers that unite a variety of academic disciplines conducting investigations. Archives of daily videos, patient records, and testimonials are kept and are available to researchers, health care professionals, skeptics, and the general public.

Rather than deal with different institutions, the casa accommodates the patient's multidisciplinary needs under one roof. An ailing mind or diseased body is treated while the soul is nurtured. As a nonprofit health care facility, the casa is fully operated by a volunteer staff and offers a place where individuals can participate in such a gratifying setting. Working with patients whose conditions are grave helps volunteers see their own sometimes ungrateful, indifferent, unforgiving, and unfaithful dispositions as trivial.

While doctors, patients, and visitors compose most of the demographic makeup of the casas, members of the paranormal national and international community also represent a significant population. Genuine members of the paranormal community have the important mission of removing barriers between human-kind and the spirit realm; they are the guardians of sacred wisdom. In this respect the casa is not only a teaching institution for doctors, patients, and visitors, but also serves as the site for potential mediums to receive inspiration and guidance. In serving as transcendental teaching institutions for future generations of healing mediums and medico-espiritas, casas are helping new generations of integrative health professionals who will complete the monumental work of transcendental medicine.

NONSURGICAL TREATMENT
MODALITIES AND REGIMENS

It is interesting to note that none of the nonsurgical treatment modalities used in spiritual healing are utilized in the traditional biomedical model. The classic model, marked by a high degree of impersonalization, at the present time uses *maintenance*-oriented care, and when needed, a prescription drug regimen that tends to be mostly suppressive in nature.

Activating the soul is done by diagnosing the patient's ailment with a spiritual consultation, where the healing medium reads the patient's electromagnetic spiritual framework: the aura, chakras, mind, and soul, ultimately detecting any energy and spiritual imbalance. A healing medium can see beyond the patient's physical body to also read a blueprint of the patient's past lives (the patient's soul), and can detect whether illness originated in this lifetime, if it is karmic (from past existences), or whether it originated from a spiritual imbalance in this lifetime. (This is not to be misinterpreted; not all ill conditions or individual suffering indicate a person has bad karma that needs atonement; sometimes disguised as problems, these may be the path that leads the patient to new knowledge, and experiences that will also contribute to his evolutionary progress.) Depending on the individual case, healers may recommend simultaneous allopathic treatment.

With a realigned and reenergized electromagnetic spiritual framework, the patient—having received a type of perispirit adjustment—has unclogged and improved the condition of and access to his means of communication. Once treated, a patient's extrasensorial channels should allow for optimal performance in the flow of energy between the patient and cosmos.

The patient at this point has been prepared and is now ready to undergo intensive therapeutic intervention utilizing an essential educational regimen that proposes a new type of learning. This type of education is not necessarily found within the usual boundaries of an institution or classroom, nor is it one found in an already existing curriculum; instead, it is one that goes with the pace and the willingness of the individual.

Education of the soul is an education that awakens human consciousness to potential values, goodness, altruism, and solidarity. It helps develop the positive human attributes originally planted within us that have, for a host of reasons, either been neglected or forgotten. Faith as taught by the doctrine is both human and divine; through faith one can accomplish miracles of love, devotion, and sacrifice. It is a most powerful tool in correcting any negative impulses of the soul, and has incredible power to release internal healing energy. World-recognized quantum physicist Amit Goswami (2001) posits that the presence of the subtle fields in the human electromagnetic structure allow us to receive the energy vibrations of prayers.

Identifying negative emotions, ways of thinking, and ways of acting can help patients make the connection between their ailing spiritual system and their symptoms of physical illness. Educating and purifying the soul then becomes the pivotal treatment in the course of patients' healing, since this is the divine inspiration and guidance that patients require in order to obtain healing, and consequently regain physical health. Regular meditation, prayer, and charitable works are essential to the healing process as they are the essential elements in maintaining a state of spiritual equilibrium. Without activating this important internal power to heal, disease will continue to have its way with the physical body.

The importance of becoming strong in faith, hope, and love in order to protect the soul from harming or destroying itself is found in many different world spiritual traditions and teachings. Fear, being the opposite of faith, transgresses human trust in divine guidance. By constantly wearing an armor of genuine love and faith (through constant prayer) a vigilant and disciplined soul cannot be disturbed. The mind, when vibrating in elevated tonality, blocks the approximation of less-evolved spirits and is more receptive to more highly evolved spirit influences that positively affect human intelligence and emotional behavior (Brolio, 1999). There exists a reciprocal exchange between human beings and spiritual entities: humans acting on spirit help (through prayer and through mental vibrations/frequencies), and highly evolved spirit entities acting equally on them (intuitively clarifying, and orienting them) labor together toward the realization of good acts. And by the same token, if the spirit world senses a vibrational tune that consists of negative thoughts or feelings, the lower-evolved spirits can negatively influence the individual, causing him to do wrong or bringing upon him a mental distrurbance such as an obsession or mental subjugation (Brolio, 2000). Charity also has great implications in a patient's recovery. Serving for the common good allows love to become the predominant energy, a most vital elixir in a patient's recovery.

SPIRITUAL SURGERIES

Spiritual (visible and invisible) operations are quite common procedures in Brazil. Spiritual surgery, psychic surgery (visible and invisible) refers to a nonphysical therapeutic technique that removes deep rooted negative and stagnant energy that is almost always the root cause of many diseases in the physical body. It can also potentially remove or regenerate pathological matter. In Brazil, invisible spiritual surgery involves surgery that is done without the medium ever physically touching the person. It is done with the application of spiritual passes with the final objective of harmonizing the patient's ill energy. A spiritual pass can be done either in visible or invisible spiritual surgeries. Coming from superior spirits, the fluids that are transmitted to a healer during a spiritual pass have greater healing power than those transmitted during magnetic passes (which involve no help from a spirit being, are done entirely by a living physical being). While the spiritual pass is magnetic in nature, it is believed that the quality of the fluid that is transmitted is definitely more invigorating than those transmitted during magnetic passes. Furthermore, magnetic passes address physical ailments with a physical remedy, by first removing negative energy from the physical body, but spiritual passes address spiritual ailments requiring spiritual healing.

With invisible spiritual surgery, a surgery is done without the use of any physical surgical instruments because there is no need for physical incision. Furthermore, nonphysical instruments that are utilized in invisible spiritual surgery do not have the physical density which would allow a person with normal senses to see or feel them. Nonetheless, patients have reported movement within the auric field and manipulation of material under the skin while undergoing a spiritual surgical intervention.

In both visible and invisible spiritual surgeries, it is believed that radiant fluids interpenetrate the healer's spiritual body. The healer then transmits these fluids to the auric field, skin, tissue or organ of the patient and subsequently reaches the cellular life field, bombards the atoms elevating their intimate vibration and gives cells a more intense vitality. The healer with the guidance of spirit entities extirpates diseased growths, regenerates atrophies, unties obstructed circulation, reduces stenosis (an abnormal condition characterized by the constriction of an opening or passageway), and regenerates irreparable organs. Once a visible or invisible spiritual surgery is complete and a particular organ or tissue has been regenerated or excised, the medium sends healing energy directly to the specific area to recompose the affected organ or tissue. By doing so, its function is reestablished. The spirit entities channel spiritual energies and principles to support the patient's own internal healing process. This is how healing is achieved, the function of the organ is recuperated, and the patient's aspect of the disease is modified.

By treating the patient's perispirit, the medium alters the patient's disturbed constitution, reestablishing the patient's natural organization. This realigning of the perispirit with the physical body reestablishes the necessary harmony for the patient's recovery, thus explaining spiritual passes and surgeries as the natural Law of Equilibrium taking place during the exchange of essential body fluids. These visible and invisible surgeries have shown pain is absent in most cases, despite the lack of (chemically) sterile procedures and anesthesia—although "astral" anesthesia and antiseptics are used. The "spirit anesthesia" allows a patient to stand while undergoing the surgical intervention, and has enabled patients to speak clearly when they are asked a question, signaling an active consciousness on behalf of the patient. With those surgeries involving physical (visible) spiritual surgery, very little bleeding from the physical incisions or removal of tissue has been documented, thus demonstrating they are a most unique and noninvasive form of surgery.

Traditional surgical procedures remove the "blocked energy" at the physical level—the tissue, organs, or any other type of physical anomaly generated by the process of disease. Physical surgery only addresses the physical area of the body.

On the other hand, both visible and invisible spiritual surgery acts directly upon the root of the problem, the primary cause of the problem. Traditional medical surgery is significant within the sphere of the physical body and spiritual surgery (unlike traditional surgery) performs beyond that conventional therapeutic (physical) arena—reaching the "energetic organs," chakras, "bioplasmic body," and the aura [done by removing blocked energy, negative feelings, "miasmas energeticas" (a type of psychic parasite that has been formed by heavy and dense energy)]—areas not addressed by conventional therapies and that require a transcendental approach to understand in their entirety. Therefore, healing can be seen as an attunement to Divine love and energy that a healing medium passes on to his patients to rebalance their own physical, emotional, and spiritual energies, something allopathic doctors are not trained to do.

WHY OUTDATED MODELS MUST CHANGE

Our current health care system is, unfortunately, still modeled on disease patterns that were predominant in the first half of the 20th century. From treating acute conditions (beginning with the epidemics of the latter half of the 19th century) to trauma and infectious diseases (in the first half of the 20th century) to treating chronic illness (from 1950 to the present), the current system has never modified the therapeutic interventions of the health care model. A system originally designed to treat acute, short-term, and individual episodes of illness that were discontinuous in nature was also used to treat chronic illness (characterized as long-term and continuous) as if it, too, was a series of acute and separate episodes. If chronic illness is and will continue to be the prevalent health problem, the current model demands attention and modification. Chronic illness—often beginning early in life, long before overt symptoms appear and before medical treatment is directed toward them—allows disease to become firmly implanted. Unlike acute conditions, chronic illness once present usually remains with the patient forever, meaning that our classic model of medicine does not include treatment modalities aimed at completely healing the disease but instead treats only its more prominent symptoms or external manifestations. Short intensive interventions that may effectively treat acute illness episodes have not been able to provide appropriate or effective treatment modalities for chronic illness. The case of cancer in the United States demonstrates that survival rates after diagnosis have made a slight improvement in the past few years, but nothing significant thus far, despite the vast medical and pharmaceutical interventions and tremendous financial resources directed toward research. The prospect for the future, if nothing is fundamentally changed within the current paradigm, is bleak (Williams & Torrens, 2002). Obviously, when an entirely different set of health conditions arose these required an entirely different array of services and interventions to ensure a health care system that would be appropriate and responsive to the changing health problems of the times. When this did not occur, it created increased frustration compounded by the complexity, bureaucracy, and escalating expenses exacerbated by increasing morbidity and mortality rates—as is seen in our current health crisis.

America is experiencing an epidemic of chronic diseases that it doesn't know how to heal. As reported in the Annual Report to the Nation on the Status of Cancer, 1975–2004: Overall cancer death rates decreased by 2.1% per year from 2002–2004, but the incidence rate was *higher* for stomach, liver, cervix, kidney, and gallbladder (SEER, 2007). While some may interpret these findings as individuals are now living longer with cancer and with an improved quality of life (comparatively speaking), it should not be taken out of context. The truth is that there are still increasing numbers of patients affected by malignant neoplasms, which our current healthcare system does not properly address. And while there may be others who may be completely beating the disease, there is still much room for improvement. There are important repercussions, as they are evident in our nation's overall health. This type of "wake up" call to the inefficiencies of our current health system should encourage classic medicine to first identify the need for fundamental change, and second to look at other paradigms that offer more effective and less costly outcomes.

In comparing Brazil's health status to the United States, specifically deaths caused by malignant neoplasms, the following observation is made from the reports of the World Health Organization (WHO). In The Deaths Caused by Malignant Neoplasms last reported for 2002, the United States reported 558,643, The death rate per 100,000 individuals was 191. The amount of money the United States expended on health per capita was three times more than the amount spent by Brazil per capita. The United States spent $6,096 per capita, while Brazil spent $1,520. When .19% of the American population dies due to malignant neoplasms versus .1% of the Brazilian population, we find a noteworthy and alarming difference in mortality rates, .18% to be precise. Keeping in mind that the United States spends three times as much money on the resources directed to reduce the number of deaths related to cancer, the results call for a fundamental change in the way treatment is directed (WHO Global InfoBase, Deaths Caused By Malignant Neoplasms, 2002).

Dr. Len Saputo believes that the training he received at Duke University was impersonal, detached, competitive, and adversarial; he was trained to look at each person as a number, a diagnosis, and a prognosis. He was trained to speak to people with a detached analysis—to fix, not heal. Medical school, he feels, taught him the opposite of what he should be doing. And while medical schools teach many positive things, there are also many facets of that education that need to be unlearned, beginning with treatment modalities that have been developed to plug a patient into an established conventional theoretical orientation rather than to design a treatment modality that will suit his *individual* needs. Saputo is one of the many doctors who have visited the Casa de Dom Inácio and is convinced that health care practitioners need to be more open to the spiritual realms of healing: "'The Casa definitely has a role to play in redefining health and helping us to restructure health care delivery systems. This place is a model'" (Saputo, quoted in Bragdon, 2002, p. 38).

BUILDING NEW HEALTH PARTNERSHIPS WHILE IMPROVING SOCIAL CONDITIONS

Preparing for the future requires an expansive vision that will enable the humanistic and transcendental medical model of the future to be characterized by a wide-ranging representation of healing traditions, faiths, nationalities, and ethnic and traditional points of view; in short, a vision that demands a delicate look at the web of life in its entirety. The invaluable cooperation of world spiritual and healing wisdom offers the medical community a new constellation of conceptions, values, perceptions, and practices that can assist it in forming a new world model of social health that will offer a *universal code of human ethics* in the practice of humanistic and integrative medicine.

Mediumistic, humanistic, transcendental, or spiritual medicine—however one prefers to term it—will help individuals recognize the importance of moral health in the context of complete health; it requires a multidisciplinary cooperation between spiritual science and traditional science.

While there are many definite health benefits to be gained from adapting the dualistic Brazilian model of health, not all will embrace it. Perhaps after the relatively young field of parapsychology (and particularly mediumistic healing) gains stronger academic and scientific support and validation it can influence a new perspective on the scientific, medical, and legal arenas. Not until then will it be permitted to coexist with traditional medicine. In the meantime, there is still much that can be done to improve our current health crisis.

To begin with, traditional medicine must admit that the current model is outdated and requires major modification, recognizing the importance of preventative-oriented care and adding much-needed emphasis on the importance of patient education. That alone is a start. Biomedicine would also benefit from acknowledging important contributions coming from all healing and spiritual traditions and therapies, and that these can aid in healing.

The concept of casas as healing sanctuaries is extremely important to replicate here in the United States, as it has proven success that would likely also replicate anywhere outside of Brazil. Establishing health care facilities that serve the same purpose—to educate, spiritually guide, and heal both the spiritual and physical ailments of a patient—offers great potential in reducing mental illness and in significantly changing current morbidity and mortality rates. These health care facilities could also serve as research centers—collaborative working environments that would permit many different world healing and spiritual traditions to come together.

FINAL THOUGHTS

Undoubtedly, Brazilian spiritual/psychic healing requires an understanding of Brazilian culture: the particular way in which Brazilians view the world, their unique position in the general progress of humanity, and their passion for the continuous evolution of the world's soul. Brazilians, believing their land and people have been given the task of alleviating human suffering, humanizing medicine, and Christianizing humanity, may turn out to be the light bearers in a project involving major world progress. When the objectives of medicine are no longer overshadowed by the interests of insurance

companies nor the larger medical, economic, and political con-
glomerates and instead are met with a most basic and practical
application of the pedagogical Christian principles of spiritual
and physical health, then medicine will reach a greater level.

Working to create a better world where wisdom, faith,
reason, and love are fully integrated involves a grand effort.
Important spiritual hearts and minds of the ancient world
showed humanity the way. Christ, as well as other enlightened
minds, brought greater and clearer understanding of the way.
And today, the current humanistic health movement in Brazil
will help humanity complete its transcendental and evolutionary project of integrative medicine. These Brazilians are acting upon a most honorable oath to defend God's creation, even
when their messages do not conform with those of our time.

If humanity had never allowed new, revolutionary ideas to
coexist with those of the paradigms of its time, and had simply discarded the ideas because they were beyond the thinking parameters of the time, the evolutionary progress made in
all areas would have never reached present heights. Each idea
from all disciplines comprises the whole. Notes Kardec, "The
fact that honorable and highly accomplished individuals, after
extensive inquiry, have come forth in defense of these new
ideas, makes those ideas at least a distinct possibility" (2003,
p. 19). Undoubtedly, spiritual healing offers both great spiritual value and intellectual worth.

REFERENCES

Almeida, A. M. de, Almeida, T. M. de, & Gollner, A. M. (2000).
    Cirurgia espiritual: Uma investigacao [Spritual surgery:
    An investigation]. *Revista da Associacao Medica Brasileira,*
    46(3), 194–200. Retrieved July/September 2000 from http://
    www.scielo.br/scielo.php?script=sci_arttext&pid=S0104-
    42302000000300002.

Bragdon, E. (2002). *Spiritual Alliances: Discovering the roots of*
    health at the Casa de Dom Inacio. Woodstock, VT: Light-
    ening Up Press.

Brolio, R. (1999). *Educaçao da alma* [Education of the soul].
    Sao Paulo: FE Editora Jornalistica Ltda.

Brolio, R. (2000). *Doenças da alma* [Disorders of the soul]. Sao
    Paulo: FE Editora Jornalistica Ltda.

Costa, V. (2001). *Enfermidades da alma, e a proposta terapeu-*
    tica espirita [Diseases of the soul, and a spiritual therapy
    proposal]. São Paulo, Brazil: DPL Editora.

Cherry, R. (1999). *Healing prayer: God's divine intervention in medicine, faith, and prayer.* Nashville, TN: Nelson.

Dossey, L. (1993). *Healing words: The power of prayer and the practice of medicine.* San Francisco: Harper.

Dowling, L. (1979). *The aquarian gospel of Jesus the Christ.* Marina del Rey, CA: De Vorss.

Estrich-Pellegrino, R. (1997). *The miracle man: The life and story of João de Deus.* Cairns, Queensland, Australia: Triad.

Finkler, K. (1994). Sacred healing and biomedicine compared. *Medical Anthropology Quarterly 8*(2), 178–197.

Goswami, A. (2001). *Physics of the soul: The quantum book of living, dying, reincarnation, and immortality.* Charlottesville, VA: Hampton Roads.

Kardec, A. (1978). *O Evangelho Segundo o espiritismo* [The Gospel According to Spiritism]. São Paulo, Brazil: Instituto de difusão espirita.

Kardec, A. (2003). *The spirits' book.* Philadelphia: Allen Kardec Educational Society. (Original work published 1857.)

Krippner, S. (1987). Cross-cultural approaches to multiple personality disorder: Practices in Brazilian spiritism. *Ethos, 15*(3), 273–295.

Krippner, S. (1998). *Psychic and spiritual healing with Stanley Krippner, PhD.* Interview by J. Mishlove. Thinking Allowed: Conversations on the Leading Edge of Knowledge and Discovery Series. Retrieved October 23, 2007, from http://www.williamjames.com/transcripts/krippner.htm.

Kulcheski, E. (2001). Os mecanismos da cura espiritual [The mechanisms of spiritual cure]. *Revista Crista de Espiritismo, 2,* 8–11.

Larson, D., Milano, B., & Lu, F. (1988). Religion and mental health: The need for cultural sensitivity and synthesis. In S. O. Okpaku (Ed.), *Clinical methods in transcultural psychiatry* (pp. 191–210). Washington, DC: American Psychiatric Press.

Mishlove, J. (1998). *Psychic and spiritual healing with Stanley Krippner, Ph.D.* [Online]. Transcript of an interview. Available at: http://www.intuition.org/txt/krippner.htm

Nuñez, S. (2008). *Brazil's Soulful Medicine.* West Conshohocken: Infinity Publishing.

Povoa, L. (1997). *João de Deus, fenomeno de Abadiania* [João de Deus, phenomoenon of Abadania]. Uberaba, Brazil: Editora Vitoria.

Schroeder, G. (2003). Bezerra de Menezes: O medico dos pobres [Bezerra de Menezes: The doctor of the poor]. *Espiritismo e Ciencia, 5*, 4–7.

Schubert, S., (2004). *Os Poderes da mente* [The powers of the mind]. Sao Paulo: EDM Editora.

Sherwood, K. (1995). *The art of spiritual healing.* St. Paul, MN: Llewellyn.

Smith J. (1973). The influence on enzyme growth by the "laying on of hands." In California Academy of Parasychology and Medicine (Ed.), *Dimensions of healing: A symposium.* Los Altos, CA: California Academy of Parasychology and Medicine.

Souza, O. de. (2001). Curas Espirituais. *Revista Crista de Espiritismo, 2*, 8–11.

Voeks, R. (1997). *Sacred leaves of Candomblé: African magic, medicine, and religion in Brazil.* Austin: University of Texas Press.

Williams, S., & Torrens, P. (2002). *Introduction to health services* (6th ed.) Albany, NY: Thomson Delmar.

Xavier, F. C. (1938). *Brasil, Coracao do Mundo, Patria do Evangelho* [*Brazil, Heart of the World, Land of the Gospel*]. Rio de Janeiro, Brazil: Federacao Espirita Brasileira.

Chapter Six

La Limpia de San Lazaro as Individual and Collective Cleansing Rite

KAREN V. HOLLIDAY

Limpias son para purificar a la persona, para abrirle el camino, y para dar mejor suerte.

[Cleansings are to purify a person, to open the road, and to give better luck]

—Aurora, the 26-year-old daughter of a Colombian botánica owner

INTRODUCTION

The ameliorative effect that the *limpia*, or ritual cleansing, promises is one of the main reasons why botánica patrons seek this form of treatment.[1] If physical maladies are understood not solely as products of an unsound body, but also as manifestations of socially derived conditions, then a limpia proves to be a body technique that addresses physical discomfort in relation to social conditions.[2] In this chapter I suggest that the limpia represents a body technique that allows an individual to address and negotiate socially derived physical problems. In this case, *socially derived* refers to the emotional exchanges that occur in social relationships as emotions, such as envy, and are cited as sources of illness in Latina/o ritual healing practices. In this chapter the physical expression of envy as a source of illness is analyzed within the context of collective action embodied in the form of ritual healing. Consequently, the limpia described in detail in this chapter represents a language that provides a syntax for the articulation and negotiation of illness.

La Limpia de San Lazaro, as witnessed by this author on December, 17, 2001, is the focus of this chapter.[3] In the African-based religious tradition of Santería (or, La Regla Lucumi),[4] San Lazaro, the Catholic patron saint of the sick, is syncretized with the Santería *Orisha* (deity) Babalú Ayé.[5] Research participants referred to this ritual as La Limpia de San Lazaro and La Entrega a San Lazaro. Although legends and folk tales claim that San Lazaro is as much revered for his ability to heal as much as his ability to cause "the most dreadful diseases, from cancer and paralysis to syphilis, leprosy, and epidemics

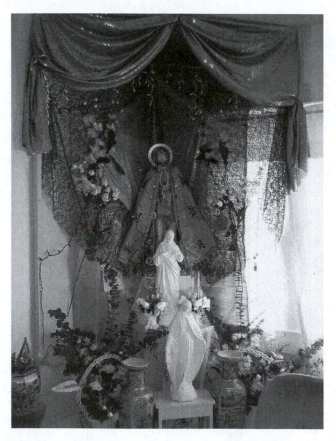

Figure 6.1

of all kinds" (Gonzalez-Wippler, 1998, p. 54), research participants in this study emphasized that the saint's redemptive
qualities supersede his ability to harm. For example, Tomas,[6]
a 65-year-old Cuban *Santero* who has been working with the
Santos (saints) for more than 40 years, described San Lazaro
as a benevolent entity who has the extraordinary capacity to
heal the most impossible of health-related maladies. What follows is an ethnographic account of La Limpia de San Lazaro
as performed in Santa Ana, California, in 2001.

DESCRIPTION OF THE RITUAL

Preparations for the ritual resembled those of any other ordinary festive celebration, with a number of people congregat-
ing at Botánica Luna by 7 P.M. Those present included Mario,
the 48-year-old Salvadorian botánica owner and *padrino*, or
godfather, and a number of his *aijados*, or godchildren—most
notably Antonio, a 28-year-old Mexican man who is credited
with encouraging Mario to commence Santería initiations in
Orange County.[7] Mario's own initiation took place in April
2000, and within one year he had welcomed 30 people into the
religion as ordained Santería priests and priestesses (*Santeros*
and *Santeras*).

Within an hour, a number of people simultaneously speaking Spanish and English arrived, crowding the small botánica.
The majority of those in attendance were uninitiated individuals who had received referrals from friends and family,
encouraging them to consult Mario about their life challenges.
Reflecting geographic sensibilities, immigrant and nonimmi-
grant attendants from Central America, Cuba, Mexico, South
America, and the United States commingled and did their
best to not obstruct the flow of the movement of the Santeros
and Santeras. As a service-oriented religion based on hierarchy and rank, recent initiates, who symbolize the spiritually
young, were primarily responsible for ensuring that objects
used in the ritual were properly assembled, and in doing so
provided the main form of manual labor. These preparations
included numerous plates referred to as *minestras* that were
filled with beans and grains for each of the *santos* as well as
the symbolic objects associated with each of them.[8]

Amid the flurry of activity, I joined a group of other noninitiates when a recent initiate named Laura began describing
a physical problem she was experiencing. Upon seeing her
grimace and touching what seemed to be the left side of her

abdomen, I inquired about her pain. She responded, *"Tengo dolor en el ovario"* (I have a pain in my ovary), and that she had not gone to a clinic or biomedical physician for diagnosis or treatment because she is more interested in having her *"Santo hecho,"* her "saint made"—a reference to becoming initiated into Santería as a priestess by going through the weeklong process of initiation—than in receiving a biomedical diagnosis. In her opinion, the Santo, along with the relationship she will develop with her deity, will completely alleviate all her physical problems, including the pain she is experiencing during the ritual. While in the process of accumulating the monetary amount necessary for initiation,[9] she is satisfied attending La Limpia de San Lazaro, which, she believes, will stave off the onslaught of illness until she is able to be integrated fully into Santería. In the midst of Laura's explanation regarding her preference for religious healing, Antonio approached us and motioned for the noninitiates to retreat to the rear of the store because it is believed that the lack of spiritual preparation on the bodies of noninitiates carries with it the potential for physical harm when exposed to certain mysteries of the religion. As we joined others in the rear of the botánica, we were forced to stand, since all the folding chairs were taken. Through the constant flow of people, Mario ceremoniously placed *cascarilla* (powdered eggshell) on each person's forehead, forming a straight line beginning at the top of the forehead and ending in the space between the eyebrows.

Once the ritual congeries met the required standards of the senior Santeros, Antonio and the Cuban Santero who had initiated Mario joined the senior Santero in the back room, walking directly to the *boveda* (altar[10]) while chanting in Yoruba.[11] A rhythmic melody developed, with the initiated chanting a verse and those familiar with the response responding while a communal drink called *omiero*, a ritually processed fluid believed to have medicinal properties and comprised of a number of herbs and grains, was passed around in what seemed to be half of a coconut shell. The chanting became frenzied as the Yoruba verses melted into the Spanish command *¡Tómalo!* (Drink it!), encouraging each of us to imbibe the ritual drink. The first woman to receive the coconut shell was Mercedes, an elderly woman who was going to include San Lazaro in her personal Orisha pantheon during an elaborate part of the ritual referred to as "receiving the saint."[12] Ironically, she explained later that the drink had caused her to vomit. Admittedly, the drink did not have the most pleasant flavor, especially with its distinct maize taste, and I along with others frowned after drinking it. It was during this ecstatic moment in the ceremony that the botánica was about to receive unanticipated visitors: the police had been called because the adjacent parking lot was illegally overflowing with an abundance of cars belonging to ritual participants. Mario moved around the botánica with lightening speed, directing initiates to place ceremonial accoutrement in boxes to be transported to a another house, where the ceremony would continue. As we were all leaving the botánica, Mario declared, "*Esto no es nada malo. Es religion pero no van a entender*" (This isn't bad. It's religion, but they're not going to understand).

LA LIMPIA DE SAN LAZARO

At the sponsor's house, the ceremony was immaculately arranged in the garage, the only space large enough to include physical and metaphysical bodies. A large basket was placed in the center of the garage with the different minestras, which contained various beans, grains, rice, salt, and butter, decoratively arranged around the large basket. In adhering to the hierarchical status ranking of the religion, initiates were the first to participate in the *limpieza* (cleansing) while the uninitiated waited in the adjoining kitchen. The process of purification commenced in a rhythmic motion, with participants entering the garage through the doorway that joined the consecrated space to the mundane kitchen. As a ritual of performance, the sacred space had been transformed through the placement of objects and physical bodies. Those versed and initiated in the art of healing occupied particular roles that night, and engaged with participants in a series of body techniques meant to elicit individual and communal healing. As a symbol of the influence he had exerted in augmenting Santería participation in Orange County, Antonio was the first to greet participants as he passed a live rooster over each person's head and torso, beginning with the front and continuing down the backside. This initial salutation prepared congregants to participate in an intersubjective exchange of bodily techniques meant to elicit health and well-being. After gaining entry into the sacred space, each person was directed toward the minestras in the center of the garage, where the flow of individual movements became rhythmically synchronized with the germinal act of placing a monetary amount in a medium-sized bowl, symbolically representing reciprocity as well as reflecting capitalist sensibilities whereby financial capital is exchanged for anticipated social capital. Following the individual placement of varying sums and reflecting the movements of a choreographed dance, each person grabbed fistfuls of the various beans and grains as they walked in a counterclockwise direction in the room, passing these ceremoniously officinal objects around individual arms and legs to allegorically absorb that which ails, and culminating with the casting of sullied articles into the large basket in the center of the garage. In this large basket personal harmful contagions were corralled through collective action in a penultimate exercise of purification.

With the completion of the central portion of the ritual, each person faced Sofia, a 36-year-old Santera who, with a live hen instead of a rooster, performed the very same procedure that Antonio had executed upon commencement of the ritual. The concluding act took place with Claudia, a Santera next to Sophia, tapping each person's shoulders with two large wooden rods. With this portion of the limpia completed, those who were uninitiated were asked to leave while the initiated remained for the subsequent part of the ceremony where Mercedes, the elderly woman in the botánica who had experienced the ill effects of drinking the omiero, would receive San Lazaro. Mario explained that without going through the intense purification rituals performed during the initiatory year, a person's body would be too weak to witness the sacred event of calling down the saint. Nonetheless, the senior Santeros assured all participants that San Lazaro's blessings would reach all as long as one had *fe*, or faith. Having faith and working in a communal manner to address individual concerns marks the bedrock of this ritual, whereby shared interactions provide the cornerstone for the healing process to unfold.[13]

ANALYSIS: INDIVIDUAL BODY, SOCIAL BODY

In this chapter, La Limpia de San Lazaro is not analyzed in terms of efficacy of treatment as biomedically defined by the elimination or reduction of unwanted disease from a person's body. Instead, this particular ritual is analyzed as a language or method of articulation that allows for the negotiation and contestation of socially derived physical inconsistencies. To accord an overall sense of the processual and fluid nature of bodily and social interpretation, ritual analysis here interlocks with information collected during fieldwork conducted from

July 2000 to June 2002, with primary emphasis placed on the location of illness in relation to social relationships. Of particular interest in terms of locating the individual experience of health in relation to the social is the following description by Lock and Scheper-Hughes, provided in their seminal work on the differentiations among the individual body, the social body, and the body politic[14]:

> Social relations are also understood as a key contributor to individual health and illness. In short, the body is seen as a unitary, integrated aspect of self and social relations. It is dependent on, and vulnerable to, the feelings, wishes, and actions of others, including spirits and dead ancestors. The body is not understood as a complex machine but rather as a microcosm of the universe. (1996, pp. 58–59)

In emphasizing the relationship between the self as both localized in the individual body and in relationship to a community in the form of social relationships, it is necessary to elaborate on the conceptualization of the body as framed by research participants. As with other studies of nonbiomedical views of the body (Finkler, 1994; Last, 1996; Loustaunau & Sobo, 1997; O'Connor & Hufford, 2001; Rubel & Hass, 1996; Worseley, 1982), research participants described their bodies as a conglomeration of elements and as transactional entities. Avoiding Cartesian dualisms of mind/body separations, research participants described the body as a manifestation of spiritual life in which the body's physical state is a reflection of, and closely intertwined with, the spiritual realm. Consequently, addressing physical maladies requires addressing the spiritual nature of illness, making the Limpia de San Lazaro an effective means of assuaging illness. In this sense, this ritual serves as a therapeutic process defined by Csordas and Kleinman as "all the meaningful activity that mediates procedure and outcome" including diagnosis (1996, p. 8), administration of the therapy, and successful outcome in that it includes administration of therapy in direct relation to the spiritual cause. While biomedical success measures success through the elimination of disease or disorder, a Parsonian sociological approach would argue that success is determined through the termination of the "sick role." La Limpia de San Lazaro allows participants to conceptually abate thoughts of illness and disease, including the experience of pain, and envision themselves as active actors in promoting their own well-being. As McGuire explains, "Ritual practice may be effective precisely because of its ability to metaphorically address and transform the unitary body/mind/self" (1988, p. 114).

Through ritual activity, the body is perceived as an instrument to be used by the Orishas as well as the individual. For the uninitiated, as Mario explained, communion with the Orishas can be too powerful, hindering the achievement of physical well-being. The initiated, however, are permitted, through the yearlong preparatory process, to experience an extreme form of body manipulation through possession. As explained by research participants, possession entails an individual's own spirit, which acts as a guardian to the physical body, allowing for another entity, ideally that of an Orisha or other high-order spirit, to occupy the individual's physical body for divination or healing.[15]

While the possession experience provides a very vivid and extreme sacred body technique, the experience of supplicating spiritual entities in a communal effort provides a less dramatic but also demulcent body technique that addresses, articulates, and negotiates pain. In this interpretation, the body serves as the binding concept between health and religion in understanding individual experience in relation to the social. Through the communication of bodies in choreographed movements, individual bodies are worked alongside the social body of congregants.

ROLE OF EMOTION IN RELATION TO ILLNESS EXPERIENCE

Mario provided a complex rationale about the relationships among the body, emotion, and illness during the course of fieldwork activities. As he practiced Santería he would explain that the physical body experienced in daily life is made meaningful because of human dependence on the five senses. Perception of pain as interpreted through the senses diminishes the connection between disease and emotion—which, in his opinion, is the primary source of illness. Thus, manifestations of illness have an emotional cause and negative emotional states can be triggered through inharmonious social interaction. Melding beliefs in reincarnation with his Santería practices, Mario elaborated that global illness experience reflects the current evolutionary process of the human race where illness serves as a means of karmic purification. He believes that although this macrolevel interpretation provides a feasible rationale for the experience of pain, as a healer he is committed to providing instruments of relief, such as La Limpia de San Lazaro, to help provide meaning and understanding to those who seek help from him. While he does not advocate the experience of pain as an ideal method for evolutionary progress, he provides this explanation to patrons in an attempt to provide an alternative outlook that growth, perception, and advanced understanding of self can be possible through pain.

The pivotal components in determining evolutionary progress and the source of disease are social relationships. In Mario's worldview, emotion is linked to thought so that the process of thinking negatively about another can potentially manifest as illness if the vibration generated through thought is conveyed through emotion, which Mario frames through the discourse of energy: "Bad energy can enter a person simply when someone sees you poorly, as in the case of mal de ojo or envy. Then, the bad energy stays and produces discomforts in the physical body."[16]

During the ritual, Laura had revealed a pain she experienced and surmised that it was located in her ovary. She later revealed that she had experienced this sharp pain for about three months, and that the diagnosed source was *envidia*, or envy. She elaborated:

> Well, this woman left me her bad luck, her bad vibes. When she came to visit me she was very envious. She left me her bad—well, more than bad—her envy that is for me—well, instead of visiting me, right, and leaving love, leaving peace, she left me with this pain.

Envy has commonly been identified as a cause for misfortune in studies of witchcraft (Evans-Pritchard, 1976; Rasmussen, 2001) and Latina/o interpretations of illness experience (Chavez, 1984; Gomez Beloz and Chavez, 2001; Jacobson, 2003; Kearney, 1978; Keefe, 1981; Nuñez Molina, 2001; Perez y Mena, 1998; Rubel 1984).[17] Laura specifically described her neighbor's feelings toward her as full of ill will because of her current life state:

> That woman would enter my house and harm me with her envy. Because I don't have problems with my children, I have a job, I don't have a man, but besides this I don't have problems. But, what can you do? People don't like to see you without problems—content, right, happy.

The relationship between the subjectively experienced body and the socially defined person is confronted with the possibility of physical ramifications with the onset of symptoms associated with disease. As a result of this exchange, Laura identifies her physical illness, located in her left ovary, as the end result of an emotion that another feels toward Laura because of her life circumstances. Laura conceptualizes the pain she experiences as a direct result of the emotion of envy her neighbor projects onto her physical body, resulting in the experience of pain. The exchange is described as spontaneous and unconscious, arising from the self-determination of another.

THE ROLE OF RITUAL PERFORMANCE IN ADDRESSING SOCIALLY DERIVED PAIN

In order to adequately address the experience of pain, Laura turns to the limpia as an effective body technique that gives meaning to disease location as well as providing the method by which to performatively address an unharmonious social relationship. As Csordas and Kleinman (1996) eloquently indicate, the cure utilized is dictated by the determined source of the disease. The limpia provides Laura with a language through which she is able to speak to the source of illness in the act of ridding her body of the unwanted agent of disease while relying on the communal support made available through the limpia performance. While not being able to adequately address the negative perception of another directed toward her at the moment of emotional exchange, Laura is able to give meaning to the pain she experiences, as well as giving voice through ritual to speak against feelings of misunderstanding experienced with her neighbor, and is provided with symbolic harmonious relationships through the very act that offers hope for physical well-being (Newman, 1999).

In conceptualizing ritual performance as a form of therapeutic process (Csordas, 1996), La Limpia de San Lazaro provides a method of addressing life's ills, including illness manifestation. In thinking about ritual as performance, individual actors are provided a venue in which experiences of pain associated with illness are given a voice, as Laura's case indicates. The mercurial nature of the act "alters moods, attitudes, social states, and states of mind" (Scheiffelin,

1996, p. 59) providing individual performers with a stage for cathartic release. La Limpia de San Lazaro is best perceived as a performative act that addresses social conditions within the context of religious perception. The ritual activity is not a psychodrama that symbolically and collectively re-creates social problems as a method of addressing them.[18] Instead, the limpia serves as a petition to a particular deity, San Lazaro, where the collective intention drawn from a constructed sense of community, loosely defined by the experience of pain, provides a support system as a means of addressing the presence of illness in individual bodies. However, to relegate ritual to religion is a disservice in the sense that ritual activity is a form of address and negotiation of material social conditions, whether they are health or finance related. As well, different religious affiliation does not preclude participation.

Through the communal performance, where individual bodies address individual concerns in a communal format, the idea of purification is at the forefront of activity. Individual actions intermingled with relational experiences provide a continuum by which personal agency is directionally tied with the collective experience. Mario sets the stage by symbolically marking each person's forehead with cascarilla. In this act he both acknowledges the individual need for protection and the collective endeavor of preparation for seeking help from divine sources. Everyone who is greeted by Antonio and Sofia establishes a relationship within the community of health seekers, where it is understood that assistance will be provided to alleviate pain produced by illness. The entire ritual takes the form of one entire body, where the movement of each individual action to reduce pain and illness is part of a collective purpose legitimizing the ability of the group to alter individual and social status. The individual end goal is reduction and eradication of pain and illness. By performing this act together, participants are able to create a space in which the effort of all strengthens each personal goal. The emphasis on unity of motion, as illustrated by the orchestrated hand and body movements throughout the event, accentuates the reliance on social bonds in order to achieve a heightened state of well-being. Community is at the forefront of this ritual performance, whereby each participant has an important and required role that offers personal satisfaction as well as neighborly support.

CONCLUSION

The primary promise of healing is at the forefront of the limpia experience. In thinking about the limpia as a therapeutic process, the healing received supersedes an interpretation based on a biomedical expectation of disease eradication. It can be understood as a process by which an individual attempts to improve her life conditions, including social, emotional, physical, and psychological well-being (Brodwin, 1996). For some, magical and spiritual care addresses a variety of illnesses as well as certain social and psychological problems (Brown, 1991; Gonzalez-Wippler, 1982; Lefley, 1998; McGuire, 1988; Newman, 1999; Nodal 1992). Essential in this analysis is recognizing that the individual physical imbalance is caused by social conditions.

In the Santería pantheon San Lazaro's prominence hinges on the faith that adherents have in his ability to alleviate physical pain and illness. The specific ritual described in this chapter offers a magnification of the Santo's perceived powers in that the communal supplication made for improved physical status provides a venue to address and heal socially derived illnesses. In a popular image of San Lazaro he is feeding a scraggly dog instead of feeding himself, a symbol of selfless love and concern for another being above and beyond himself; communal ritual in part honors this aspect of helping each other and thinking of self in relation to others.

In the attribution of illness to social tensions (Lock and Scheper-Hughes, 1996), contradictions and hostilities (Foster, 1965), and folk idioms of witchcraft (Scheper-Hughs and Lock, 1996; Young, 1980), La Limpia de San Lazaro can be interpreted through the anthropological paradigm of embodiment in terms of perception and practice, whereby perception refers to the thinking of the self as an "object in a world of objects" and practice refers to "orientation with respect to self, objects, space and time, motivations and norms" (Csordas, 1990, p. 6). By taking the two principle concepts of perception and practice, the ritual performance described in this chapter collapses both in a process of redress. First, the perception of self through the body as an "object in a world of objects," equally susceptible to life's inconsistencies—or, as Finkler (1994) describes it, life's "lesions"[19]—is made evident. Second, the performative act clearly orients the self "with respect to self" as individual pain experience, "with respect to objects" in relation to other people, "with respect to space and time" in the ceremonial configuration of sacred space, and "with respect to motivations and norms" as defined by envy and energy. In using interpreting this ritual through the paradigm of embodiment as outlined by Csordas (1990), the social significance of the act is accentuated. At the heart of embodiment analysis is the configuration of the body as an active subject in the world as opposed to a passive object of ideological representation through which emotion offers the means by which "the intersection of individual order and social order may be most clearly seen" (Lyon and Barbalet, 1994, p. 63).

The allure of the performative ritual of La Limpia de San Lazaro lies in the active engagement of adherents, as opposed to a passive form of participation in the process of healing (Joralemon, 1986; Lanford, 1998; Schneirov & Geczik, 1998). The act of performing healing can reshape an individual's perception and consciousness of an illness condition (Bourguignon, 2003) and transform the individual through the physical act of addressing pain (Finkler, 1994). In essence, performing an act to address illness offers an individual the opportunity to actively transform her perception of illness and to occupy the position of active agent.

NOTES

1. There are two types of limpias that can be performed—the simple and the more elaborate. The most common one, which is well documented in Latina/o religious healing literature is the limpia that is performed with an egg and alcohol-based colognes. The egg is passed around a person's entire body and aromatic colognes of orange, rose, sandalwood, or a variety of other fragrances are sprayed on the body. Also commonly used for the ridding of "negative energy" as experienced by unwanted physical symptoms are herbal spiritual baths. These can be self-prepared, prepared by a specialist, or purchased through commercial vendors. While the focus of the baths, or *baños*, are also cleansing in nature, I do not elaborate on them in this chapter since they are an individual endeavor and not intersubjective in practice.

2. As Jackson explains, "bodily movements can sometimes do more than words can say. In this sense techniques of the body may be compared with musical techniques, since both transport us from the quotidian world of verbal dis-

tinctions and categorical separations into a world where boundaries are blurred and experience transformed" (1989, p. 132).

3. This ritual is taken from the larger study on botánicas in southern California conducted by the author from July 2000 to June 2002 (Holliday, 2002).

4. Research participants used both terms interchangeably. See McNeill, Esquivel, Carrasco, and Mendoza, "Religious Healing and Biomedicine" (chapter 9 of the present volume) for a historical account of Santería.

5. I use the term *syncretized* here to designate that these two religious entities are mutually acknowledged in the ritual.

6. All names of participants herein are pseudonyms.

7. See McNeill, Esquivel, Carrasco, and Mendoza (in chapter 3 of the present volume) for a description of the Santería initiation process.

8. The term *minestra* refers to a thick soup made with beans. Here, however, the reference is directly to the soup plate used, which in the limpia is filled with the dry ingredients that would be included in the hearty soup. Research participants also referred to Santería deities—authentically known as *Orishas*—as saints, or *Santos*.

9. During my fieldwork activities in Orange County from 2000 to 2002, the cost for the weeklong ceremony ranged from $10,000 to $15,000.

10. Research participants explained the *boveda* to be an altar for one's ancestors and "friend" spirits, serving as a physical portal that intersects with metaphysical reality, allowing for the expression of familial and fraternal relationships therein.

11. Feld and Brennis (2004) emphasize the connection between sound and place in orienting one's knowing and being in the world. Here, sound serves as a means of articulating collective identity and membership.

12. To "receive a saint" translates to participating in a ceremony in which such receiving has been determined through an oracle to be a necessary step in an individual's personal development in the religion. The term *to receive* is used because the person is ritually prepared for possession whereby the deity will enter the person's body through the topmost portion of the head.

13. As Silver and Wilson (1988) note in their study of Lakota and Sioux sweat lodge ceremonies, the process of purification that ensues in the ritual has physical, symbolic, and metaphysical elements. For a detailed account of the conceptualization of self in relation to environment as it informs health, see Farella (1984).

14. Del Vecchio Good, Brodwin, Good, and Kleinman (1992) argue that while the experience of pain—especially chronic pain—is created in or generated by the individual body, it is also constituted in the individual body's relationships to society and its local worlds.

15. Bourguignon (2004) and Ong (1987) argue that possession provides women with a means of resisting positions of powerlessness. Of importance here is the theme of empowerment that emerges from having the ability to commune with the divine in the intimate manner that possession suggests.

16. My translation.

17. *Merriam-Webster's Online Dictionary* defines *envy* as "painful or resentful awareness of an advantage enjoyed by another joined with a desire to possess the same advantage." Retrieved October 26, 2007, from http://www.merriam-webster.com/dictionary/envy.

18. As such, this interpretation counters Turner's (1997) idea of the social drama in that the social space created in the ritual described in this chapter emphasizes cohesion instead of providing a venue for reenacting social unrest.

19. Finkler defines life's lesions as "perceived adversities of existence, including inimical social relationships, and unresolved contradictions in which a human being is entrenched and which gnaw at the person's being" (1994, p. 15).

REFERENCES

Bourguignon, E. (2003). Faith, healing and "ecstasy deprivation": Secular society in a new age of anxiety. *Anthropology of Consciousness, 14*(1), 1–19.

Bourguignon, E. (2004). Suffering and Healing, Subordination and Power: Women and Possession Trance. *Ethos, 32*(4), 557-574.

Brodwin, P. (1996). *Medicine and morality in Haiti: The contest for healing power.* Cambridge, England: Cambridge University Press.

Brown, K. M. (1991). *Mama Lola: A Vodou priestess in Brooklyn.* Berkeley: University of California Press.

Chavez, L. (1984). Doctors, curanderos, and brujas: Health care delivery and Mexican Immigrants in San Diego. *Medical Anthropology Quarterly, 15*(2), 31–37.

Csordas, T. J. (1990). Embodiment as a paradigm for anthropology. *Ethos, 18*(1), 5–47.

Csordas, T. J. (1996). Imaginal perfomance and memory in ritual healing. In C. Laderman & M. Roseman (Eds.), *The Performance of Healing* (pp. 91–113). New York: Routledge.

Csordas, T. J., & A. Kleinman. (1996). The therapeutic process. In C. F. Sargent & T. M. Johnson (Eds.), *Medical anthropology: Contemporary theory and method* (pp. 3–20). Westport, CT: Praeger.

Del Vecchio Good, M.-J., Brodwin, P. E., Good, B. J., & Kleinman, A. (1992). *Pain as a human experience: An anthropological perspective.* Berkeley: University of California Press.

Evans-Pritchard, E. E. (1976). *Witchcraft, oracles, and magic among the Azande.* Oxford, England: Clarendon Press.

Farella, J. (1984). *The Main Stalk.* Tucson, AZ: University of Arizona Press.

Feld, S., & Brenneis, D. (2004). Doing anthropology in sound. *American Ethnologist, 31*(4), 461–474.

Finkler, K. (1994). *Women in pain: Gender and morbidity in Mexico.* Philadelphia: University of Pennsylvania Press.

Gomez-Beloz, A., & Chavez, N. (2001). The botánica as a culturally appropriate health care option for Latinos. *Journal for Alternative and Complementary Medicine, 7*(5), 537–546.

Gonzalez-Wippler, M. (1992). *The Santeria Experience.* St. Paul: Llewellyn Publications. (Original work published in 1982).

González-Wippler, M. (1998). *Santeria: The religion.* St. Paul, MN: Llewellyn.

Holliday, K. V. (2002, November). Limpiando energía negativa: Issues of self and identity at la botánica. Paper presented at the the American Anthropological Association Annual Conference, New Orleans, LA.

Jackson, M. (1989). *Paths toward a clearing: Radical empiricism and ethnographic inquiry.* Bloomington: Indiana University Press.

Jacobson, C. J., Jr. (2003). "Espiritus? No. Pero la maldad existe": Supernaturalism, religious change, and the problem of evil in Puerto Rican folk religion. *Ethos, 31*(3), 434–467.

Joralemon, D. (1986). The performing patient in ritual healing. *Social Science and Medicine, 23*(9), 841–845.

Kearney, M. (1978). Spiritualist healing in Mexico. In P. Morley & R. Wallis (Eds.), *Culture and curing: Anthropological perspectives on traditional medical beliefs and practices* (pp. 19–39). Pittsburgh: University of Pittsburgh Press.

Keefe, S. E. (1981). Folk medicine among urban Mexican Americans: Cultural persistence, change, and displacement. *Hispanic Journal of Behavioral Sciences, 3*(1), 41–58.

Kleinman, A. (1992). Pain and resistance: The Deligitimation and relegitimation of local worlds. In M.-J. Del Vecchio Good, P. E. Brodwin, B. J. Good, & A. Kleinman (Eds.), *Pain as a human experience: An anthropological perspective* (pp. 169–197). Berkeley: University of California Press.

Langford, J. M. (1998). Ayurvedic Psychotherapy: Transposed Signs, Parodied Selves. *Polar, 21*(1), 84–98.

Last, M. (1996). The Professionalization of Indigenous Healers. In C. F. Sargent & T. M. Johnson (Eds.), *Medical Anthropology*, pp. 374–395. Westport, CT: Praeger.

Lefley, H. P., Cros, M. & C. Charles. (1998). Traditional Healing Systems in a Multicultual Setting. I. A. O. Okpaku, (Ed.) *Clinical Methods in Transcultural Psychiatry*, pp. 88–110. Washington, DC: American Psychiatric Press, Inc.

Lock, M., & Scheper-Hughes, N. (1996). A critical-interpretive approach in medical anthropology: Rituals and routines of discipline and dissent. In C. F. Sargent & T. M. Johnson (Eds.), *Medical anthropology: Contemporary theory and method* (pp. 41–70). Westport, CT: Praeger.

Loustaunau, M. O. & Sobo, E. J. (1997). *The Cultural Context of Health, Illness, and Medicine.* Westport & London: Bergin & Garvey.

Lyon, M. L., & Barbalet, J. M. (1994). Society's body: Emotion and the "somatization" of social theory. In T. J. Csordas (Ed.), *Embodiment and experience: The existential ground of culture and self* (pp. 48–66). Cambridge, England: Cambridge University Press.

McGuire, M. (1988). *Ritual healing in suburban America.* New Brunswick, NJ: Rutgers University Press.

Newman, D. (1999). The Western psychic as diviner: Experience in the politics of perception. *Ethnos, 64*(1), 82–106.

Nodal, R. (1992). The concept of *ebbo* (sacrifice) as a healing mechanism in Santería. *Journal of Caribbean Studies, 9,* 113–124.

Nuñez Molina, M. A. (2001). Community healing among Puerto Ricans: Espiritismo as a therapy for the soul. In M. F. Olmos & L. Paravisini-Gebert (Eds.), *Healing cultures: Art and religion as curative practices in the Caribbean and its diaspora* (pp. 115–129). New York: Palgrave.

O'Connor, B. B. & Hufford, D. J. (2001). Understanding Folk Medicine. In *Healing Logics: Culture and Medicine in Modern Health Belief systems,* pp. 13–35. Logan: Utah State University Press.

Ong, A. (1987). *Spirits of resistance and capitalist discipline: Factory women in Malaysia.* Albany: State University of New York Press.

Pérez Y Mena, A. I. (1998). Cuban Santeria, Haitian Vodun, Puerto Rican Spiritualism: A multiculturalist inquiry into syncretism. *Journal for the Scientific Study of Religion.* 37(1), 15–28.

Rasmussen, S. (2001). Betrayal or affimation? Transformations in witchcraft technologies of power, danger and agency among the Tuareg of Niger. In H. L. Moore & T. Sanders (Eds.), *Magical interpretations, material realities: Modernity, witchraft and the occult in postcolonial Africa* (pp. 136–159). London and New York: Routledge.

Rubel, A. (1984). *Susto, a folk illness.* Berkeley: University of California Press.

Rubel, A. J., & Hass, M. R. (1996). Ethnomedicine. In C. F. Sargent & T. M. Johnson (Eds.), *Medical anthropology: Contemporary theory and method* (pp. 113-130). Westport, CT: Praeger.

Schiefflin, E. (1996). On Failure and Performance: Throwing the Medium Out of the Séance. In C. laderman & E. Roseman (Eds.) *The Performance of Healing,* pp. 59–89. New York & London: Routledge.

Schneirov, M. & Geczik, J. D. (1998). Technologies of the Self and the Aesthetic Project of Alternative Health. *The Sociological Quarterly, 39*(3), 435–451.

Silver, S. M. & Wilson, J. P. (1988). Native American healing and purification rituals for war stress. In J. P. Wilson, Z. Harel & B. Kahan (Eds.), *Human adaptation to extreme stress: From the Holocaust to Vietnam,* pp. 337–355. New York: Plenum Press.

Turner, V. (1997). *The ritual process*. New York: Aldine de Gruyter. (Original work published in 1965.)

Wilson, D., & Csordas, T. J. (2003). "Now you got your answer..." Healing talk and experience in the Navajo lightning way. *Ethnography, 4*(3), 289–332.

Worseley, P. (1982). Non-Western Medical Systems. *Annual Review of Anthropology*, 11, 315–348.

Chapter Seven

Resé un Ave María y Encendí una Velita

The Use of Spirituality and Religion as a Means of Coping with Educational Experiences for Latina/o College Students

JEANETT CASTELLANOS AND ALBERTA M. GLORIA

The first in her family to go to college, Maribella is a sophomore who is for the first time living away from home while attending a large predominately white university. She is the oldest in the family; five brothers and sisters still live at home with their parents. Struggling to find connections on campus and with faculty, Maribella feels particularly lonely when she has to stay at school to study on the weekends knowing that her family (including her grandmother and aunts) gather to eat dinner and spend time together. Growing up in a fairly traditional Mexican household, she has always known her family to be religious, with her mother attending church, praying regularly, and lighting candles to *La Virgen*. She fondly remembers attending mass with her mother and grandmother almost every Sunday, and lighting candles as offerings—particularly when a family member was sick. It was also on the weekends that she would say prayers to help protect the family and their home. Now at college, Maribella finds it difficult to attend mass as she does not like the masses in English, and even more so, does not like attending services alone. She has attempted to create her own alter in her dorm room with *La Virgen de Guadalupe* (the Virgin Mary), a prayer book, and a *veladora* (prayer candle). Because lit candles are against dorm regulations, Maribella feels unable to make proper prayer offerings to help her with school and to help provide support for her father, who was recently laid off at work. Maribella has struggled to keep present her spiritual practices, yet as she has been less able to engage in them she feels out of balance and less connected with her family.

This scenario is an all-too-frequent experience of many Latina/o college students who come from families whose religious and spiritual traditions are part of their daily home lives. Given the importance of Maribella's faith-based activities, she may experience feeling isolated and alienated from others given her practices. Unfortunately, as many Latina/o students in higher education find that their values, customs, and beliefs are held deviant or suspect, the struggle to maintain who they are ethnically, culturally, or spiritually is often challenged (Castellanos, Gloria, & Kamimura, 2006). Despite the challenges, many Latina/o students find means and sources to cope with their academic difficulties as they pursue their educational degrees. Literature points to a range of different coping responses college students have implemented that reflect both positive and healthy activities, such as creating academic families (Segura-Herrera, 2006) or finding mentoring relationships, as well as to more detrimental or negative processes such as substance abuse or harm to oneself (Bishop, Weisgram, Holleque, Lund, & Wheeler-Anderson, 2004; Delva et al., 2004). Yet, studies have yet to examine explicitly how Latina/o students call upon their sense of spirituality or religious practices as coping responses to their educational challenges and experiences.

From a larger student body perspective, this chapter will examine the milieu of college that students encounter in developing their sense of selves as cultural and spiritual beings. Next, to contextualize the issues that Latinas/os encounter, a brief review of values and beliefs is provided. Central to this discussion is the presentation of data from Latina/o students about their individual and familial practices of spirituality and religion. Finally, practice implications and directives for those individuals who provide counseling or support services for Latina/o students are discussed.

THE CONTEXT OF HIGHER EDUCATION

Without doubt, the college years are aptly described as a time of personal search and exploration during which students find a sense of purpose or civic belonging. Similarly, universities and colleges serve as the context and framework within which students often explore and solidify different aspects of their socially ascribed (e.g., gender, sexual, ethnic) identities. In particular, many universities and colleges strive to educate "the whole person" by emphasizing the value of human development and citizenship and character development in the learning process (Chickering & Associates, 1981). Although higher education attempts to create contexts and venues through which students might understand their inner selves, Astin (2004) contends that academic institutions remain focused on the outer development, with few substantial attempts to assist students in developing a sense of meaning or purpose. Higher education curriculum primarily focuses on cognitive and analytical thinking, yet there exist alternate ways of knowing (through self-knowledge, self-exploration, life purpose, and other existential explorations) by which individuals can experience learning and develop scholarship. Despite educational scholars having called for the integration of multiculturalism, diversity, and pluralism into the all aspects of higher education (see, e.g., Banks & Banks, 2001; Sleeter & Grant, 1994), only more recently has the emphasis on including various dimensions of student development such as character development, personal insight, and social consciousness been more readily emphasized.

This increased focus on students' inner lives and their well-being is reflected in recent research efforts that examine students' perceptions and importance placed on different identities. Described as a "community of imagination," higher education has been touted an institution of preference in which young adults who are "engaged in the activity of composing a self, world, and 'God' adequate to ground the responsibilities and commitment of full adulthood" (Parks, 1991, p. 133) are in effect formulated in their identities. For example, research has expanded to focus on meaning and importance of one's ascribed gender, sexual orientation, ethnicity, or spiritual and religious dimensions as part of exploring one's inner focus and self-development. As a case in point, the Higher Education Research Institute at the University of California–Los Angeles recently conducted a national study of college students' search for purpose and the role of spiritual within their lives (Astin, Astin, Lindholm & Bryant, 2005). Surveying more than 100,000 students on their spiritual and religious development and involvement, findings revealed that students have high spiritual interest, with 80% of the student sample believing in God. As a topic of conversation that is infrequently broached within academic settings (classrooms or faculty offices), the spiritual and religious dimension of students' lives is an area of development that practitioners and student-affairs professionals should be aware of and knowledgeable about as regards how to best support and foster it as a means for coping within the educational setting.

College Life: Changes, Challenges, and Stressors

At a time of self-growth and exploration, college students encounter numerous changes and challenges as they enter the realm of higher education after coming from secondary institutions or community colleges (Noel, Levitz, & Saluri, 1985; Pascarella & Terenzini, 1980; Pratt, 2000). From being away from home for the first time, to juggling compacted schedules and deadlines, paying bills, taking care of themselves, developing new relationships and exploring or experimenting with their sense of self, students are challenged to meet the demands of the educational system while balancing school and family needs (Gloria & Castellanos, 2003; Larose & Boivin, 1998).

In the process of balancing home, work, school, and friends, students manifest various degrees of stress (Hammer, Grigsby & Woods, 1998; Sax, 1997). Some students feel nervous or have varying levels of anxiety (Tobey, 1997), while others may feel depressed (Ndoh & Scales, 2002) as a result of life transitions associated with college life. Similarly, many students experience difficulty with the increased social demands and interpersonal skills requisite to engage fluidly in social gatherings or navigate professional encounters with faculty or staff (Chickering & Reisser, 1993). For example, students who feel socially unprepared to engage with faculty and staff often experience feelings of isolation, marginalization, and inadequacy (Boyer & Castellanos et al., 2006). Further, as students negotiate their academic setting, they simultaneously must balance the amount of time and energy that they can spend with their families while maintaining focus on their academic roles and responsibilities. Unfortunately, students often experience family conflict as a result of being unable to make time for family engagements and not meeting parental expectations. Such conflict has been related to students' decreased ego strength and increased feelings of loneliness and even depression while at school (Adams, Ryan, & Keating, 2000; Mounts, 2004; Wintre & Yaffe, 2000).

Although the college years are deemed difficult and challenging for all students, it is well-documented qualitatively and quantitatively that the educational experiences of racial and ethnic minority college students have added and intensified challenges and stressors (see, e.g., Hernandez, 2000; Hurtado & Carter, 1997; Rodriguez, Guido-DiBrito, Torres, & Talbot, 2000). In a setting that is often unwelcoming to difference and is not reflective of multiple cultures (Gloria & Pope-Davis, 1993), students of color frequently report feeling marginalized, alienated, and a sense of normlessness in their university settings (Castellanos & Jones, 2003; Jones, Castellanos, & Cole, 2002; Orozco, 2003). In particular, the educational experiences of Latinas/os who are frequently first-generation college students are fraught with challenges such as having few Latina/o faculty or staff mentors, needing to work full- or part-time to address limited financial resources, contending with racism and discrimination and negative stereotypes, experiencing cultural isolation and defamation, reshaping cultural gender roles, balancing values of home and school, and often living in the borders of two worlds ("code switching"). Typically, a few Latinas/os on college campuses and within individual classroom settings, these students are frequently overscrutinized as representatives of the entire Latina/o population while simultaneously being asked to serve as cultural ambassadors or sources of connection to local Latina/o communities (Gloria & Castellanos, 2003). Further, the mismatch (i.e., cultural incongruity) of values between the educational setting and the individual leads to increased stress, feelings of alienation, despondence, and isolation (González, 2002; Orozco, 2003; Segura-Herrera, 2006). The stressors frequently feel insurmountable, as many Latinas/os choose to stop out or even drop out of school as a final recourse to coping with their educational challenges.

Coping through It All: Strategies and Responses to Educational Difficulties

As students successfully complete their degrees every year, it is obvious that they work to mobilize their internal and external resources and energies to various degrees as they successfully navigate their educational settings (Kariv & Heiman, 2005). The coping responses implemented, however, range in scope (e.g., emotional or instrumental) as well as utility and practicality to aid in daily life functioning (Guinn & Vincent, 2002; Lazarus & Folkman, 1984). Research on coping responses for college students reveals that many students are proactive as they frequently generate a list of alternatives for their challenges or identify active ways to alleviate their stress (Kirkpatrick, 1998; Lee, 2000). Less productive coping responses to educational challenges unfortunately include withdrawal, avoidance, anger, substance use and misuse, violence, and occasionally even suicide (Bishop et al., 2004; Delva et al., 2004; Lenz, 2004; O'Hare, 2001).

In examining the degree to which they use spirituality, religion, or some faith-based activity (e.g., prayer or talking with a priest), several research studies have found that students pray and call upon their religion and spirituality as a means of resilience during trying times (Kirkpatrick, 1998; Lee, 2000; Zern, 1989). As the practice of one's religion or spirituality has been associated with stress reduction (Schafer, 1997), it seems logical that such activities might be used by students as a coping response. Notably, however, the limited research on Latina/o student coping reveals that prayer or consultation with a priest is an infrequently reported coping response. For example, in separate gender-focused studies of Latina/o undergraduates (see, e.g., Castellanos, Gloria, Scull, & Villegas, 2006; Gloria, Castellanos, & Orozco, 2005), both male and female students cited taking a planned and active response to the situation as their most frequently reported coping response. The second most frequently reported coping response for female students was to rely on one social network (peers and friends) to talk about the concern. For male students, however, the second most frequently reported response was to draw upon past experiences. That is, the men took a more individualistic approach to their coping. It is interesting to note that few students from either study reported seeking psychological services (e.g., seeing a counselor) or praying or consulting with a priest as a means for coping. However, the degree to which these and previous quantitative studies fail to capture fully the deeper rooted beliefs and manifestations of Latina/o students' cultural and familial values and traditions within their educational coping processes and, ultimately, adjustment to college and well-being can be called into question.

Cultural Contextualization for Latina/o College Students' Coping

To understand how Latina/o students negotiate their educational challenges within the higher-education context, a brief discussion of a guiding philosophy or perspective, common cultural core values, and practices for many Latinas/os is warranted. Although the presentation of these values can lend some explanation and insight into the coping process for Latina/o students, they are not intended as causal or to have direct attribution of the educational negotiation. What is important to recognize, however, is how core cultural values play a role within the daily lives of students and the degree to which they influence the way students view the world and the manner they interact or cope within it.

For example, the degree to which students endorse the *mestiza/o* or indigenous value of interconnectedness with all of the things around them can moderate the way in which they understand their role and place within the world (Ramirez, 1999). That is, many Latinas/os believe that the individual is inseparable from the physical and social environments in which he/she lives. Central to this worldview is the belief that knowing oneself is the key to understanding the spiritual world. It is through the belief that a strong identity with the group or family is central to maintaining a proper balance between the individual and the supernatural (Ramirez, 1999). The values of *familismo* (familism) and *comunidad* (community) are centralized in the belief that individuals are embedded within the context of the family or group, which is a central Latina/o cultural value (Santiago-Rivera, Arredondo, & Gallardo-Cooper, 2002). As many Latinas/os emphasize collectivism, cooperation, and intergenerational familial ties as core tenets of family, it is not surprising that Latina/o students consistently identify their families as their propelling force and source of cultural and emotional connectedness (Gloria & Segura-Herrera, 2004; Hernandez, 2000). Ultimately, the value of connection and interconnection—in particular, for those who share common values, traditions, and beliefs—is central to many students.

In achieving harmony and reconciliation with oneself and the higher powers, a frequently held concept of giving oneself over to higher powers and all that comes with it is evident. It is through the trust or the practice of *resignarse* (resignation) that an everyday assurance of faith is placed. For example, a frequent practice of Latinas/os is that of *encomendarse*, or entrusting or turning over to God or *La Virgen de Guadalupe* a particular issue, concern, or life difficulty. In doing so the individual resigns or releases the difficulty, turning it over to a higher power and process, with the knowledge that the individual is centrally connected with others (Ramirez, 1999). This process is similarly reflected in the frequently stated and importantly held belief of *si Dios quiere*—That is, if God wants, wills, or allows it, only then will it or can it be. Within this statement, the individual is resigned to God's higher power, will, and wisdom. Although this may unduly implicate the idea of fatalistic beliefs for Latinas/os, the *mestiza/o* worldview that the individual is part of the larger system and has influence and affect on the environment lends way to the different spiritual engagements or even folk traditions practiced by Latinas/os in their daily lives (Ramirez, 1999).

An Overview of Latina/o Students' Family Practices

As the primary socialization for individuals often occurs within a family context, a glimpse into personal and familial spiritual practices was assessed for Latina/o college students. To inform this chapter about current practices and spiritual engagements of students, the authors conducted a small-scale study with current undergraduates attending a research type institution. Specifically, students in an undergraduate class addressing ethnicity in America agreed to complete a 10-minute pen-and-paper survey consisting of six demographic items (e.g., gender, ethnicity, class standing) and several open-ended questions regarding personal and family spiritual practices. Specifically, students were asked about family folk beliefs, about their personal spiritual beliefs, and to recount a specific story that highlighted their spiritual traditions. Each of the questionnaires was transcribed and analyzed using line-by-line analyses to develop themes that were enumerated and subjected to descriptive analyses per Bogdan and Biklen (1992) and Le Compte and Schensul (1999).

Intended as an exploratory investigation of spiritual practices of Latina/o undergraduates, a total of 59 students completed the surveys. Of these, 42 self-identified as Latina/o and

16 were non-Latina/o. Focusing on Latina/o student familial experiences, only information from the 42 Latina/o students is presented for consideration here.

The Latina/o students included 11 men and 31 women who ranged from first generation to fourth generation; the majority, however, were either first or second generation. More than three-quarters of the students ($n = 33$) were juniors or seniors, and all but two students reported being either Catholic ($n = 36$) or Christian ($n = 4$). One student reported not having a religion, and one did not answer the question. Almost two-thirds of the student sample (64%; $n = 27$) indicated that their families believed in cultural-bound syndromes, such as *mal de ojo* (the evil eye), *susto* (fright or extreme fear), or *empacho* (abdominal ailment). As a result, it is not surprising that more than half of the students (55%; $n = 23$) indicated that they similarly believed in cultural-bound syndromes. For a more complete description of cultural-bound syndromes, see Harris, Velasquez, White and Renteria (2004).

Assessment of the open-ended student responses yielded interesting insights into personal and familial beliefs. In particular, of the students who provided written responses, they not only addressed their personal and familial knowledge of the issues but their current experiences with spiritual activities in their daily home lives. Although students again reported families and parents to believe in different concerns—*vista fuerte* (fixed stare), *mal de ojo, empacho, susto, and nervios* (nervousness)—than they did, the students addressed how their families and individual family members engaged in the activities within their households. For instance, students indicated how their families knew of the importance of touching a baby in order not to give the child *mal de ojo*, and others reported how their mothers perform *limpias* or *limpiesas* (spiritual cleanings or cleansings) to purge their living spaces of negative energies or "bad vibes." Several of the students reported having witnessed family members having *empacho* and the subsequent remedy of an intense massage and pulling of the skin on the family member's back performed by *curaderasos* or *sobadores* (traditional faith healers) within their households. It is interesting to note that a few students revealed that their grandmothers had the gift of healing powers to attend appropriately to such concerns. For these students, emphasis was on the importance, to them and their families, of having appropriate respects for these beliefs and practices in their homelands and within their cultural upbringing.

In addition to those spiritual and folk tradition-based experiences within students' families, many of the students relayed their own personal experiences with such concerns. First, students reported having experienced firsthand cultural-bound syndromes such as *empacho* or having had a *limpia* performed on them. As part of this and other rituals, students revealed that they had engaged in activities such as having had cards read for personal guidance and direction, using teas and natural herbs for healing (in particularly for *ataques de nervios*, or anxiety), lighting candles and making prayer offerings to saints, wearing an *asabache* (spiritual protection amulet) or keeping trinkets for protection from negative energies, being visited by past family members through different forms (e.g., as doves or visions), and having prayed to particular saints for specific needs and concerns (e.g., to St. Anthony for a relationship).

Although each of the spiritual activities named were varied and the subsequent adherence of the beliefs were diverse, it was evident from the student responses that the role of prayer and the centrality of a higher power (primarily named as God) were also considered primary to maintaining balance and harmony in students' families and households. Although not specifically stated, the students further indicated that it was during times of distress or specific need that either their family members or they themselves would engage in such practices. Although the activities were not specifically church-related, the activities were relayed as key activities that were important to the well-being of their families and those around them.

APPROACHING SPIRITUALITY AND COPING FROM A HOLISTIC PERSPECTIVE: A PSYCHOSOCIOCULTURAL FRAMEWORK FOR LATINA/O STUDENTS

Given the importance of integrating all components of Latina/o students' experiences, a psychosociocultural (PSC) approach should be considered (Gloria & Rodriguez, 2000). This framework is multidimensional, fluid in its inclusion of concepts, and specifically developed for Latina/o undergraduates. Specifically developed as a counseling model for these students at predominately White institutions, Gloria and colleagues (Gloria & Castellanos, 2006; Gloria & Rodriguez, 2000; Gloria & Segura-Herrera, 2004) have extended and expanded its application for student service personnel, faculty, and researchers, as well as clinicians. Central to this framework is the premise that the context (university environment, campus and classroom climate) must be considered in conjunction with the *psychological* (personal agency to succeed, coping responses), *social* (connections with others who can provide both academic and nonacademic information), and *cultural* (congruity of beliefs, values, and behaviors that are rooted in familial and ethnic traditions) dimensions of each individual. Neglect of any of these dimensions severely limits the understanding of the whole person in context—or, as it would be here, the whole Latina/o within the university setting.

Although the PSC may seem a simplistic framework to address Latina/o student issues, current literature that examines educational concerns rarely takes a dimensionalized approach. That is, impact of the campus milieu or climate on a student's sense of adjustment or well-being while simultaneously knowing sources of support to manage the environment and their cultural connections (both internal and external) have yet to be fully explored. Such a framework provides direction to assess from a "whole student" perspective, one in which familial and cultural traditions are centralized, relationships and social connections are emphasized, personal capabilities and strengths are accentuated, and environmental challenges and barriers are considered.

Voces de los Estudiantes (Student Voices)

Utilizing this framework, a qualitative study was conducted at a large research type institution to assess the challenges Latina/o students encounter in college, their subsequent coping mechanisms, and the specific role of religion and spirituality in their daily lives as a specific coping response and means to college adjustment. A total of six Latina/o college students, all of whom were of Mexican heritage, seniors, and ranged between 20 and 24 years of age, agreed to answer several open-ended questions via e-mail. The student sample— four women and two men—reported closely identifying with their Mexican heritage, speaking Spanish, and identifying as active students on campus. Five of the six students reported being employed part-time by the university and three of the six students lived on campus while the other three lived off campus (but nearby). Each of the students reported having been raised Catholic, and two of the six reported attending Bible study on a regular basis. Participation in the study was voluntary, and the Latina/o students were not provided compensation or incentive.

Using a line-by-line analysis to identify emerging themes, the researchers employed a color-coding process that allowed each theme to be placed into different categories for a comparison of the interviews through themes. Results were categorized by emerging patterns, and direct quotes were extracted to exemplify the interrelationship between spirituality and coping in determining college adjustment among Latina/o undergraduates.

Challenges Experienced by Latina/o Students

The students unanimously reported having a difficult time adjusting to college. The primary challenges to their adjustment were limited preparation for entering college and a lack of knowledge about the college system. Additional barriers included campus climate, limited ethnic affirmation, irrelevance of the curriculum to their culture and history, and limited social support. In particular, students' lack of social support was reflected in their perceptions that they could not relate to their peers, experiencing low expectations from their professors, and having limited access to and implementation of mentorship. Central to their daily adjustment difficulties was the need to constantly navigate school and the different contexts while also balancing school and family demands. For example, one student poignantly summarized this challenge of this balance, writing:

> I've always found it hard to balance school and family. As a Latina, family is very important. When I started my undergraduate career I found myself having to choose between going home for the weekend and staying to get my work done. I quickly learned that in order for me to stay on top of my studies I had to stay and I had to give up family visits. I knew this was something I had to do if I wanted to do good in school but I also felt that I grew more apart from my family the more educated I became because I was spending less and less time with them and because I was being exposed to all this knowledge that they didn't really care for. Of course they still valued my education and saw my university degree as very important for my future; they just didn't care to know the details of it.

Examination of the challenges across the students' responses revealed gender differences. The Latina undergraduates highlighted the socially and culturally ascribed aspects of being Latina as a challenge to being in college. More specifically, they each expressed their incongruence of feeling liberated and less restricted to conform to traditional rules and mores when at college while simultaneously having to fight against the gender-based expectations and restrictions from home (from their parents and male siblings). For example, one Latina described being able to come and go as she pleased while on campus, but when she returned home having to readjust to the expectations that she always let her family know where she was and who she was with. In contrast, the male participants reported feeling isolated and invisible within their different educational settings. Marked by a sense of disrespect and accompanying low expectations from faculty, the males reported that their presence was readily and frequently dismissed. For example, one Latina/o described the lack of interest his professor had in him, stating, "I visited during [his] office hours and [he] did not have high expectations and did not take me seriously when I approached him regarding research."

Coping Responses

As expected, the range of coping responses from these six students was considerable; however, the primary means for coping was that of social support. Almost all (five of the six) noted that family and friends served as their chief source of strength and support in contending with their educational challenges. Particularly with regard to family, students uniformly reported visiting home, calling parents, bringing parents onto campus whenever possible, and maintaining a high level of contact with siblings (who were both in and out of the family household). Relative to peers or friends, five of the six students were members of Latina/o student organizations (e.g., the *Movimiento Estudiantil Chicano de Aztlán*), with four of these five students reporting to be active members in their organizations. Less frequently did the students (one woman and one man) report connecting with individuals other than family or friends. Only one student indicated seeking out her faculty mentor, and the other reported utilizing the university counseling services as a means of coping and navigating educational stresses.

When gender was considered, Latinas and Latinos also identified implementing different coping responses. Specifically, Latinas reported increasing their level of social engagement as a means to navigate their educational concerns. For example, three of the four Latinas expressed the intrinsic and recentering value of relaxing with female friends, dancing, watching movies, and "being silly" together. It was during this time together that the Latinas indicated that they were able to gain support and validation from one another. Additional coping responses were avoidance, over- or undereating, and crying as a means of sorting out their emotions. One student indicated that she sometimes avoided her emotions by compartmentalizing her problems and attempting to be logical rather than emotive in her problem solving.

Both of the Latinos implemented more individualistic approaches in their coping. In contrast to gathering with others, the Latinos identified engaging in solo activities (i.e., working out and playing the guitar). Notably, the men reported isolating themselves as their primary means of coping. For example, one of the Latina/o students indicated that he would find spaces where no one could find him, stating that "in some instances, I submerge myself in isolation." One of the two Latinos, however, reported playing group sports (e.g., soccer) as a means of coping.

The Use of Religion and Spiritual Practices as Coping Responses

After addressing a general question about coping with their educational challenges, the students were asked to specifically consider the degree to which they used religion and/or any spiritual practices as coping responses. It is important to note that each of the six students reported coming from families that had a specific religious (i.e., Catholic) affiliation, and that religion was integrated into their daily home lives. Although each of the students indicated that they were raised in homes in which their families went to church and believed in God, only four of the six students (three women and one man) viewed themselves as religious. Yet, when asked about the role of religion in their daily lives, each student indicated that God was a primary source for their resilience and problem solving on a day-to-day basis. It is important to note, however, that all of the students qualified whether they believed themselves to be spiritual or religious, with four of the six students reporting being spiritual.

Two Latinas reported not having "this type of relationship with God" but at some point hoping to be more spiritual.

Notably, all of the students reported that going to college had somehow hindered their church involvement, but that their religion and spirituality ultimately assisted their college adjustment. For example, one student indicated that as a first-year student she joined a Latina/o religious group (i.e., *Jóvenes Para Cristo*, or Young Adults for Christ), but in actuality she attended the group to gain support as she adjusted to college rather than for religious replenishment. As she progressed educationally, she no longer had the time nor need to participate in the group's gatherings. Another Latina similarly affirmed this process by her statement that "[my] religious practices have diminished since attending college" but "[I] preserve important rituals like Ash Wednesday." Similarly, one Latina/o reported attending mass, being part of a church choir, and facilitating catechism early in his undergraduate career, yet his current involvement was now limited due to time restrictions. Although each of the students reported no longer attending mass regularly or having more limited affiliation and activity, each still identified as being religious.

However, the students reported being interested in attending church services when time permitted. For example, five of the six students reported going to mass with their family and finding satisfaction and reprieve from stress when they visited home. For example, one student wrote:

> I can't say that I am extremely religious as in I attend mass or other religious events every Sunday, partly because mass was something that I did with my family (more specifically my mother) and now that I am away it's just not the same. When I come home to visit it's one of my favorite things to do with my mother.

Similarly, when students were able to attend church services, their enthusiasm was somewhat limited. For example, two students indicated that they attended mass while at the university, but because the mass was offered only in English, which it made it difficult to attend regularly. Both students reflected that attending English masses just "did not feel the same" as it did when attending mass in Spanish.

Despite reports of having limited time or feeling uneasy about the English services, weekly mass attendance was cited by three of the four women as a coping response. Going to mass was referred to as "a safe haven" where students felt "replenished and able to gain the strength needed" to confront their educational stressors.

All six students attributed aspects of religion and spirituality as having a significant role in their college adjustment. Using slightly different working definitions for religion and spirituality, all of the students nonetheless made cogent and direct remarks as to how they used these faith-based activities to help them cope with their educational stressors and concerns. For example, as one student reflected, "Spirituality helps me think beyond the present and makes me realize that there are more important things than work, like family and friends, and it also gives me strength under hard circumstances." Another wrote:

> With every year of my undergraduate career I have become less and less involved with my religion. I still attend weekly mass and use it as a time of reflection and when I can allow myself to feel peace after a week of chaos and nonstop [school]work.

Prayer was cited as the most common religious practice for the students. This practice of prayer was described by one student as providing "hope, help to overcome barriers and [to] provide a sense of strength." As might be expected, the times, duration, and frequency of prayer varied for the students. For example, some students reported praying in the morning, others on a daily basis. Only two of them, however, indicated that they prayed only during difficult or stressful times. Notably, the students indicated that they prayed about their education. For example, one student indicated:

> I pray to God every morning when I wake up and every night before going to bed that He will help me in my educational endeavors. I pray at church every Sunday that God will help me during the school week ahead.

Another student emphasized the importance of prayer relative to her education:

> Prayer and a sense of my being have definitely helped me adjust in college. I continue to pray for others and continue to ask Christ to help me become an instrument of love and peace, and [to] continue to assist humanity.

Without prayer, I do not know what other mechanism will help me during my times of distress in college.

It is important to note that prayer was not only conducted on an individual basis, but with others, such as friends, room-mates, or mentors.

Discussion

Although this was a small study, the findings were consis-tent with current educational and psychological research on Latina/o college students. Reporting educational challenges similar to those currently found in the literature (Jones et al., 2002), the Latina/o students were challenged to balance home and school concerns, and often struggled with the resulting incongruity of their familial/cultural and university values (Gloria & Segura-Herrera, 2004). The reported coping responses were consistent with research findings that Latinas take a more social approach to their coping (Gloria et al., 2005) whereas Latinos take a more individualistic approach to cop-ing with their educational challenges (Castellanos et al., 2006). Contrary to this same research, however, these six Latina/o students unanimously identified how both spirituality and religion were central and salient aspects of how they managed their educational pursuits. From daily prayer to finding spiri-tual succor and fellowship in others' company, these students relayed how their spiritual and faith-based practices were a central component of who they are as students in higher edu-cation. Notably, however, these students did not identify reli-gion or spirituality as a coping response for their educational pursuits, but as an integral component to who they are as cul-tural and ethnic beings who happen to be college students.

Indeed, there is a need for all aspects of the individual to be well in order to be most effective as a student. As it was perhaps best stated by one of the students:

> To me, spirituality is being in touch with your inner core, having the ability to introspect and ask, What do I need to do as a human being to improve my faith, my persona, and my life? I have come to understand that my prayer will be strong if I pray inside a Catholic Church, how-ever, it will be stronger if I pray with all my energy and spirit. It is interesting because now, if I do not feel well spiritually, I find ways to meditate. For example, if I feel that my behavior creates dissonance with my values, I

will record my feelings in a journal and meditate. I will
ask myself, what went wrong? Why was I not strong? Or
why did I do the contrary of what I value? My spirituality
plays a major role in my education. If I try to study while
feeling guilty or my dissonance [is] bothering me, I do
not concentrate and I am not as focused. Thus, in order
to be productive in school, I must be both physically and
spiritually well.

In effect, this statement and the other students' reflections
on needing to be wholly integrated lends further support to
taking a dimensionalized approach when providing mentorship (Gloria & Castellanos, 2006), psychoeducational support
(Gloria, 1999), or counseling services (Gloria & Rodriguez,
2000) with Latina/o students. That is, addressing an individual from the context of a larger system (e.g., family, university
setting), in which the individual influences and is influenced
by the balance of the person and environment connection
(Ramirez, 1999) is necessary to address the whole Latina/o—
person or student.

PRACTICE IMPLICATIONS

In assessing where and how Latina/o students manage themselves and ultimately cope within the university context and
contend with their educational challenges and stressors (with
particular emphasis on the use of spiritual or faith-based
activities), the following framework of PSC questions is provided as a beginning point for practice considerations.

Dimension	Questions for Consideration
University	Where and how have you been able to practice your spirituality, faith, or religion since coming to campus? How are your spiritual or faith-based practices accepted in your surroundings (e.g., the residence hall)? What faith-based activities or services (attending mass, Bible study) are offered here on campus that you might consider being a part of?
Psychological	How important is it for you to practice your family faith? When you engage in your spirituality or faith-based practices, how do you feel about yourself? To what extent is your spirituality or religion a source of comfort for you?

Social	Who on campus do you spend time with that helps you feel spiritually rejuvenated or reconnected? Who do you talk with about your spirituality or religion on campus? What relationship do you have with those in your spiritual or religious community?
Cultural	What spiritual practices or rituals do you do at home or with your family that you could you also do here at school? When you are having a stressful time at school, how do your family's spiritual and faith-based practices help you cope? What access do you have to spiritual or religious items that allow you to engage in your faith-based practices here at school?

At the structural level, universities and colleges must first address the climate and impeding obstacles that Latina/o students encounter in higher-education settings. Only with continued investment and commitment to creating an inclusive learning setting for Latina/o students, at the institutional and personal levels, will the experiences of Latinas/os become less fraught with difficulties. In encouraging students to negotiate and explore who they are as young adults, there are several suggestions that have emerged from this chapter's studies.

First, the struggle to negotiate a home and school balance continues to be central to the Latina/o students' experience. In particular, the balance of transporting familial and cultural traditions and faith-based practices into the university setting is challenging. As a result, universities need to provide church services in different languages, such as Spanish. Doing so can allow students to connect to a part of themselves and to their families even when they are physically apart. Further, it is evident that universities and colleges need to create formal mechanisms (along with financial assistance) in order for families to be more consistently incorporated into the daily lives of Latina/o students. As family is a primary source of support for many Latinas/os, it behooves the university not to overlook and to underutilize a built-in retention and well-being mechanism for students.

Second, it is evident that service providers must provide outreach or informal conversations with Latina/o students to address their adjustment and sense of personal exploration. As students look inward and to their peers for their primary source of support, reaching out to them (and into their learning and living spaces) to provide information and suggestions and to establish connections and relationships is warranted. Although many university counseling centers provide outreach and workshops for students, offering one-self as a community member, supporter, or academic family member (Gloria & Castellanos, 2006) can only serve to create the sense of care and connection that Latina/o students often seek. Establishing connections and creating a sense of purpose within a group is central to the *mestiza/o* worldview and could be appropriately integrated into any programming provided for Latina/o students. Also any activities offered should reflect the given gender differences in coping. For example, support groups assisting Latinas could address their gender identity development and values incongruence, whereas groups for Latinos could focus on establishing connections and socialization.

Perhaps the most important implication of this study's findings is the importance of clinicians and university personnel acknowledging and addressing the multiple dimensions of who students are as cultural beings—that is, the role of spirituality and religion are paramount to these students as individuals negotiating their educational settings. Although it may be difficult to create programming that specifically addresses or creates a religious or spiritual focus for students, university personnel can focus on internal growth and self-awareness activities. Posing self-reflective question such as, "How are you taking care of your inner self?" prompts and dimensionalizes students in their self-discovery.

As is evident from the findings of this chapter's studies, there is considerably more to be known about how Latina/o students' spirituality and religion play a role in their educational experiences. From examining different practices to particular faith-based beliefs, it is evident that intentional and focused examination can provide insight into Latinas'/os' interpretation of religion and spirituality in comparison to their practice of culture. Similarly, a more in-depth exploration of the centrality of religion and spirituality in Latina/o students' lives relative to their educational coping and subsequent college adjustment is warranted. Finally, examination of Latina/o undergraduates' gender roles, familial and cultural traditionalism and practices, and daily practice or religious or spiritual engagement could inform their negotiation of educational experiences and ultimately their personal well-being.

REFERENCES

Adams, G. R., Ryan, B. A., & Keating, L. (2000). Family relationships, academic environments, and psychosocial development during the university experience: A longitudinal investigation. *Journal of Adolescent Research, 15*, 99–122.

Astin, A. W. (2004). Why spirituality deserves a central place in higher education. *Spirituality in Higher Education Newsletter, 1*(1), 1–12.

Banks, J. A., & Banks, M. J. (2001). *Multicultural education: Issues and perspectives* (4th ed.). New York: Wiley.

Bishop, D. I., Weisgram, E. S., Holleque, K. M., Lund, K. E., & Wheeler-Anderson, J. R. (2005). Identity development and alcohol consumption: Current and retrospective self-reports by college students. *Journal of Adolescence, 28*, 523–533.

Bogdan, R. C., & Biklen, B. (1992). *Qualitative research for education: An introduction to theory and methods.* Boston: Allyn and Bacon.

Castellanos, J., Gloria, A. M., & Kamimura, M. (Eds.). (2006). *The Latina/o pathway to the Ph.D.: Abriendo caminos.* Sterling, VA: Stylus.

Castellanos, J., Gloria, A. M., Scull, N. S., & Villegas, F. (2006). *Sobreviviendo la universidad*: Latino male undergraduates' educational barriers, coping, congruity, and psychological well-being. Manuscript submitted for publication.

Castellanos, J., & Jones, L. (Eds.). (2003). *The majority in the minority: Expanding the representation of Latina/o faculty, administrators and students in higher education.* Sterling, VA: Stylus.

Chickering, A. W., & Associates (1981). *The modern American college: Responding to the new realities of diversity and a changing society.* San Francisco: Jossey-Bass.

Chickering, A. N. & Reisser, L. (1993). *Education and Identity* (2nd Ed.). The Jossey-Bass Higher and Adult Education Series. San Francisco, CA: Jossey-Bass.

Delva, J., Smith, M. P., Howell, R. L., Harrison, D. F, Wilke, D., & Jackson, D. L. (2004). A study of the relationship between protective behaviors and drinking consequences among undergraduate college students. *Journal of American College Health, 53*(1), 19–26.

Gloria, A. M. (1999). *Apoyando estudiantes Chicanas*: Therapeutic factors in Chicana college student support groups. *Journal for Specialists in Group Work, 24*, 246–259.

Gloria, A. M., & Castellanos, J. (2003). Latino/a and African American students at predominantly white institutions: A psychosociocultural perspective of educational interactions and academic persistence. In J. Castellanos & L. Jones (Eds.), *The majority in the minority: Retaining Latina/o faculty, administrators, and students* (pp. 71–92). Sterling, VA: Stylus.

Gloria, A. M., & Castellanos, J. (2006). Sustaining Latina/o doctoral students: A psychosociocultural approach for faculty. In J. Castellanos, A. M. Gloria, & M. Kamimura (Eds.), *The Latina/o pathway to the Ph.D.: Abriendo caminos* (pp. 171–189). Sterling, VA: Stylus.

Gloria, A. M., Castellanos, J., & Orozco, V. (2005). Perceived educational barriers, cultural congruity, coping responses, and psychological well-being of Latina undergraduates. *Hispanic Journal of Behavioral Sciences, 27*, 161–183.

Gloria, A. M., & Pope-Davis, D. B. (1997). Cultural ambience: The importance of a culturally aware environment in the training and education of counselors. In D. B. Pope-Davis & H. L. K. Coleman (Eds.), *Multicultural counseling competencies: Assessment, education and training, and supervision* (pp. 242–259). Thousand Oaks, CA: Sage.

Gloria, A. M., & Rodriguez, E. R. (2000). Counseling Latino university students: Psychosociocultural issues for consideration. *Journal of Counseling and Development, 78*, 145–154.

Gloria, A. M., & Segura-Herrera, T. M. (2004). Ambrocia and Omar go to college: A psychosociocultural examination of Chicanos and Chicanas in higher education. In R. J. Velasquez, B. McNeill, & L. Arellano (Eds.), *Handbook of Chicana and Chicano psychology* (pp. 401–425). Mahwah, NJ: Lawrence Erlbaum Associates.

González, K. P. (2002). Campus culture and the experiences of Chicano students in a predominantly white university. *Urban Education, 37*(2), 193–218.

Guinn, B., & Vincent, V. (2002). A health intervention on Latina spiritual well-being constructs: An evaluation. *Hispanic Journal of Behavioral Sciences, 24*(3), 379–391.

Hammer, B. L., Grigsby, D. T., & Woods, S. (1998). The conflict demand of work, family, and school among students at an urban university. *Journal of Psychology, 132*(2), 220–226.

Harris M., Velasquez, R. J., White J. & Renteria, T. (2004). Folk healing and curanderismo within the contemporary Chicano community: Current status. In R. J. Velasquez, L. M. Arellano, & B. W. McNeill (Eds.), *The Handbook of Chicana/o Psychology and Mental Health*, pp. 111–125. Mahway, NJ: Lawrence Erlbaum Associates.

Hernandez, J. C. (2000). Understanding the retention of Latinos. *Journal of College Student Development, 41*, 575–588.

Hurtado, S., & Carter, D. F. (1997). Effects of college transition and perceptions of the campus racial climate on Latino college students' sense of belonging. *Sociology of Education, 70*(4), 324–345.

Jones, L., Castellanos, J., & Cole, D. (2002). Examining the ethnic minority student experience at predominantly white institutions: A case study. *Journal of Hispanic Higher Education, 1*, 19–39.

Kariv, D., & Heiman, T. (2005). Task-oriented versus emotion-oriented coping strategies: The case of college students. *College Student Journal, 39*(1), 72–84.

Kirkpatrick, L. A. (1998) God as a substitute attachment figure: A longitudinal study of adult attachment style and religious change in college students. *Personality and Social Psychology Bulletin, 24*(9), 961–974.

Larose, S., & Boivin, M. (1998). Attachment to parents, social support expectations, and socioemotional adjustment during the high school–college transition. *Journal of Research on Adolescence, 8*, 1–27.

Lazarus, R. S., & Folkman, S. (1984). *Stress, appraisal, and coping.* New York: Springer.

Le Compte, M. D., & Schensul, J. J. (1999). *Analyzing and interpreting ethnographic data: Ethnographers tool kit* (Vol. 5). Walnut Creek, CA: AltaMira.

Lee, J. J. (2000). Changing religious beliefs among college students. Paper presented at the Annual Meeting of the Education Research Association, New Orleans, LA.

Lenz, B. (2004). Tobacco, depression, and lifestyle choices in the pivotal early college years. *Journal of American College Health, 52*, 213–221.

Mounts, N. S. (2004). Contributions of parenting and campus climate to freshmen adjustment in a multiethnic sample. *Journal of Adolescent Research, 19*(4), 468–491.

Ndoh, S., & Scales, J. (2002, February). The effects of social economics status, social support, gender, ethnicity and grade point average on depression among college students. In

An imperfect world: Resonance from the nation's violence (pp. 170–184). 2002 Monograph Series, Proceedings of the Annual Meeting of the National Association of African American Studies, the National Association of Hispanic and Latino Studies, the National Association of Native American Studies, and the International Association of Asian Studies, Houston, TX. (ERIC Document Reproduction Service No. ED477960.)

Noel, L., Levitz, R., & Saluri, D. (1985). *Increasing student retention: Effective programs and practices for reducing dropout rate.* San Francisco: Jossey-Bass.

O'Hare, T. (2001). Stress and drinking context in college first offenders. *Journal of Alcohol and Drug Education, 47*(1), 4–18.

Orozco, V. (2003). Latinas and the undergraduate experiences: *No estamos solas!* In J. Castellanos & L. Jones (Eds.), *The majority in the minority: Expanding the representation of Latina/o faculty, administrators and students in higher education* (pp. 127–128). Sterling, VA: Stylus.

Parks, S. (1991). *The critical years: Young adults and the search for meaning, faith, and commitment.* San Francisco: Harper.

Pascarella, E. T., & Terenzini, P. (1980). Predicting freshman persistence and voluntary dropout decision from a theoretical model. *Journal of Higher Education, 51*, 60–75.

Pratt, M. W. (2000). The transition to university: Contexts, connections, and consequences. *Journal of Adolescent Research, 15*, 5-8.

Ramirez, M. (1999). *New development in mestizo psychology: Theory, research, and application.* (Occasional Paper No. 46.) East Lansing, MI: Julian Samora Research Institute, Michigan State University.

Rodriguez, A. L., Guido-DiBrito, F., Torres, V., & Talbot, D. (2000). Latina college students: Issues and challenges for the 21st century. *NASPA Journal, 37*(3), 511–527.

Santiago-Rivera, A. L., Arredondo, P., Gallardo-Cooper, M. (2002). *Counseling Latinos and la familia: A practical guide.* Thousand Oaks, CA: Sage.

Sax, L. J. (1997). Health trends among college freshman. *Journal of American College Health, 45*, 252–262.

Schafer, W. (1997). Religiosity, spirituality, and personal distress among college students. *Journal of College Student Development, 38*(6), 633–644.

Schneider, M. E., & Ward, D. J. (2003). The role of ethnic iden-
    tification and perceived social support in Latinos' adjust-
    ment to college. *Hispanic Journal of Behavioral Sciences,*
    25(4), 539–554.

Segura-Herrera, T. A. (2006). *Querer es poder*: Maintaining
    and creating familía as a doctoral student. In J. Castel-
    lanos, A. M. Gloria, & M. Kamimura (Eds.), *The Latina/o*
    pathway to the Ph.D.: Abriendo caminos (pp. 223–233).
    Sterling, VA: Stylus.

Sleeter, C. E., & Grant, C. A. (1994). *Making choices for mul-*
    ticultural education: Five approaches to race, class, and
    gender (2nd ed.). Englewoods Cliffs, NJ: Prentice Hall.

Tobey, P. E. (1997). Cognitive and noncognitive factors as pre-
    dictors of retention among academically at-risk college
    students: A structural equation modeling approach. *Dis-*
    sertation Abstracts International A: The Humanities and
    Social Sciences, 57(7-A), 2907.

Wintre, M. G., & Yaffe, M. (2000). First-year students' adjust-
    ment to university life as a function of relationships with
    parents. *Journal of Adolescent Research, 15,* 9–37.

Zern, D. S. (1989). Some connections between increasing reli-
    giousness and academic accomplishment in a college
    population, *Adolescence, 24*(93), 141–154.

Part Three

CONTEMPORARY ASPECTS OF MESTIZA/O AND INDIGENOUS HEALING PRACTICES: RECLAMATION AND INTEGRATION

Chapter Eight

Los Espiritus Siguen Hablando
Chicana Spiritualities

LARA MEDINA

The spiritual practices of many Chicanas emerge from a purposeful integration of their creative inner resources and the diverse cultural influences that feed their souls and their psyches. Accepting their estrangement from Christianity, many Chicanas return to an *Indígena-* (indigenous-) inspired spirituality, learn to trust their own senses and bodies, look to non-Western philosophies, and re-create traditional and new cultural practices, all of which offers them a (re)connection to their selves, their spirits, and to the ongoing process of creating *nuestra cultura* (our culture). As they journey on paths previously prohibited by patriarchal religions, Chicanas redefine and decide for themselves what images, rituals, myths, and deities nourish and give expression to their deepest values.

Chicanas venturing into often undefined spiritual arenas continue a tradition of religious agency as lived by many of our *anteparados* (ancestors), *abuelas* (grandmothers), *madres* (mothers), and *tias* (aunts). Our *consejeras* (advisors), *curanderas* (healers), *rezadoraras* (prayer leaders), *espiritistas* (spritists), and even *comadres* (intimate friends) practiced and still practice their healing ways in spite of, in lieu of, or in conjunction with the sacraments and teachings offered by the Christian traditions. Likewise, contemporary Chicanas, either as self-taught healers or as trained officiates, follow in the footsteps of our foremothers to provide spiritual nourishment for themselves and their communities.

This chapter provides a glimpse of how 22 Chicanas define, live, and express their spirituality as individuals and as members of communities. Through these voices we hear the ways they have learned to supplant patriarchal religion with their own cultural knowledge, sensibilities, and sense of justice. Their experiences differ widely, yet they share a common desire for healthy and creative lives, with their spirits intact and a willingness to teach and share their thoughts and practices with others.

Unknowingly, this manuscript began in the late 1980s, when I actively began to explore my spirituality outside of institutional religion. Like many Chicanas, I grew up in a strict Catholic environment, reciting the memorized prayers, receiving the Sacraments, internalizing the infamous Catholic guilt. My rebellious years led me away from the faith and a spiritual awareness to life. Little did I know that, years later, I would return to the church with tears on my face, in need of answers to life's crises. I found comfort at the time, and ministers (both men and women) willing to listen to my story and my seeking. My questions led me to study theology, as I wanted to know more of "the truth." Ironically, my three years spent studying church teachings, scripture, ritual, and ministry exposed me to the contradicitons of the religion, and it was liberating! What freedom to learn that patriarchy cast Mary as a virgin, and that Jesus died not to forgive sins but because of his resistance to the power of the state. Liberation theology and feminist theology enabled me to revisit the religion I inherited from my parents. Although a liberating experience, I groped to find a place for my voice and emerging identity as a Chicana feminist liberationist—a Chicana committed to a religion only if it addressed the economic and political struggles of her people, only if it dealt with its own inherent sexism, homophobia, and racism, and that of the society in which it functioned.

After graduating I became a lay minister, preacher, counselor, and ritual leader, but because of my gender I was unable to bless the folks or the Communion bread they came to consume on Sundays. Unwilling to accept these limitations, I began meeting with a group of Chicanas/Latinas in a spiritual circle or community outside of the church. They were *mujeres* (women) like me, wanting more than what the church offered them. We wanted to know our own spirits, our own goddesses, our own ways of blessing and praying.

I eventually left the patriarchal Eurocentrism of the Catholic Church, as the contradictions were too great to reconcile. However, I continue to identify as a "cultural Catholic," as one who appreciates and at times practices many of the popular religious expressions of Mexican Catholicism. The next few years introduced me to other Chicanas engaged in creating spiritual circles based on their own authority. Many of these *mujeres* had been working on their spirituality for years. What struck me was their commitment to inner growth and the building of *nuestra cultura* based on feminine wisdom as a natural evolution of their keen political awareness. These *mujeres* involve themselves in a variety of spiritual practices that reflect not only their diversity but the different arenas they have chosen to "locate their spirituality."' Utilizing their intuition, gut, and intellect, they discern the multiplicity of ways they can decolonize their spirits in order to heal and be healed.

The voices who help shape this narrative have committed themselves to developing a spiritual perspective to life and the realization that as Patricia Parra says, "we are the generation to teach healing." We have our elders and our curanderas in our communities, but often they are not easily accessible as they age or choose to live very private lives. These Chicanas have had to seek out the teachers, traditions, and unlearned knowledge, combined with their own sensibilities, to do *"la tarea, nuestro trabajo* (the task, our work)—changing culture and all its oppressive interlocking machinations" (Anzaldúa, 1990, p. xviii). Formal interviews, spontaneous dialogues, and my own participation in and facilitation of *ceremonias* informed my writing and affirmed my understanding. The mujeres quoted through out this chapter have honored me with their integrity and their power. Representing various educational levels from high school graduate to PhD candidate, and ranging from ages 23 to 55, most were born in the United States, are of the second and third generations, and reside either in Los Angeles or San Francisco. All are from working-class origins and range in occupations from educator, artist, therapist, and student to community organizer, writer, and entrepreneur. All of the women concern themselves with political issues facing the Chicana/Latina community. Their levels of political activism vary and occur in a variety of arenas, from the classroom to city hall to the streets. Three of the women identify as lesbian, nineteen as heterosexual. Fourteen of the women participate in spiritual circles on a regular basis. Two of the women own and operate healing spaces for the public, one a botánica in

San Francisco and the other offering *alternativas espirituales y practicas* (spritual alternatives and practices) from her home.

SPIRITUALITY

Spirit and *spirituality* can be somewhat mysterious words. Western thought separates spirit from body, mind, and woman. We are taught to find spirit outside of ourselves rather than finding spirit within ourselves. In order to begin to heal, we must first reformulate dichotomous and wounding understandings of spirit or God. Lisa Duran says very accurately how, like so many of us, she:

> grew up with the image of God as a white man in a robe on a throne in the clouds. I didn't realize how alienating this was until I understood issues of gender oppression and power relations.... I give thanks that things change and that I have sisters who collectively resist male oppression.... The language and images I use to speak of God have changed. Spirit as creator is a power incorporating both female and male power, or at times I want to call to my source of strength as a woman, and that is Goddess or Great Mother.[1]

For María Elena Fernandez, God or spirit is defined as "truth, energy, love ... the impulse or essence of life ... spirit feels like the energy of life." Toni Garcia speaks of God or spirit as a very intimate "source of strength rather than condemnation.... I have learned to search for that source inside of me." (Re)locating and (re)naming spirit as energy, power, love, mother, or source of strength within us as well as among and beyond us transcends the dichotomies between spirit and woman, spirit and humanity.

Spirituality, then, becomes our own individual but also communal way of connecting with the spirit within us as well as with those around us. As Antonia Villaseñor states:

> Spirituality is about connection. Connecting to our feelings, emotions, our own bodies, our own integrity, our own sexuality, our own intellect. It is also understanding the connections between each other, whether we like it or not. Realizing our connectedness requires me to be respectful of myself as well as others. The isms in our societies, like racism or homophobia, set up

others as being different than ourselves, that they are bad. But understanding connections acknowledges we are all human and requires us to examine our isms.... Respect and integrity are the behaviors resulting from these connections. My spirituality informs how I see others.... It has to do with coming into contact with the sacred in us.

Zosi, who identifies herself as a *consejera intuitiva* (intuitive advisor), believes that spirituality is "life essence." For her it goes beyond our relations with other humans:

It is not only how you deal with other people every day, but with plants and animals as well. It is your outlook, what keeps you going, where your faith lies. It is knowing that something connects us to each other and to the earth. Sea water is almost the same as placenta liquid. We are of the earth and there are many connections from ourselves to the earth, yet there is something beyond the earth as well.

In an essay by Audre Lorde, "Uses of the Erotic," the spiritual as the erotic is identified in the myriad of human experiences that moves what is "deepest, and strongest and richest within each of us" [Lorde, 1989, p. 210], that which provides a deep sense of satisfaction and connection to our capacity to feel, to create. Naming this creative energy, power as the erotic, Lorde challenges the patriarchal definition of the erotic as a nonspiritual, nonrational aspect of women to be controlled unless utilized in the service of men. In order to control this power in women, and thus its potential to create change, patriarchy separates the erotic from anything other than sex. In (re) claiming the erotic/the spiritual in that which allows us to fully experience the depth of our creative power, we experience its force in activities ranging from delivering a speech we feel passionate about, sharing deeply with a friend, taking a walk, organizing a campaign, as well as "writing a good poem to moving into sunlight against the body of a woman I love" [Lorde, 1989, p. 212]). The erotic, the spiritual redefined becomes that which moves us, tantalizes us, that which brings forth our energy, our power, our creativity. Settling for nothing less, our work, our relations, our art become sites holding erotic spiritual power.

Healing the split between the spiritual and the physical also challenges patriarchy's division of spirituality and sexuality. Antonia comments:

> Sexuality is not just about our sexual behavior. My sexuality is about my strongest felt feelings. For example, I am an artist, but there are moments when I am not doing my art yet I am still being creative. [Likewise,] my sexuality is not restricted to the moments I am in bed with someone. I think creativity, sexuality, and spirituality are all connected. They come from the same place in me that acknowledges who I am and celebrates that with someone else. I may do it intellectually, or in political action, or over good conversation with a friend. Western thought says only artists are creative people, sex only belongs in bed. We become disconnected from our own sexuality, our own creativity. Sexuality is about exploring your own intuition, trusting and expressing your knowledge about things. Creativity is another way of expressing our sexuality merged with our spirituality.

Antonia speaks of the interconnections among spirituality, sexuality, and creativity, and broadening our understanding of how each can be expressed. Toni speaks of how sexual behavior and spirituality can merge as well:

> Spirituality and sexual behavior are not in conflict with one another, but it takes a lot of soul-searching to bring the two together. When intimacy, trust, respect, and commitment are present in sexual behavior then the sexual act can be a spiritual experience.

Understanding these connections between spirituality and sexuality challenges the requirements to be honored as a saintly or spiritual woman within patriarchal religions. As Carolina Saucedo points out:

> The worst thing [patriarchy] can say about a woman is that she is lustful. So they take her sexuality away and create virgin madonnas who are seen as good, powerful women. Powerful, as their sexuality is in control.... We are taught to venerate the Virgin Mother but not the woman.

Making the connections reinscribes the creative/sexual/spiritual power we carry in our daily lives. For the lesbians interviewed, making the connections or healing the split takes on a particular urgency, as they have had to battle not only sexism but the threat of eternal damnation. Antonia explains:

> When I was 18 and realized I was lesbian, it horrified me because I thought it literally meant I was going to Hell! There was a significant spiritual crisis. Not until I considered trusting my identity, risking the consequences and living with integrity, could I step away from my Catholic upbringing.

For mujeres rendered completely invisible by homophobic doctrine, (re)capturing one's own spiritual authority and autonomy becomes not only a creative act but a political one as the systems of domination are circumvented. (Re)defining "where we locate our spirituality" subverts dominant cultural norms that traditionally place spiritual authority in the hands of male mediators who can easily orchestrate a monopoly over the sacred.

(Re)claiming one's spiritual power as an act of self-determination can directly affect our politics. Lisa, a community organizer, comments:

> The work I engage in every day is about liberation and resistance. This has great spiritual significance for me. It is very tied into my conception of who I am. Spirituality no longer remains a non-rational aspect of life, but rather the power of energy behind creative, sexual, political activism.

CULTURAL AND POLITICAL INFLUENCES

The spiritual practices of the women interviewed are informed by a mestiza consciousness. Being a product of many cultures—African, Asian, European American, Meso American, Spanish—the mestiza stands at the crossroads where she can choose to balance the multiple and diverse cultures that inform her daily experiences and psyche. The effort to work out a synthesis requires the ability to live in more than one culture, to make sense out of contradictory values, and to create a way of life that transcends opposing dualities (Anzaldúa, 1987).

When the Chicana/o civil rights movement began in the 1960s, activists looked to their indigenous ancestral roots to reclaim values and philosophies that would unify and solidify their emerging Chicana/o consciousness. Alienated from their Christian heritage, their efforts represented a spiritual renaissance rooted in *indigenismo* (indigenousness), a worldview and way of life that understands the interconnections among all of life (Martinez, 1993). Artists and community workers assigned themselves the responsibility of recreating Mesoamerican traditional ceremonies that would "nurture and sustain ethnic pride and cultural solidarity as a necessary first step toward the formulation of a new cultural resistance" (Ybarra-Frausto, 1993, p. 64).

Five of the women interviewed for this chapter were among the originators of some of the first communal ceremonies that not only solidified a Chicana/o consciousness but offered emotional and psychic healing against the weight of colonization. From 1979 to 1984, Flores de Aztlán, a group of six women under the artistic direction of Josefina Gallardo, a Mexicana trained in Mayan and Mexica *danza* (dance), met once a week to develop danza based on Mesoamerican traditions and values "while incorporating present day spiritual growth and reality" (Espinoza, 1995). As a collective, they extended traditional concepts with members doing the research and designing their ceremonial garb. Chicano/Indígena music by the group Kukulkán accompanied the danza. Presenting at various community events, these mujeres participated in the enhancement of a culture determined to regain a silenced heritage.

At the same time, other spiritual circles had begun in California—circles that developed communal ceremonies such as the Fiesta de Maíz in Los Angeles and San Diego, the Fiesta de Colores in Sacramento, and the Día de los Muertos statewide. Calmécac, meaning school of learning in Nahuátl, organized in Los Angeles due to the efforts of Chicana and Chicana/o mental health workers who understood the need to heal the spirit in their work with the community. As a collaborative effort between Calmécac, Flores de Aztlán, and Kukulkán, the first Fiesta de Maíz was held in Los Angeles on June 5, 1979. This first fiesta included the participation of Esplendor Azteca, the *danzante* troupe of the now deceased maestro Florencio Yescas of Tacuba, Mexico. It also brought together artists involved at Self-Help Graphics, a community art center in East Los Angeles. Similar efforts nationwide served to communicate and implant the spiritual, political, and cultural ideals of the emerging Chicana/o consciousness during this "cultural nationalist phase of the Chicana/o Movement" (Ybarra-Frausto, 1993, p. 64. According to Linda Vallejo, a member of Flores de Aztlán:

We were developing a Chicana/o calendar of ceremony.... Through the ceremonies we acknowledged the different [cardinal] directions and the continuation of the cycle of life. Fiesta de Colores honored spring, Fiesta de Maíz honored summer, and Our Lady of Guadalupe celebrated the new year. We were also learning the full moon ceremony and the sweat lodge ceremony.

Other artistic endeavors also helped to transmit cultural knowledge. In reflecting on the influence of these early community efforts, Carolina Saucedo, who was involved in *teatro* (theater) groups, comments, "We were alive and growing, talking about Tonantzin, learning to drum, being politically active, learning from Native American brothers and sisters, sharing our commonalities." These initial experiences of women immersing themselves in ancestral indigenous knowledge provided the stage for further spiritual growth and development. Patricia Parra comments:

In the 1960s and 1970s I started grasping my spiritual power. I wanted to go back to who my people really were and what they did before the imposition of Christianity.... We began to give ourselves the structures and foundations to have our own strength.

Mexicano elders such as Arnaldo Solis transmitted knowledge through oral tradition, as did elders and teachers of North American native peoples. The process of forging a spiritual path informed by northern and southern indigenous ways resulted in Chicana/mestiza/Indígena ceremonial practices. Becky Bejar, one of the founding members of Calmécac in Los Angeles, speaks of this process as "my effort to bring together the various traditions of the Indígena of the continent to create the ceremony we think needs to continue." Linda Vallejo now facilitates the sweat lodge ceremony for Chicanas and Latinas in Los Angeles. Taught the tradition by her participation in sweats run by Lakota, Navajo, Chicana/o, and California Indian tribes (the Chumash, Gabrieleño, and Tule River people), Linda explains:

I have not had a hierarchy of teachers. They have all been at the same big table ... giving me responsibility. The ways I have been taught to pray are Indígena, the way I play the drum, stand, the language I use is Indígenia. The tools I use are from my experiences in the different fiestas, danzas, sweat lodges, sun dances. The multiple experiences are specific to the Indígena of this continent.... I open and close the sweat ceremony in a Sioux tradition taught to me by Beverly Littlethunder, but I incorporate a mixture of traditions. I sing Chicana/o, Sioux, Seneca, California Indian, and Navajo songs in the sweat. Each leader follows her spirit. I use my creative intuition and am comfortable with the rhythm of the lodge. It is understanding the rhythm of things. We can't get it from a book.

As mestizas living between the north and the south, these women act as bridges between groups. Their concerted efforts to learn from northern native peoples but through their own lenses and experiences as Chicanas result in specific and unique ceremonies. This time the bridges lead to their own power, their own identity as mestiza women of the Americas.

Participating in ceremonies not only shares healing knowledge but builds political alliances between Chicanas and northern Indígena peoples. Analuisa, a founding member of Calmécac and member of Flores de Aztlán, reflects on her participation in the Sun Dance ceremony and what it has taught her about struggle:

The Sun Dance requires great sacrifice and dedication. Dancing for four days for the sacred renewal of the earth and the people.... I learned to make sacrifice on behalf of the people protesting at Big Mountain and for Mother Earth. In the ceremony, the water we would normally drink we instead give up to the earth. The ritual allows for the concrete as well as the symbolic sacrifice necessary to transcend the secular and become immersed in the sacred.

For Lisa Duran, her exposure to Chicana/Indígena ceremonies "incorporates our visceral understanding of what it means to live in the U.S. under constant cultural oppression. The sharing is very liberating politically, psychologically, and emotionally." Chicanas seeking to reclaim their indigenous ancestry by learning from northern native peoples often receive criticism from those who believe Chicanas/os should limit themselves to the indigenous traditions of Mesoamerica. While encouraging mestizas to return to indigenismo, critics often ridicule the efforts of Chicanas to learn from northern

Indígena. For example, some critics incorrectly believe that the sweat ceremony is not indigenous to Mesoamerica, and this is contrary to historical and contemporary documentation that places the sweat bath as a tradition that is indeed rooted in Mesoamerica. Chicanas refusing to accept dichotomous understandings of where they find spiritual strength accept their geographical location in history. Identifying as mestiza women, these Chicanas "learn from where we are at and what we have access to. The spirit would laugh if we couldn't have access to our spirituality because of our experience in multi-cultural living." Like the Indígena of the continent, different tribal people historically shared food, shelter, ideas, and culture when the environment or politics necessitated exchange. In reflecting on intertribal relations, Linda Vallejo comments:

> I don't think drawing from many traditions is specific to Chicanas. It is specific to ceremony. For example, the major ceremonies are intertribal. You will hear songs from different peoples. I have danced at a Sioux Sun Dance on Navajo land singing songs from different tribes. Tribal people meet people from different areas and share their songs. The mixture becomes indigenous. I have heard Yaqui songs in the middle of a California Luceño Ghost Dance. It is not a Chicana/o urban reality but an indigenous reality.... Chicana/os are becoming indigenous.

While many elders have been brought up in a specific tradition, they share their spirit with those they meet. Linda continues, "Eventually you must go out of your barrio and meet people from other places and integrate it into your style of living. Learn to sing other songs; the oral tradition shares knowledge." While it remains important for the Chicana to know her unique indigenous history, "to feel the spirit of her own people as there is strength for her there, to sing her own songs," she can connect with the multiple realities that resonate with her spirit. Combining these experiences with Chicana/o and Meso-american Indígena traditions results in a meaningful expression of ritual or ceremony that seeks to heal, strengthen, affirm, and build *la cultura Chicana*. As Virginia Espino notes:

> When I began to connect with traditional [indigenous] practices, I felt like I was at home.... I felt like I went back 500 years. I could feel the spiritual connection to those

original ceremonies, and I never felt like that before. I really felt a spiritual, deep, inner connection.

While indigenismo provides a source of balance and nourishment for these women, the romanticization of indigenous people and their practices can occur at the popular level, as with the image of the male Mexica warrior. Often depicted wearing a full *penacho* (feathered headdress) and supporting a dying Mexica woman, the image became a predominant one depicting Chicana/o ancestry and gender relations at the beginning of the Chicana/o movement. Though the image represents a romantic legend about two young lovers from different social classes, it represents and validates the all-too-familiar gendered roles of the strong, active male and the weak, passive female. The image persists in some sectors of Chicana/o communities on murals, T-shirts, and calendars, or even within the danza of many Mexica troupes who "don't present a balance of feminine and masculine powers in their danza." The persistence of the warrior, limited to military or domineering power, reinforces a distortion of the values of interconnectedness, balance, gender equality, and humility that traditionally characterize indigenous values. In reflecting upon the warrior image, Linda Villanueva coments:

The image of the Aztec warrior has been misused and created misunderstanding about Nahua culture. The warrior caste was only part of the culture, but it has received primary attention. It would be as if all [U.S.] humanity perished and the only thing left was the Army or the Marines. We are not going to pass on the traditions of the military as representing the entire culture. This is what has happened for the Aztecs, which has misguided a lot of people. A lot of Chicana/os have glorified the warrior Azteca.

What appears as indigenous spirituality through the uncritical appropriation of popular images becomes a way to encourage patriarchy and cultural nationalism. Glorifying spiritual power as domination becomes a way to hide from the hard work of creating gender equality and cross-cultural dialogue. Indigenismo, as practiced by the Chicanas interviewed herein, rejects hierarchies of power, redefines a warrior as "a constructor," and commits to the deconstruction of dualities, all of which lead to "healing the split that originates in the very foundation of our lives, our culture, our languages, our thoughts" (Anzaldúa, 1979, p. 80).

While indigenismo plays a vital role in the lives of these women, so do additional cultural influences such as African-inspired spirituality. Petra Martinez grew up in Montana and eastern Oregon as a daughter of a Mexican father and Blackfoot mother. She owns and operates a botánica called La Sirena. Her great-grandmother was a curandera and spiritualist, and her grandfather had "his own candle rituals and meditations." The spiritual tradition she resonates most with now is Ifa, one of the oldest religions in the world, originating in Nigeria. Aspects of Ifa include the worship of ancestors and *Orishas,* or deities who offer guidance and protection. Petra comments:

> Ifa offers a magical ritual that I feel very comfortable with as a result of my childhood experiences.... It is about learning to trust your mind, body, instincts, and spirit guides. Spirituality is a very individual thing. It has to do with how you feel about something and how you choose to use it.

While practicing an African religion, Petra still draws from the spiritual traditions taught to her by her family. "My spirituality comes from both sides of my family and it comes together, she notes. "For example, doing candle ritual along with using herbs or burning sage and standing over it naked after childbirth for purification."

Zosi, the daughter of a Yaqui mother and a Turkish-Iraqi father, was raised Catholic but now practices a combination of these influences: performing egg cleansings to purify one's energy (from her Yaqui grandmother), praying to Our Lady of Guadalupe (from her Mexican Catholicism), and reading coffee grounds for direction (from her Middle Eastern father). She offers her private clients a specific tradition or combination of traditions most appropriate to their needs and life experiences.

Patricia Parra experienced much of her healing through African American woman-centered ritual and metaphysical teachings. She integrates these experiences with Indígena practices and feels strongly that Chicanas should integrate cross-cultural knowledge into their lives.

Eastern thought, through Buddhism, also has influenced some of the women. For Linda Villanueva, her research into Buddhism occurred as a result of an early attraction to India:

As a child I was fascinated with the life of Christ. I thought he was from India, so I started exploring the history of India.... I became very interested in Buddhism and how they perceived the divine. It made sense and related to my American Indian values. I was initiated into Buddhism and lived in India for two years.

Toni Garcia, who calls herself a "lapsed Mexican Catholic with Buddhist tendencies," has experienced healing to her spirit through channeling with Tibetan monks, African drumming, Native American healing rituals, and performance art. Dolores Chávez also practiced Buddhism for several years and is now "learning how my abuela, a Tarahumara Indian, learned through her dreams ... how to communicate in silence."

Catholic ritual also continues to resonate with some of the women. While they do not adhere to Catholic doctrine, the religious practices of their ancestors continue to have their place at certain times. Monica Rodriguez y Russel comments:

I feel Catholic in a cultural way. I don't follow the rules.... Seeing members of my family baptized, going to weddings, funerals, and novenas, has kept our family together. In my home I have the image of Our Lady of Guadalupe along with elements that identify me with my indigenous culture. I have a *nicho* [a small sacred box] for Santo Niño de Atocha because he was important to my grandfather. I want to carry on the tradition even though I don't have a particular relationship with this saint.

Hilda Escalante visits Catholic churches "when they are empty, to see the lighted candles and to smell the incense. There is something about it that comforts me."

For a few of the women, learning a "radical Catholic vision" has led to a positive recognition for the role Christianity has played at certain points in their development. Maria Elena Fernandez states:

The roots of my politicization are from a Catholic youth group I belonged to in high school. I learned that everyone is equal and that the Gospels demand justice. I was taught to see Jesus as an older brother. My political consciousness comes from this.

Mona Devich-Navarro reflected on the impact liberation theology made on her during her travels in El Salvador:

> I experienced life and death with the *campesinos* [farm-workers] on a daily basis.... I saw them make a connection to Christ and the land through liberation theology. I was able to make a spiritual connection with Christ. The Mayas are able to integrate their indigenous beliefs and Christianity. This is a path, a process for me.... I don't know where I will come out.

Many of the women interviewed participate in spiritual circles of small communities for the purpose of learning healing traditions or creating new ones for the overall goal of healing themselves and the larger Chicano/Latina/o community. Many of their efforts reflect the evolution of their earlier involvement with communal celebrations during the Chicana/o movement. For others, their efforts reflect a more recent exposure to ceremony.

CEREMONIA

Many of the women participating in ceremony during the 1970s realized early on "that we must develop for ourselves how to conduct ceremonias that will provide us and the gente (people) with a sense of purposeful belonging and spiritual connection," as stated by Analuisa Espinoza. Lacking female teachers among the elders coming from Mexico, these women combined knowledge of traditional ways learned through oral history and archival research with their own intuition, experience, values, and objectives. Their creation of ceremonia exemplifies the process mestizas engage in as they participate in the making of meaning and the production of knowledge. Inés Hernandez captures this experience when she comments:

> *O sea, hemos tenido que recobrar y revalorizar lo que es nuestra cultura no sólo por medio de investigaciones formales sino tambien y en gran parte según nuestra intuición y los mandatos del corazon.* [We have had to recover and revalidate that which is our culture not only by means of formal research but also in great part according to our own intuition and mandates of our heart.] (Hernández, 1988, p. 263)

The work of creating ritual articulates not only a spirituality but an identity, and the ritual itself becomes a political
act. The creation of ceremony by the Chicanas interviewed
herein is not merely for personal pleasure. Unlike the indi-
vidualism within New Age spirituality and ritual, Chicanas
develop ceremonies as tools for daily survival within a society
that seeks to silence them. As tools or strategies of resistance
for personal and communal healing, they challenge the norms
of the dominant culture. Much like generations of Mexicanos
living a synthesized Christian/indigenous faith, mestizas create their own religious spaces, implement their own language
and gestures to name what has deepest meaning to them, to
express "a language of defiance and ultimate resistance" (Elizondo, 1994, p. 116).

Ritual as an act of resistance lies within the ceremony of
the Fiesta de Maíz in Los Angeles. Seven of the women interviewed participated in this annual ceremony between the
mid-1970s and the mid-1990s. Under the direction of Calmécac, women and men joined together to honor the importance
of *maíz* (corn) in Chicana/o culture and the importance of adolescence in the life cycle. The process of growing up is likened
to the process of harvesting maíz. Attention and honor given
to our youth supplants Euro-American societal norms, which
fail to provide young people with rites of passage acknowledging their importance for the future of Chicana/o communities.
According to Calmécac:

> Today's youth, especially, is [*sic*] in need of acknowl-
> edgment and spiritual integration into the fabric of our
> community. They need our individual and collective
> nurturance, teaching, comfort, guidance, protection,
> and examples of living in balance and harmony. This
> year's Fiesta de Maíz is dedicated to the spiritual healing
> and strengthening of the youth and their families, and
> the commitment by all to walk together in *Flor y Canto*
> [flower and song]. (Fiesta de Maiz, 1993, p. 1)

The ceremony consists of the community gathering to
build altars in honor of the four directions of the universe
and the four stages of life, and forming a large circle around
the young boy and girl chosen to represent all of the youth of
the community. Participants ask permission of the spirits to
perform the ceremony, followed by an honoring of the four
directions of the universe and elders offering a blessing for

the ceremony. The youth sit in the south, the direction of children and innocence. Representatives from the various directions offer *consejos*, or advice, to the youth. The youth become visually transformed through the donning of ceremonial garb that symbolizes their maturity and affirms the native dress of their ancestors. They then sit in the west, the direction of adulthood, growth, and integration. They receive gifts from the community, which emphasize their particular strengths and how they might be used for self-empowerment and the empowerment of the community. For example, a talking stick is given to the young woman to encourage her to publicly voice her ideas. A sketchbook is given to the young man to encourage his artistic abilities for the benefit of the community. The youth then address the community with their own consejos and lessons. Prayers of thanks are directed to the community and the ancestors.

Calmécac's focus on the healing tradition seeks to fill the spiritual vacuum existing for many Chicanas/os who no longer practice any type of spiritual tradition. Linda Villanueva, a member of Calmécac, states:

> Even though many parents are Catholic or Protestant, they no longer practice it, so the children are not being taught to have a spiritual sense of themselves. If something as socially acceptable as Christianity is not being taught or practiced, much less indigenismo... there exists a real vacuum.

While efforts to fill this spiritual vacuum take on a very public nature for Calmécac, more private (yet communal) endeavors are undertaken by several of the women interviewed. Meeting monthly, these women gather to share ritual, beliefs, and ceremonial knowledge. In discussing her participation in a spiritual circle named Corazón, Carolina Saucedo comments:

> Women find that there is power as they come together to discuss and share what they believe ... to talk about magic, mystery, our bodies and how we relate to the universe. This grows into something political.... We gather to discuss our ways.

Corazón also meets on a monthly basis to participate in a sweat lodge ceremony, or *baño de temazcal*. Over the past five years they have built and managed the sweat house, or *temazcalli*, on land owned by one of the members, gathering the wood, rocks, sage, and other resources needed for the ceremony. While some of the members are more knowledgeable in the tradition than others, the style of leadership empowers each member to assume more responsibility when she feels ready. Considering themselves a leadership circle, their purpose is to "pass on knowledge to lead. We must walk away from our ego as we do not want only one leader." Before each sweat ceremony, the women take time to talk about themselves and particular challenges they face. During the sweat, the women pray together, purify themselves, and build endurance to face life's challenges. For Patricia, the temazcal "helps me be aware of my weaknesses but also harness power." For Raquel Salinas, a fire keeper, "The fire has taught me about myself... that I am a strong woman but my strength does not have to be a physical strength." Carolina notes, "The more we do the ceremony, our bonds grow tighter, we grow together. As leaders in our jobs, our communities, we gain strength from sharing in the experience."

Four of the women interviewed participate in another spiritual circle that has been meeting for the past four years. Four to six mujeres meet monthly to create ritual around the events taking place in their lives. Pregnancies, engagements, deaths, and the variety of life's transitions are ritualized. Much of what they do comes from the desire to create expressions for their spirituality rooted in a quest for self-determination and the liberation of their communities. Most of the women received Catholic formation. All have rejected its constraints and contradictions, with some maintaining a Catholic identity in a cultural way. All of the women are activists, whether in the community or in the academy. They consider themselves warriors. As member Lisa Duran states, "A warrior fights for her people. War is waged in many ways... from resistance against oppression to organizing or promoting a vision of what should be. A warrior is a constructor."

Filling a spiritual vacuum, creating ritual and community comprised the goals of the group at their initial gathering. Lisa Durán expressed her desire for meditations so that "she can do political organizing with love." Other women wanted to reconcile their traditional religious formations that no longer made sense to them. Space to express doubts, fears, and hopes and to discover ways to pray created a common bond. A general consensus arose that they would be embarking on a journey. After four years, the women express enthusiasm and commitment to the circle. Teri Gomez comments:

It was an amazing experience.... As a scholar I can move away from the academy and have a spiritual connection to my life, to my work. I sometimes get caught up in intellectualizing, so it [enables me] to feel things on a different level... it is cultural production. It is the mixing of different influences. I see people doing that in their research and I see us doing that with spirituality.

Soon after forming the circle, the women acknowledged that growing up in a patriarchal society does not provide essential affirmation to young women at the time of puberty. Their decision to create a puberty rite for themselves, with the assistance of a member of Calmécac, served to regain a sense of the power they hold as women, particularly at the time of menstruation. As Teri adds,

For those of us who have had a miserable time with our periods... never able to claim it as something powerful, we gave it new meaning. Every month now when I go through tremendous PMS, I remember what we did and that the cramps are the way of the goddesses telling us we need to be alone, to reflect. At times this isn't easy to do, but I try and find the space to light my candles, pull out my journal, and write about what I am feeling. I am able to take what we do in the group and do it in a private setting.

The spiritual work these women engage in enables them to take control over their lives. By reclaiming traditions that have their well-being in mind (such as puberty rites), the women gain a sense of balance and power. The lack of such ritual in patriarchal societies results in women often having to struggle to gain the confidence to take positions of leadership. If women experienced rituals focusing on their abilities throughout their development, they would be prepared to assume positions of authority quite naturally. Talamantez (1993) affirms this in her discussion of the ceremonies for young females among the Mescalero Apache people: "Any post-patriarchal tradition must incorporate ceremony that specifically links girls and women to the knowledge and use of power that will be required of them when they assume responsible roles of leadership and authority" (p. 132).

Chicanas purposefully gathering to plan and carry out rituals in honor of significant transitions in their lives exemplify what Anzaldúa (1990) describes as "cultivating our ability to affirm our knowing. Jauntily we step into new terrains where we make up the guidelines as we go" (xxvii). Never taught rituals to honor a woman's life cycle, her sexuality, or her intellectual and emotional decisions, these Chicanas have decided to shape and form their own healing ways. The rituals they have developed can serve as models for other Chicanas in search of their own healing. "New ways, feminist ways, mestiza ways" are injected into our culture (Anzaldua, 1987, p. xxvii).

A woman from the wider community of activists requested a blessing ritual for her journey to the East Coast, where she would live for two years to finish her dissertation. At a gathering of supporters, women from the circle ritualized this significant point in her life. After invoking the goddesses Coyolxauhqui and Tonantzin through poetry, we encircled her with ground maíz as a symbol of nourishment and blessing of the space. The circle symbolically provided protection from disempowering hierarchical structures. We then offered her gifts of *velas* (candles): a red one in honor of her female power, a blue one symbolizing balance, a white one requesting guidance, and a purple one honoring her *mestizaje*, her mixed-blood heritage. Prayers said in her honor accompanied a water blessing as we touched her forehead in praise of her intellect, her heart for her love and creativity, her hands for the labor she would engage in and the new people she would touch, her feet for the walking of new paths. Maíz marked her path as she left the circle and began her journey.

The public acknowledgment of the task ahead of this woman validated her intellect and her emotions. She received the affirmation of the community. Though this was a very simple ritual, it served to position the woman in the center of the community as an agent of her intellectual pursuits. Using cultural symbols such as the maíz and colored velas we drew from the sensibilities of home practices. Combining intellect, intuition, and gut, we inscribed the ritual space with the language and actions that would highlight the resourcefulness and inner strength this woman exemplified.

As the healing work this spiritual circle engages in becomes known to the wider Chicano/Latina/o community, they receive requests to honor the variety of life's turning points, such as births, adoptions, house blessings, and deaths. In responding to a request to honor the passing of a young man, members of the circle facilitated the building of a community altar in his honor. The ritual involved an honoring of the four directions and invoking the spirits of the ancestors. A close friend of the soul who had passed read a letter addressed to him. Others shared their feelings or explained the symbols they brought to the altar. Music carried our thoughts and prayers. *Pan* (bread) and his favorite drink, tequila, were shared by everyone who gathered. The ritual closed with a prayer of thanks to the spirits. Many of the participants expressed their gratitude to those who facilitated the ritual, as they "would not have known what to do. It gave us the opportunity to grieve together and say good-bye to our friend." The work of these women filled the spiritual vacuum experienced by men and women and represented the significance that empowering ritual plays for the entire culture. As new ways to renew ourselves are discovered, a culture regenerates itself.

Not all of the women interviewed for this chapter participate in spiritual circles, yet all have found ways to nourish their spirituality. The decision to identify and practice what strengthens them speaks to their self-determination and what Moraga (1993) calls "a deeper inquiry into ourselves as a people" (71). For Antonia:

> working with a healer who has the ability to read energy in my body and adjust, increase, or balance it… attending a poetry reading or walking down the street breathing and being aware of the divine all around me nourishes my spirituality. On a good day, all my waking moments are sacred.

Maryann finds nourishment for her spirituality inside of herself as well as through the faith she sees in others:

> I have learned to trust what is inside of me. I've been able to find my spirituality in the little miracles that happen every day. The good things but also the negative things that I walk through with someone or that someone walks through with me… My spirituality is very much linked to my grandmother, who has a tremendous amount of faith. I used to limit her faith to what the Catholic Church teaches, but now I understand it is her faith and she merely uses the building of the church to meditate and be alone.

As Chicanas act individually or within groups to discover and create their regenerative powers, they consciously produce culture. Our multiple ways of connecting with self, spirit, and others results not in a singular spirituality but in spiritualities emanating from the ability to "navigate across cultural boundaries" (Ruiz, 1994, p. 311). Living on borders, living in the centers of our own spaces, Chicanas "pick, borrow, retain, and create distinctive cultural forms" (Ruiz, 1994, 311). Perceiving the world in ways that include rather than exclude differences serves our need to integrate the multiple realities we emerge from and the cross-cultural alliances we must build.

When asked what *consejos* advice could be given to Chicanas and mestizas embarking on a spiritual journey, several of the women stress the need to gravitate toward other women also on the same search, women wanting to question, seek, grow, and read. Linda Vallejo emphasizes the importance of finding people:

> who will allow you to think and learn according to your own personality, psyche, and spirit.... Look for people who will say, "I will be happy to share with you, but you will have to find your own road eventually." This is how your songs will come to you.

Carolina Saucedo shares the importance of not being afraid to question and not relying on others for all the answers:

> If you find a person whose ideas you feel comfortable with, continue to seek them out and go forward, but don't put all your faith in one person. We all have spirituality within us. Talk with others; reading helps along the path, but it comes from within. It is a process of getting to know yourself.

Petra Martinez emphasizes the need to nurture oneself and, above all, use one's power:

> Women must believe they have power within themselves and find ways to access it. Nurture yourself, listen to stories, call on your ancestors, listen to your dreams... sit down and figure out the rituals... Just know you have power within.

The process of creating alternative spaces for expressing a mestiza-inspired spirituality demands that we ask ourselves "questions about what types of images subvert, pose critical alternatives, transform our worldviews and move us away from dualistic thinking about good and bad" (hooks, 1992, p. 4). Retaining the *Santos* (saints) revered by our abuelos/as; renewing silenced relationships with indigenous goddesses such as Coyolxauhqui, Tonantzin, Ixchel, Yemaya, or the Corn Mother; lighting candles, as well as sage or copal; meditating; chanting; making prayer ties; and sweating in ceremony removes the limitations placed upon us by Western Christianity, which teaches us that religious practices should not be mixed. As mestizas, our very nature calls us to cross borders, to make sense out of contradictory values, to "pick up the fragments of our dismembered womanhood and reconstitute ourselves" (Moraga, 1993, p. 74). We must be able to shift our perspectives so that new knowledge can be created. This knowledge must serve the purpose of making strategic change not only in our thinking but in the ways *la cultura Chicana* expresses its deepest values. In the process of developing our own strategies, Chicanas bring to life centuries of strong and spirit-filled women and men—*y los espiritus siguen hablando*, the spirits continue speaking.

POSTCRIPT

Since the first publication of this article in 1998, I have seen the reclamation of *Indígena* values and spirituality continue to grow within Chicana/o communities. In Los Angeles, where I am located, numerous temazcal circles have become more visible and relationships are being developed with cultural workers in Mexico seeking to maintain and document the temazcal tradition among indigenous and mestizo *pueblos* (Sánchez Morales, 2003). La Red Xicana, a collective of indigenous–identified Xicanas in the Los Angeles area, gathers at an annual retreat to share knowledge, learn from elders, and create ceremony together. An indigenous consciousness informs much of Chicana/o art, theater, and activism and has expanded within academic circles as well. With white and black America becoming more and more anxious about the increase of the U.S.-born Mexican population and undocumented brown immigrants, a consciousness and activism rooted in historical memory about the land and its inhabitants is increasingly necessary to defend its native people from legislative and vigilante attempts to silence them. *¡Que viva los espiritus!* Long live the spirits that continue to speak to us, guide us, and protect us!

NOTE

1. The quotes herein come from women I have interviewed personally, except where noted as from a published source.

REFERENCES

Anzaldúa, G. (1987). *Borderlands/La frontera: The new mestiza*. San Francisco: Spinsters/Aunt Lute.
hooks, b. (1992). Black looks: Race and representation. Boston: South End Press.
Elizondo, V. (1994). "Popular religion as the core of cultural identity in the Mexican American experience." In A. M. Stevens-Arroya & A. M. Diaz-Stevens (Eds.), An enduring flame: Studies on Latino popular religiosity. New York: Bildner Center.
Hernandez, I. (1988). "Cascadas de estrellas." In C. Moraga & A. Castillo (Eds.), *Esta puente, Mi espalda*. San Francisco: Ism Press.
Lorde, A. (1989). "Uses of the erotic: The erotic as power." In J. Plaskow & C. Christ (Eds.), *Weaving the visions: New patterns in feminist spirituality*. San Francisco: Harper.
Martinez, E. (1993). "Seeds of a new movimiento." *Z Magazine*, pp. 52–56.
Fiesta de Maiz. (1993). Program booklet, privately published.
Medina, L. (2006). "Nepantla Spirituality: Negotiating multiple identities and faiths among U.S. Latinas," In Miguel De La Torre and Gastón Espinoza (Eds.), *Rethinking Latino(a) Religion and Identity*. Cleveland, OH: Pilgrim Press.
Moraga, C. (1993). "En busca de la fuerza femenina." In The Last Generation (pp. 79–76). Boston: South End Press.
Ruiz, V. (1994). Dead ends or gold mines? Using missionary records in Mexican American women's history. In V. L. Ruiz and E. C. DuBois, (Eds.), *Unequal sisters: A Multicultural Reader in U.S. Women's History*. New York: Routledge.
Sánchez Morales, P. (2003). *El temazcal: Uso ceremonial y terapéutico*. (Mexico City, Mexico: Instituto Tlaxcalteca de La Cultura.
Talamantez, I. (1993). "Images of the feminine in Apache religious tradition." In P. M. Cooey, W. R. Eakin, & J. B. McDaniel (Eds.), *After patriarchy: Feminist transformations of the world religions*. Maryknoll, NY: Orbis.

Ybarra-Frausto, Y. (1993). Arte Chicano: Images of a community. In H. Barnet-Sánchez, (Ed.) with an introduction by Eva Sperling Cockcroft and Holly Barnet-Sánchez, *Signs from the heart: California Chicano murals*. Albuquerque: University of New Mexico Press.

Chapter Nine

Religious Healing and Biomedicine in Comparative Context

KAREN V. HOLLIDAY

SANTERÍA

Santería, as a religion emerged from Cuba as a direct result of the slave trade (Brandon 1997; Conniff and Davis 1994; Efunde 1996).[1] It developed as a syncretic religious practice resulting from the Catholic colonialists prohibiting African slaves from practicing their Yoruba-based religious tradition because the worship of the Yoruba deities, known as *Orishas* (see Table 9.1), was considered idolatrous and sacrilegious (Brandon 1997; Cabrera, 1980, 1986, 1994; Canizares, 1994; Efunde, 1996, Gregory, 1999, Murphy, 1988, 1995; Vega, 2000).[2] In response to this, the slaves drew correlations between their Orishas and the Catholic saints, and Santería was born.[3] Pérez y Mena (1998) argues that the similarities drawn between Catholic saints and Orishas served as a means to viably practice a Yoruba-based religion and that Catholic saints merely represent aspects of the Orishas. Consequently, Orishas and saints are not interchangeable; they simply share particular characteristics. For example, Saint Barbara became associated with Shango (or Chango) because of the principle of force and thunder (Lefever, 1996). Pérez y Mena (1998) believes that this clarification demonstrates that African slaves did not simplify their religion to mirror Catholicism, but instead they understood both practices as two different religious ideologies that

Table 9.1 The Most Commonly Cited and Used Orishas in Santería

Orisha	Saint	Feast Day	Function or Power	Representations in Nature	Weapon or Symbol
Eleggua	Saint Anthony of Padua, Anima Sola, or Niño de Atocha	January 6 or June 13 (contested)	Delivers messages; controls fate, the unexpected; "road opener"; trickster	Corners; crossroads	Cement head with cowrie shells representing eyes and mouth
Obatalá	Jesus of Nazareth, or the Virgin—Our Lady of Mercy	September 24	Peace; purification	Fatherhood, all white substances	Iruke (horsetail with a beaded handle)
Changó	Saint Barbara	December 4	Power; passion, control of enemies; one of the warriors (guerreros)	Fire; thunder and lightening	Mortar castle; double-edged axe
Ogún	Saint Peter	June 29	Blacksmith; one of the warriors (guerreros)	Iron; steel	Metal weapons including knives
Ochosi	Saint Norbert	June 6	Hunter; justice; one of the warriors (guerreros)	All game animals	Crossbow
Babalú-Ayé	Saint Lazarus	December 17	Causes and cures illness	Smallpox; leg ailments	Crutches
Yemayá	The Virgin—Our Lady of Regla	September 7	Maternity; womanhood	The ocean	Seashells, canoes, corals
Oshún	The Virgin—Our Lady of Charity	September 8	Love; marriage; sensuality	Rivers	Fans, mirrors
Oyá	The Virgin—Our Lady of La Candelaria or Saint Teresa	February 2	Guardian of the gateway of the cemetery; protection against death	Wind, cemeteries/burial grounds	Horsetail
Orúnmila	Saint Francis of Assisi	October 4	Divination		Table of Ifá

share similar characteristics. Therefore, African slaves developed the religion Santería in order to maintain the complexity of their Yoruba-based religion by masking their belief system under that of Catholicism.

Because of this legacy of persecution, Santería has been a tradition cloaked in secrecy where knowledge is conveyed through tightly knit kinship relations formed between novices (defined as godchildren or *aijadas/aijados* and called *Iyawos*), and initiated priests and priestesses (defined as godparents and called *Santeras/os* (Gonzalez-Wippler, 1998; Gregory, 1999; Vega, 2000). It is important to note that the kinship ties that develop as a result of the initiation process create a social and metaphysical family, and "the relationship between godparent and godchild lies at the core of the social organization of Santería" (Gregory 1999, p. 39). This relationship is based on reciprocity, where the godparent directs the spiritual development of the godchild, and in return the godchild provides support in the form of labor and/or resources (Vega, 2000). As a predominantly oral tradition, the knowledge system of the religion is engaged in and developed through social activity that requires the existence and maintenance of strong social ties (Cohen, 1989; O'Connor and Hufford, 2001).

Santería developed in Cuba as a full-fledged religion in the late 19th and early 20th centuries (Brandon, 1997). Its presence in the United States can be traced to the historically catalytic moment of the Cuban Revolution (1959–1962), when Cubans sought refuge from the government of Fidel Castro. Immigration patterns concentrated on the U.S. East Coast, leading to the first emergence of this religion in areas such as Florida, New Jersey, and New York (Brandon, 1997; Gonzalez-Wippler, 1992; Lefever, 1996; Masland & Larmer, 1998; Murphy, 1988; Pérez y Mena, 1998). This religious practice provided Cuban immigrants with a flexible support system for newcomers in a similar fashion to what it provided the slaves who created it, offering practitioners sacrosanct approaches to life's ever-changing problems (Barnes, 1989).

A predominant reason given for seeking counsel from a Santera/o is that one is facing an unanswerable problem in life. As Gregory (1999, p. 67) states, "Frequently, a person's first contact with Santería is prompted by a personal problem which leads to a referral, through an acquaintance or a botánica, to a santero or santera." This concise statement clearly traces the manner in which this religion is customarily approached. Health problems—in particular, those that have not been satisfactorily addressed—are a primary reason people may seek counsel from Santeras/os. Their assistance is valued because they are able to identify spiritual aspects of physical problems and provide advice that relies on intimate social and spiritual kinship ties. The conceptual imagination of kinship superseding the "here and now" is one of the powerful beliefs that provide Santería practitioners with a form of agency in facing challenges in life, including those that are health related.

Divination, the "the art or practice that seeks to foresee or foretell future events or discover hidden knowledge usually by the interpretation of omens or by the aid of supernatural powers,"[4] is the method by which problems are uncovered and resolved with particular emphasis placed on uncovering sources of misfortune (Turner, 1977; Worseley, 1982). A predominant system of divination is called *Dilogun* and consists of an ordained diviner called an *Oriate* throwing 16 cowrie shells on a mat while asking the Orishas, on behalf of a supplicant, about the source of specific problem(s) the supplicant is encountering in her life. The pattern formed by the configuration of the shells is interpreted by the *Oriate* through *pataki* (short stories or myths), and prescriptions are made to assist the supplicant with her problems (Vega, 2000; Gonzalez-Wippler, 1998). In this sense, divination is used as a form of social analysis by exploring unharmonious relationships an individual may have and providing spiritually sanctioned prescriptions for tangible maladies.

If a potential practitioner decides to join the religion, she must go through a complex initiation process that begins with a *misa espiritual* (séance) and culminates in *asiento* (initiation to become a Santería). The misa espiritual is held to determine which Orisha the initiate is meant to receive and be bound to for a lifetime of service. There are a number of compliances and rituals associated with each Orisha that an initiate must perform during the ceremony and for the rest of her life in order to maintain a harmonious relationship with her designated Orisha. The asiento is the actual one-week ceremony in which the initiate receives her Orisha; it is designed according to the Orisha received, including particular food preparations and colors used. The relationship formed with an Orisha is the ultimate metaphysical kinship bond an initiate has in which she agrees to devote a life of service toward her Orisha in return for a lifetime of guidance and protection. The week-long initiation process is long, arduous, and complicated.[5] A significant feature of this process is the costly nature of this ceremony (Gonzalez-Wippler, 1998; Gregory, 1999).[6]

Another aspect worth noting is the gendered component of the religion as exemplified by the roles ascribed to men and women. While the majority of initiates tend to be women (Murphy, 1995, Vega, 2000), leadership positions are held by men. In fact, only men are permitted to become high priests known as *Babalawos* in the religion, and menstruating women are denied participation in certain events. However, through spirit possession, women are allowed to circumvent some of the gendered ascriptions of the religion. Finally, Santería has probably received more attention in the United States over the controversial practice of animal sacrifice (Gonzalez-Wippler, 1998, Vega, 2000). In 1987 the Hialeah, Florida, City Council banned animal sacrifice. The case went to the U.S. Supreme Court in 1992, and in June 1993 the ruling favored the Santeros, allowing them to sacrifice animals as a component of their religious practice (Kosmin & Lachman, 1993).

SPIRITISM AND SPIRITUALISM

Spiritism and spiritualism have had different historical developments from that of Santería.[7] This section will briefly outline Kardecian spiritist and U.S. spiritualist developments and relate them to Cuban Santería.

Spiritism is traced to the teachings of French-born Leon Denizarth Hippolyte Rivail, better known by his nom de plume, Allan Kardec (Díaz-Stevens & Stevens-Arroyo, 1998; Hess, 1994; Macklin, 1974). Kardec opposed the term *spiritualism*, explaining that it was a general term that could be applied to anyone who believes in metaphysical reality but not necessarily in spirits (Macklin, 1974). In contrast, Kardec based his philosophy precisely on the belief in spirits and founded this philosophy with the name *spiritism*. Historically, spiritualists have formally distinguished themselves from spiritists by stating that their set of beliefs constitutes a religion, while spiritism deals with the occult (Macklin, 1974, p. 389; National Spiritualist Association, 1967, p. 59).

Macklin (1974) argues that the major points of Kardec's doctrine as transmitted by the spirits he communicated with were based on traditional Christianity. For Kardec, "God is seen as eternal, immutable, all-powerful, just and good, while the moral teachings of the higher spirits may be summed up in the golden rule" (1989, p. 31). Kardec's doctrine also reflects such 19th-century ideals as the importance of metaphysical reality over the physical. Using an Enlightenment-derived evolutionary model of progress, spirits climb through hierarchical ranks and advance based on their individual merits (Kardec 1989). Consequently, human effort is rewarded spiritually and is reflected bodily in existing social class-based rankings. In other words, a person's social standing also determines his spiritual level of development. This belief system spread and became widely adopted in Latin America, where the division of classes consist of a dominant petit bourgeoisie, a formal proletariat, and an informal sector (Portes & Hoffman, 2003). Given the emphasis placed on class in Latin America in determining an individual's social status, it is not uncommon to find practitioners and clients of this practice divided accordingly—as exemplified in Brazil, where mediums come from a predominantly white upper middle class and clients are ethnically diverse and poor (Hess, 1994).

Spiritualism had a distinct development in the United States in the mid-19th century in that social class did not play as much of a formative role as the promise of a new moral world in which social and individual needs could be met (Isaacs, 1983; Macklin, 1974). The genesis of this movement is traced to 1848, when the three Fox sisters reported hearing rapping on the wall of their home and the noise was identified as coming from the spirit of a dead peddler (Isaacs, 1983; Macklin, 1974; Trimble, 1995). While the advent of spiritualism as a religion is generally attributed to the mediumistic experience of the Fox sisters, other accounts claim that Andre Jackson Davis actually communicated with spirits in 1843, five years before the Fox sisters (Isaacs, 1983). While 19th-century spiritism in Latin American countries centered on personal growth, the goal of 19th-century spiritualism was instead directed toward public edification (Brown, 1997).

One particular form of social enlightenment centered on the relationship between health and spiritual development. This understanding fostered the development of a number of medicinal practices in the United States and Europe during the 19th century; these focused on the idea of the body having a vital energy (Fuller, 1989). One example is Thomsonianism, a practice developed by Samuel Thomson (1769–1843) that emphasized the value of herbs in restoring vital energy in the body (Griggs, 1981). Homeopathy, the practice established by German physician Dr. Samuel Hahnemann (1755–1843) is based on the belief that dispensing a single remedy that is the cause for producing illness symptoms in small dosages will cure the body by restoring balance ("like cures like"). Hydropathy, also referred to as the "water cure," was a practice promoted in the United States by Dr. Joel Shew, whereby the body was treated using external (e.g. baths) and internal (e.g. drinking) applications of water. Sylvester Graham (1797–1851), inspired by the vitalist theories of the Frenchman Francois J. V. Broussois, developed the theory that the stomach and intestines were the physiological agents responsible for delivering vital power in the body to overcome disease (Roth, 2000). Mesmerism, a practice founded by the Viennese physician Franz Anton Mesmer (1734–1815), and which described an invisible fluid that permeates the universe and must be kept in balance for good health as "animal magnetism," was introduced in the United States in 1836 (Schmit, 2005). Swedenborgianism, which was established by Sweden's Emanuel Swedenborg (1688–1772) and touted that a positive bodily health status is the product of harmony among an individual's spiritual, mental, and physical levels, spread in the United States in the early 1800s. Of great value in noting the connection between health and religiosity is recognizing that medicine and religious ideals intermingle in a historical Western context.

The primary difference between Kardec's spiritism (in which an individual spirit experiences a series of incarnations) and U.S. spiritualism (in which an individual spirit is only incarnated once), is the idea of multiple incarnations. At the inception of these separate 19th-century religious traditions, Macklin surmises that the English and Americans did not incorporate Kardecian spiritism because the capitalist pursuit of material interests in these countries did not lend itself to the "romantic, idealistically based, nationalistic ideology which Kardec synthesized" (1974, p. 390). As Macklin further explains, both religious practices emerged as direct responses to the 19th-century conflicting views of science versus religion and materialism versus vitalism.

In fact, the emergence of nonmainstream religious ideologies and practices otherwise defined as "the occult" are often associated historically with periods in which social inequality becomes pronounced (Finkler 1985, Geschiere 1997),[8] leading to the interpretation that social change plays a crucial role in the formation of new religious ideologies. A secondary difference between the value system of spiritualism and that of spiritism is the emphasis that spiritualism places on individual agency exemplifying its Protestant roots, specifically in achieving a state of personal physical well-being. Spiritism's value system, on the other hand, emphasizes the healing relationship that ensues between medium and client in the form of public diagnosis, exemplifying its traditional Catholic roots (Macklin, 1974, p. 405).

Within a medical context these systems are described as "folk medical systems." The next section will provide a basic overview of the logic used in interpreting the dominant biomedical system in comparison to folk systems of healing. The presentation of these religious belief systems has been with the Durkheimian notion that religion is a social fact (1995).[9]

FOLK SYSTEMS

The following characteristics are primarily used to describe folk medical systems (O'Connor and Hufford, 2001, p. 18): transmission primarily through oral means coupled with unofficial status; health as harmony or balance; interrelation of body, mind, and spirit; vitalism; magical or supernatural elements; thoughts and emotions as etiologic factors; concern with underlying causes; positive/negative energies; transference of energies; moral tone; meaning of illness. Of particular importance in the understanding of folk medical systems is the concept of *folk illness*. The most commonly identified Latina/o folk illnesses include *empacho* (food sticking to the stomach walls), *mal de ojo* (the evil eye), *susto* (soul loss), *nervios* (nerves), and *caida de mollera* (fallen fontanel; see Chavez, 1984; Rubel, 1998; Trotter, 1998). Within the framework of a folk medical system, folk illnesses are understood as illnesses "that have no apparent equivalent in bioscience ... in that their clusterings of signs and symptoms do not conform to bioscientific diagnostic categories" (Browner, Ortiz de Montellano, & Rubel 1988, p. 684). In biomedicine, folk illnesses are psychologized, making it difficult to separate disease processes from the cultural response to them (Rubel, 1984). As Csordas and Kleinman explain, "Perhaps the most frequently encountered assertion in the literature on therapeutic process is that there exists an analogy between psychotherapy and religious or folk healing" (1990, p. 24). While psychotherapy and religious traditions such as Santería, spiritism, and spiritualism share similar results in alleviating the symptoms of the patient, these religions are not concerned with a subconscious motivation since this is usually attributed to spiritual forces or with behavioral independence (Finkler, 1985). Rubel suggests that "the most fruitful approach to understanding folk ill-nesses is to seek an interaction between social and biological factors" (1984, p. 122). Folk systems are also described as uti-lized by those who have a limited access to biomedical forms of health care. Reasons cited for this supplemental form of health care are the high cost of health care, low levels of medical insurance coverage, patient dissatisfaction with conventional forms of medical care, language barriers, and undocumented immigrant status (Applewhite, 1995; Astin, 1998; Austin, 1999; Chavez, 1984, 1997; Kearney, 1978; Kreisman, 1975; Lefley, 1998; Mayers, 1989; Padilla, Carlos, & Keefe, 1976; Quesada, 1977; Vincent & Furnham, 1996).

The religious and spiritual association, described also as "magical or supernatural," is a very important element in folk systems, as Santería, spiritism, and spiritualism attest. Illness causation in Santería can be attributed to a witch, sorcerer, or other entity, whereas in spiritism it is related in capital-ist metaphors as debts due to past sins, and in spiritualism it is generally attributed to an imbalance in the body. The notion of balance, particularly with respect to the humors, is a recurrent and common naturalistic etiology in literature focusing on health and spiritual practices (Laderman, 1994). Humoral approaches toward healing look at health as a mat-ter of balance between opposites (e.g., hot/cold and wet/dry; see Rubel & Hass, 1990). The humoral theory of disease was a basic framework of Western medicine derived from Emped-olces, Galen, and Hippocrates. Humoral theories conceptual-ize the world in terms of four basic elements (fire, earth, air, and water), four qualities (heat, cold, dryness, and dampness), four humors (blood, phlegm, yellow bile, and black bile), and four personality types (sanguine, phlegmatic, choleric, and melancholic; see Rubel & Hass 1990; Turner, 1987).[10] How-ever balance is achieved, as Rubel and Moore (2001) explain in their comparative study of susto and tuberculosis among urban working-class Mexicans in Ensenada and Guadalajara, humoral systems of health perception continue to be impor-tant *alongside* biomedical interpretations.

Personalistic illness etiologies—including sorcery, witch-craft, and occult practices—can be specifically linked with health issues and thus function as a social anodyne. In a very concrete way, practitioners seek the counsel of alterna-tive religious or folk medical practitioners and practice the recommended rituals, in part, to alleviate pain (Geschiere, 1997). It is important to note, as Kleinman suggests, that folk medicine is frequently classified into sacred and secular parts, but "this division is often blurred in practice, and the two usually overlap" (1980, p. 59). Given that folk models are placed in comparison with the dominant biomedical model, measuring and defining efficacy is difficult.

One of foremost characteristics respected in folk healers is the ability to read and respond to the feelings and the needs of the person who seeks healing (McGuire, 1988, p. 179). This can be referred to as the *emotional component* associated with healing practices, and is an important reason individuals seek nonbiomedical and often religiously affiliated treatments (Dunfield, 1996; Newman, 1999). The exchange of feelings that is generated in healing activities, coupled with the relationship that develops between patients and healers, significantly influences the experience of healing (Astin, 1998; Galanter, 1997; Strathern & Stewart, 1999). In addition, folk systems actively engage adherents in the process of healing instead of expecting a passive form of participation (Joralemon, 1986; Langford, 1998; Schneirov & Geczic, 1998).

BIOMEDICINE

Biomedicine by definition focuses on the biological aspects of sickness relying on the scientific paradigm of investigation whereby disease is observable (Loustenau & Sobo, 1997). World War II served as a catalyst in defining disease as located in the body as a tangible, physical, and often aggressive agent that wreaks havoc inside the human body (Good, 1994; Martin, 1990, 1994). In the United States, biomedicine developed as a hegemonic health practice through the development of the American Medical Association (AMA), founded in 1847, and the publication of the Flexner Report in 1910.[11] The AMA developed the scientific basis for the practice of medicine and consolidated the economic position of the medical profession within society (Loustenau & Sobo, 1997). The Flexner Report standardized U.S. medical education, eliminating incompetent treatment but also leading to discrimination against women, African Americans, Jews, and other immigrants in the field of medicine. Most important, the Flexner Report "established a new medical paradigm—that of the body as machine with an emphasis on research, therapy and repair (pathology and cure)" (Loustenau & Sobo 1997, p. 118). The impact of this paradigm has led to the process of medicalization whereby pathological terminology is extended to cover new conditions (Baer, 1997). Given the emphasis placed on the discovery of malfunctioning biological components, the medical physician observes the patient during the diagnostic process in a detached manner, somehow uninvolved in the experience (Romanucci-Ross, Moerman & Tancredi, 1997). In reducing sickness to biological terms, biomedicine only addresses the physical component of illness, placing greater emphasis on curative (removing the object of disease from the biological body) over preventative (enhancing the current condition of the individual to counter the development of negative physical manifestations) approaches (Loustenau & Sobo 1997; Rhodes, 1996).

COMPARING FOLK AND BIOMEDICAL MODELS

A primary difference between the biomedical approach and the folk medical approach is the "curing of disease" endemic in the biomedical model and the "healing of illness" more prevalent in the folk model (Berlin & Fowkes, 1998; Kleinman, 1980). Illness can best be understood as "syndromes from which members of a particular group claim to suffer and for which their culture provides an etiology, a diagnosis, preventive measures, and regimens of healing" (Rubel, 1984, p. 2). In nonbiomedical healing practices the idea of health is not divorced from social relationships, including the metaphysical, while biomedicine places an emphasis on the localization of disease on the physical body and the ramifications that disease has on particular organs (Kleinman, 1980). From a medical anthropological perspective, it is important to understand that the perception of the concept of health, well-being, disease, and illness constructs the experiences associated with each, along with determining the appropriate types of treatment (Foucault, 1994; Good, 1994). For example, in Mexican spiritualism, Finkler (1994) notes that while both biomedicine and sacred healing focus on the manifestation of illness on the body, and that the role of the patient is passive in both practices, sacred healers address patients' overall experience of illness while biomedical physicians focus on particular physical symptoms. In biomedicine, disease via pathogens and behavior via poor habits are identified as the primary sources of illness, while religious healing practices can alter "the person's experience of his or her body" (Finkler, 1994, p. 189). In religiously derived models, healing is perceived as a process that involves the relationships that an individual has with metaphysical entities and, as such, requires a process of understanding the underlying rationale for the appearance of illness in the body (Fuller, 1989).

In comparing healing systems as distinct languages, it can be concluded that the degree to which an individual is fluent in a particular language will determine the level of comprehension experienced. In understanding healing practices in this manner, it becomes apparent that different systems require different "patterns of speech," leaving some symbols translatable and others not. This problem has been encountered in research conducted on humoral medical systems that "have had to face problems of translatability or commensurability" (Good, 1994). By understanding the hegemonic position of biomedicine—which emphasizes curative approaches that focus on the removal of a diseased object from a biological body rather than preventative approaches that focus on enhancing the current condition of an individual to counter the development of negative physical manifestations—religious healing practices can be valorized as distinct models in which problems of translatability do not undermine the healing aspects of the religion. As Turner explains:

> We can no longer regard "diseases" as natural events in the world which occur outside the language with which they are described. A disease entity is the product of medical discourses which in turn reflect the dominant mode of thinking (the episteme in Foucault's terminology) within a society. (1987, p. 11)

As Foucault (1983, 1995) argues, medicine is one of the primary institutions of modern life that regulates, controls, and makes subjects of individuals in defining appropriate and inappropriate methods of healing and illness classifications; he states, "rather than asking *what*, in a given period, is regarded as sanity or insanity, as mental illness or normal behaviour, I wanted to ask *how* these divisions are operated" (1991, p. 74).

CONCLUSION

By affirming the existence of another world, religions can provide an ameliorative space in which individuals are able to negotiate adverse conditions, including poor health. In the case of Afro-Latin religions such as Santería, Pérez y Mena (1998) explains that the emphasis placed on the "here and now" provides adherents with more amenable solutions than the mainstream religion of Catholicism. Lefever notes that "religion provides a counterhegemonic challenge and resistance to the existing social, economic, and political order and functions as an important source of social change" (1996, p. 318). Within this context, Santería, spiritism, and spiritualism can be viewed as counterhegemonic religions that allow participants to address health and other life problems that are not comprehensively addressed through mainstream venues such as biomedicine. As Gregory explains, "Santeria provides a philosophy or world view for acting in the world—one which encourages people to engage, interpret and respond to the novel, challenging and often paradoxical experiences of everyday life" (1999, p. x), including having the ability to affirm their ethnic identity in the process of healing. While having divergent historical developments, spiritism and spiritualism also provide a value system that relies on metaphysical knowledge and relationships to determine the source of material discomfort and disharmony. The healers in these systems play a crucial role in the healing process, just as physicians do in biomedicine. Santeras/os and mediums are recognized as having the gift (*el don*) to heal others, and communication with the spirits is considered to be a privilege (Macklin, 1974). The process of healing allows the healer to be imbued with symbolic power in that she is allowed to have the powers of God, Jesus, the saints, or the Orishas manifest themselves through her physical body.

As systems of religious healing, Santería, spiritism, and spiritualism provide alternative conceptualizations of health, illness, and the process of healing that rely on the notion that the human body is merely one aspect of an individual. Given the diverse historical developments of these systems, each emphasizes different therapeutic aspects. With its African Yoruba and Spanish Catholic roots, Santería relies on the maintenance of kinship relationships as a vital source of achieving and maintaining health. By living a life of service toward one's Orisha—demonstrated through ritual activity with one's religious family—an individual addresses health and other life predicaments. With its French Catholic heritage, spiritism emphasizes the healing relationship between a medium and his client in the pursuit of mitigating health and other problems. And spiritualism, with its English and American Protestant core, accentuates self-reliance and individual agency in achieving and maintaining health. As healing systems, these religions provide therapeutic modalities in which bodily concerns are placed in relation to social and metaphysical relationships.

NOTES

1. Practitioners argue that the legitimate name for Santería is *La Regla Ocha* or *La Regla Lucumi* (author's field notes, January 2001).
2. Shaw and Stewart argue that the term *syncretism* is contentious because it is "often taken to imply 'inauthenticity' or 'contamination,' the infiltration of a supposedly 'pure' tradition by symbols and meanings seen as belonging to other, incompatible traditions" (1994, p. 1). Their intention is to "recast" this term and to analyze the "politics of religious synthesis and the competition between discourses about syncretism" (p. 2) where authenticity is emphasized and associated with notions of purity. Or, as Van der Veer (1994) argues, syncretism is perceived as a corruption of truth historically situated with the rise of Protestantism in Europe. Herskovitz employed the term *syncretism* as an analytical tool in describing the difference between a "cultural mosaic" and an "integrative syncretism" in his study of acculturation in tracing the histories and cultures of people of African descent (1941, p. xxiii). Maldonado suggests the term *syncretization* as more appropriate because it emphasizes process instead of the notion that "one belief system continues to exist almost intact but borrows from another various trappings in order to camouflage itself," as does the term syncretism (see Díaz-Stevens, 1994, p. 18). The debate about the implications of using and defining *syncretism* centers on how authenticity becomes defined.
3. Similarly, Ortiz de Montellano (1990) discusses how curanderos masked their practice of healing by giving Christian names to their Aztec herbs to avoid persecution during the Inquisition.
4. *Merriam-Webster's Online Dictionary*. Retrieved October 29, 2007, from http://www.merriam-webster.com/dictionary/Divination.
5. For a detailed description from those who have offered public accounts of their private experiences, see Cabrera (1980, 1986); Gonzalez-Wippler (1992, 1998); and Vega (2000).

6. In Orange County, California, the cost can range between $12,000 and $15,000 (author's field notes, October 2000).

7. Mexican spiritualism is defined by Finker as a "dissident religious movement, vehemently anti-Catholic, and a nonbiomedical health-care delivery system" (1985, p. 10) founded in 1861 by Roque Rojas. While most other Latin American countries trace their practice to Allan Kardec, Finkler's informants did not. New York Puerto Rican spiritualism combines religious objects and ideologies of Cuban Santería and Kardecian spiritism (Pérez y Mena, 1991). Brandon (1997) refers to the melding of Puerto Rican spiritualism and Santería as Santerismo.

8. For a description of the occult with respect to its appeal to the French literary and artistic avante-garde during the 19th and early 20th centuries, see Eliade (1976).

9. For a description of Latino affiliation to mainstream religions (e.g. Catholicism, Protestantism, etc.), see Cadena (1995). Latinos are the largest ethnic group in the U.S. Catholic Church; in 1990 they comprised about 35% of U.S. Catholics (Cadena, 1995, p. 36). This is also an indication that Catholicism or other mainstream religions are practiced in conjunction with alternative religions, such as Santería or spiritism (author's field notes, October 2000).

10. This central notion of balance is not uncommon in other historically defined systems, as Kleinman (1980) relates the importance of attaining humoral balance in his study of Chinese folk medicine. In southern Sri Lanka, humoral discourse is associated with demons as "manifestations of the humours unbalanced, which themselves are constituted from the fundamental elements of all existence" (Kapferer 2000, p. 6).

11. Baer defines the term *hegemonic* within a biomedical context as the "process by which capitalist assumptions, concepts, and values come to permeate medical diagnosis and treatment" (1997, p. 31).

REFERENCES

Applewhite, S. L. (1995). Curanderismo: Demystifying the health beliefs and practices of elderly Mexican Americans. *Health and Social Work, 20*(4), 247–253.

Astin, J. A. (1998). Why patients use alternative medicine: Results of a national study. *Journal of the American Medical Association, 279*(19), 1548–1553.

Austin, P. (1999). *Community health: Working the puzzle.* Orange County Health Needs Assessment Spring Report. Orange County, CA: OCHNA.

Baer, H. A. (1997). What is medical anthropology about? In H. A. Baer (Ed.), *Medical anthropology and the world system* (pp. 1–36). Westport, CT: Bergin and Garvey.

Barnes, S. T. (1989). Introduction: The many faces of Ogun. In S. T. Barnes (Ed.), *Ogun: Ancient god of iron, warfare, and hunting* (pp. 1–26). Bloomington: Indiana University Press.

Brandon, G. (1997). *Santeria from Africa to the New World: The dead sell memories.* Bloomington: Indiana University Press.

Berlin, E. A., & Fowkes, W. C. (1998). A teaching framework for cross-cultural health care. In P. J. Brown, (Ed.), *Understanding and applying medical anthropology* (pp. 303–309). Mountain View, CA: Mayfield.

Brown, K. M. (1991). *Mama Lola: A Vodou priestess in Brooklyn.* Berkeley: University of California Press.

Brown, M. F. (1997). *The channeling zone: American spirituality in an anxious age.* Cambridge, MA: Harvard University Press.

Browner, C. H., Ortiz de Montellano, B. R., & Rubel, A. J. (1988). A methodology for cross-cultural ethnomedical research. *Current Anthropology, 29*(5), 681–702.

Cabrera, L. (1980). *Koeko Iyawo: Aprende novicia pequeno tratado de La Regla Lucumi.* Miami: Ultra Graphics.

Cabrera, L. (1986). La Regla Kimbisa del Santo Cristo del Buen Viaje. Miami, FL: Ediciones Universal.

Cabrera, L. (1994). Religious syncretism in Cuba. *Journal of Caribbean Studies, 10*(1–2), 84–94.

Cadena, G. R. (1995). Religious ethnic identity: A socio-religious portrait of Latinos and Latinas in the Catholic Church. In A. M. Stevens-Arroyo & G. R. C. Stevens-Arroyo (Eds.), *Old masks, new faces: Religion and Latino identities* (pp. 33–59). New York: Bildner Center for Western Hemisphere Studies.

Canizares, R. J. (1994). Santeria: From Afro-Caribbean cult to world religion. *Caribbean Quarterly, 40*(1), 59–63.

Chavez, L. R. (1997). Undocumented Latina immigrants in Orange County, California: A comparative analysis. *International Migration Review, 3*(9), 89–107.

Chavez, L. R. (1984). Doctors, *Curanderos*, and *Brujas*: Health Care Delivery and Mexican Immigrants in San Diego. *Medical Anthropology Quarterly.* 15(2), 31–37.

Chavez, L. R., & V. M. T. (1994). The *political economy of Latino health.* In N. Kanellos, T. Weaver, & C. Esteva-Fabregat (Eds.), *Handbook of Hispanic Cultures in the United States: Anthropology* (pp. 226–243). Houston, TX: Arte Público Press.

Cohen, D. W. (1989). The undefining of oral tradition. *Ethnohistory, 36*(1), 9–18.

Conniff, M. L., & Davis, T. J. (1994). *Africans in the Americas.* New York: St. Martin's Press.

Csordas, T. J., Kleinman, A. (1990). The therapeutic process. In C. F. Sargent & T. M. Johnson (Eds.), *Medical anthropology: Contemporary theory and method* (pp. 11–25). New York: Praeger.

Diaz-Stevens, A. M. (1994). Analyzing popular religiosity for socio-religious meaning. In A. M. S. Arroyo & A. M. Diaz-Stevens (Eds.), *An enduring flame: Studies on Latino popular religiosity* (pp. 17–36). New York: Bildner Center for Western Hemisphere Studies.

Diaz-Stevens, A. M., & Stevens-Arroyo, A. M. (1998). *Recognizing the Latino resurgence in U.S. religion.* Boulder, CO: Westview Press.

Dunfield, J. F. (1996). Consumer perceptions of health care quality and the utilization of non-conventional therapy. *Social Science and Medicine, 43*(2), 149–161.

Durkheim, É. (1995). *The elementary forms of religious life* (K. E. Fields, Trans.) New York: Free Press. (Original work published 1912.)

Efunde, A. (1996). Los secretos de la Santería [The secrets of Santería]. Miami, FL: Ediciones Universales.

Eliade, M. (1976). *Occultism, witchcraft, and cultural fashions.* Chicago: University of Chicago Press.

Finkler, K. (1985). *Spiritualist healers in Mexico.* South Hadley, MA: Bergin and Garvey.

Finkler, K. (1994). Sacred healing and biomedicine compared. *Medical Anthropology Quarterly, 8*(2), 178–197.

Foucault, M. (1983). Afterword: The subject and power. In H. L. Dreyfus & P. Rabinov (Eds.), *Michel Foucault: Beyond structuralism and hermeneutics* (pp. 208–252). Chicago: University of Chicago Press.

Foucault, M. (1991). Questions of method. In G. Burchell, C. Gordon, & P. Miller (Eds.), *The Foucault effect* (pp. 73–86). Chicago: University of Chicago Press. (Original work published 1980.)

Foucault, M. (1994). *The birth of the Clinic: An Archaeology of Medical Perception* (A. M. Sheridan Smith, Trans.). New York: Vintage Books. (Original work published 1973.)

Foucault, M. (1995). *Discipline and punish: The birth of the prison* (A. Sheridan, Trans.). New York: Vintage Books. (Original work published 1977.)

Fuller, R. C. (1989). *Alternative medicine and American religious life.* Oxford, England: Oxford University Press.

Galanter, M. (1997). Spiritual recovery movements and contemporary medical care. *Psychiatry: Interpersonal and Biological Processes, 60*(3), 211–223.

Geschiere, P. (1997). *The modernity of witchcraft.* Charlottesville: University Press of Virginia.

Gonzalez-Wippler, M. (1992). *The Santeria experience.* St. Paul, MN: Llewellyn.

Gonzalez-Wippler, M. (1998). *Santeria: The religion.* St. Paul, MN: Llewellyn.

Good, B. J. (1994). *Medicine, rationality, and experience: An anthropological perspective.* Cambridge, England: Cambridge University Press.

Gregory, S. (1999). *Santeria in New York City.* New York: Garland.

Griggs, B. (1981). *The green pharmacy: the history and evolution of western herbal medicine.* Manchester, England: Arts Press.

Herskovitz, M. J. (1941). *The myth of the Negro past.* Boston: Beacon Press.

Hess, D. J. (1994). *Samba in the night: Spiritism in Brazil.* New York: Columbia University Press.

Isaacs, E. (1983). The Fox sisters and American spiritualism. In H. Kerr & C. L. Crow (Eds.), *The occult in America: New historical perspectives* (pp. 79–110). Urbana: University of Illinois Press.

Joralemon, D. (1986). The performing patient in ritual healing. *Social Science and Medicine, 23*(9), 841–845.

Kardec, A. (1989). *The spirits' book.* Albuquerque, NM: Brotherhood of Life. (Original work published 1857.)

Kearney, M. (1978). Spiritualist healing in Mexico. In P. Morley & R. Wallis (Eds.), *Culture and curing: Anthropological perspectives on traditional medical beliefs and practices* (pp. 19–39). Pittsburgh: University of Pittsburgh Press.

Kleinman, A. (1980). *Patients and healers in the context of culture: An exploration of the borderland between anthropology, medine, and psychiatry.* Berkeley: University of California Press.

Kosmin, B. A. & Lachman, S. P. (1993). *One Nation Under God: Religion in Contemporary American Society.* New York: Harmony Press.

Kreisman, J. J. (1975). The curandero's apprentice: A therapeutic integration of folk and medical healing. *American Journal of Psychiatry, 132*(1), 81–83.

Laderman, C. (1994). The embodiment of symbols and the acculturarion of the anthropologist. In T. J. Csordas (Ed.), *Embodiment and experience: The existential ground of culture and self* (pp. 183–197). Cambridge, England: Cambridge University Press.

Langford, J. M. (1998). Ayurvedic psychotherapy: Transposed signs, parodied selves. PoLAR, *21*(1), 84–98.

Lefever, H. G. (1996). When the saints go riding in: Santeria in Cuba and in the United States. *Journal for the Scientific Study of Religion, 35*(3), 318–331.

Lefley, H. P., Cross, M. & Charles, C. (1998). Traditional healing systems in a multicultural setting. In S. O. Okpaku (Ed.), *Clinical methods of transcultural psychiatry* (pp. 88–110). Washington, DC: American Psychiatric Press.

Loustaunau, M. O., & Sobo, E. J. (1997). *The cultural context of health, illness, and medicine.* Westport, CT: Bergin and Garvey.

Macklin, J. (1974). Belief, ritual, and healing: New England spiritualism and Mexican-American spiritism compared. In I. I. Zaretsky & M. P. Leone (Eds.), *Religious movements in contemporary America* (pp. 383–417). Princeton, NJ: Princeton University Press.

Martin, E. (1990). Toward an anthropology of immunology: The body as nation state. *Medical Anthropology Quarterly, 4*(4), 410–426.

Martin, E. (1994). *Flexible Bodies: Tracking Immunity in American Culture from the Days of Polio to the Age of Aids.* Boston: Beacon Press.

Masland, T., & Larmer, B. (1998). Cuba's real religion. *Newsweek, 131*(3), 42.

Mayers, R. S. (1989). Use of folk medicine by elderly Mexican-American women. *Journal of Drug Issues, 19*(2), 283–295.

McGuire, M. B. (1988). *Ritual healing in suburban America.* New Brunswick, NJ: Rutgers University Press.

Murphy, J. (1988). *Santeria: An African religion in America.* Boston: Beacon Press.

Murphy, J. M. (1995). Santería and Vodou in the United States. In T. Miller (Ed.), *America's alternative religions* (pp. 291–296). Albany: State University of New York Press.

National Spiritualist Association of Churches of the United States of America. (1967). *Spiritualist Manual.* Milwaukee: WI: National Spiritualist Association of Churches of the United States of America.

Newman, D. I. J. (1999). The Western psychic as diviner: Experience in the politics of perception. *Ethnos, 64*(1), 82–106.

O'Connor, B. B., & Hufford, D. J. (2001). Understanding folk medicine. In M. O. Jones (Ed.), *Healing logics: Culture and medicine in modern health belief systems* (pp. 13–35). Logan: Utah State University Press.

Ortiz de Montellano, B. R. (1990). Syncretism in Mexican folk medicine. In B. R. Ortiz de Montellano (Ed.), *Aztec medicine, health, and nutrition* (pp. 193–235). New Brunswick, NJ: Rutgers University Press.

Padilla, A. M., Carlos, M. L., Keefe, S. E. (1976). *Mental health service utilization by Mexican Americans.* In Psychotherapy with the Spanish-Speaking: Issues in Research and Service Delivery (pp. 9–20). UCLA: Spanish Speaking Mental Health Research Center Monograph Number Three.

Pérez y Mena, A. I. (1991). *Speaking with the dead: Develpment of Afro-Latin religion among Puerto Ricans in the United States.* New York: AMS Press.

Pérez y Mena, A. I. (1998). Cuban Santería, Haitian Vodou, Puerto Rican spiritualism: A multicultural inquiry into syncretism. *Journal for the Scientific Study of Religion, 37*(1), 15–28.

Portes, A., & Hoffman, K. (2003). Latin American class structures: Their composition and change during the neoliberal era. *Latin American Research Review, 38*(1), 41–83.

Quesada, G. M., & P. L. H. (1977). Sociocultural barriers to medical care among Mexican Americans in Texas. *Medical Care, 15*(5), 93–101.

Rhodes, L. A. (1996). Studying biomedicine as a cultural system. In C. F. Sargent & T. M. Johnson (Eds.), *Medical anthropology: Contemporary theory and method* (pp. 165–180). Westport, CT: Praeger.

Romanucci-Ross, L., M. D. E., & T. L. R. (1997). Medical Anthropology: Convergence of mind and experience in the anthropological imagination. In L. Romanucci-Ross, D. E. Tancredi, L. R. Tancredi (Eds.), *The anthropology of medicine: From culture to method* (pp. 369–381). Westport, CT: Bergin and Garvey.

Roth, D. (2000). America's Fascination with Nutrition. *Food Review.* 23(1), 32–37.

Rubel, A. J. (1984). *Susto, a folk illness.* Berkeley: University of California Press.

Rubel, A. J. (1998). The epidemiology of a folk illness: Susto in Hispanic America. In P. J. Brown (Ed.), *Understanding and applying medical anthropology* (pp. 196–206). Mountain View, CA: Mayfield. (Original work published 1964.)

Rubel, A. J., & Hass, M. R. (1990). Ethnomedicine. In C. F. Sargent & T. M. Johnson (Eds.), *Medical anthropology: Contemporary theory and method* (pp. 115–131). New York: Praeger.

Rubel, A. J., & Moore, C. C. (2001). The contribution of medical anthropology to a comparative study of culture: Susto and tuberculosis. *Medical Anthropology Quarterly, 15*(4), 440–454.

Schmit, D. (2005). Re-visioning Antebellum American psychology: The dissemination of mesmerism, 1836–1854. *History of Psychology, 8*(4), 403–434.

Schneirov, M., & Geczic, J. D. (1998). Technologies of the self and the aesthetic project of alternative health. *Sociological Quarterly, 39*(3), 435–451.

Shaw, R., & Stewart, C. (1994). Introduction: problematizing syncretism. In C. Stewart & R. Shaw (Eds.), *Syncretism/anti-syncretism: The politics of religious synthesis* (pp. 1–26). London: Routledge.

Strathern, A., & Stewart, P. J. (1999). Spiritual healing: Charismatic Catholics. In A. Strathern & P. J. Stewart (Eds.), *Curing and healing: Medical anthropology in global perspective* (pp. 127–136). Durham, NC: Carolina Academic Press.

Trimble, S. M. (1995). Spiritualism and channeling. In T. Miller (Ed.), *America's alternative religions* (pp. 331–337). Albany: State University of New York Press.

Trotter R. T., II. (1998). A case of lead poisoning from folk remedies in Mexican American communities. In P. J. Brown (Ed.), *Understanding and applying medical anthropology* (pp. 279–286). Mountain View, CA: Mayfield. (Original work published 1987.)

Turner, B. S. (1987). *Medical power and social knowledge*. London: Sage.

Turner, V. W. (1977). Ndembu divination and its symbolism. In D. Landy (ed.), *Culture, disease, and healing* (pp. 175–183). New York: Macmillan. (Original work published 1968.)

Van der Veer, P. (1994). Syncretism, multiculturalism and the discourse of tolerance. In C. Stewart & R. Shaw (Eds.), *Syncretism/anti-syncretism: The politics of religious synthesis* (pp. 196–211). London: Routledge.

Vega, M. M. (2000). *The altar of my soul: The living traditions of Santería*. New York: Ballantine.

Vincent, C., & Furnham, A. (1996). Why do patients turn to complementary medicine? An empirical study. *British Journal of Clinical Psychology, 35,* 37–48.

Worseley, P. (1982). Non-Western medical systems. *Annual Review of Anthropology, 11,* 315–348.

Chapter Ten

Curanderismo
Religious and Spiritual Worldviews and Indigenous Healing Traditions

FERNANDO A. ORTIZ, KENNETH G. DAVIS, AND BRIAN W. MCNEILL

The art of healing comes from nature and not from the physician. Therefore, the physician must start from nature with an open mind.

– Paracelsus

INTRODUCTION

Recently there has been a proliferation in the utilization, publication and research of "folk medicine," "indigenous systems of medicine," and "complementary and alternative medicine" (Abbot, White, & Ernst, 1996; Campion, 1993; Pal, 2002). Folk healing alternatives had traditionally been researched by anthropologists, ethnographers, and social scientists dedicated to the study of culture (Kiev, 1968). With the advent of multiculturalism in psychology and the emphasis on multicultural competencies, mental health professionals are becoming increasingly aware of the importance of culturally sensitive therapeutic practices and have made an effort to incorporate indigenous or culture-specific therapeutic interventions in counseling (Sue, 1990; Sue & Sue, 1990). What previously had been labeled *alternative, unconventional, folk,* or *unorthodox* and considered the practice of charlatans is increasingly becoming the focus of study of multicultural psychologists and widely used by informed consumers (Arenas, Cross, & Willard, 1980; Ruesch, 1963; Ruiz & Langrod, 1976; Tan, 1988; Torrey, 1972; Van Oss Marin, Marin, Padilla, & De La Rocha, 1983). Research both in the United States and abroad has found several factors for the increasing utilization of indigenous healing alternatives, which includes holding a holistic orientation to health (Astin, 1998), having had a transformational experience that changed the person's worldview, and an interest in spirituality and personal growth (Pargament, 1997).

Curanderismo falls under the rubric of "folk healing practices" (Snow, 1974; Steiner, 1986). This indigenous system of health has been the focus of numerous anthropological and psychological investigations. The term etymologically derives from the Spanish verb *curar,* which has its roots in the Latin *curare,* "to care for, to cure" (Glannon, 2004). Thus, in defining *curanderismo* it is important to highlight the meaning of caring and healing. The dictionary of the Spanish Royal Academy provides thirteen nuanced definitions of *curar,* and includes "to successfully apply corresponding remedies to a patient for the healing of a disease or ailment," and "to heal the sorrows and pains of the soul" (Real Academia Española, 2001, p. 485) This system of folk healing holistically includes both physical and spiritual conditions. The *curandera/o* (folk healer) first appeared in the 16th century and is a product of the Spanish conquest. The Nahua *tícitl,* the Huastec *ilalix,* the Tzeltal *h'ilojel* the Tzotil *h'ilol,* the Mayan *h-men,* and the Pokoman *ah cut* were indigenous medical specialists that gradually became a homogenized group generally labeled as *curanderas/os* (Viesca-Treviño, 2001). Invariably, these indigenous specialists solved the health problems of their peoples through sacred, ritualistic, and magical practices.

The purpose of this chapter is to describe the most salient religious and spiritual dimensions of curanderismo, to explore some of the historical and cultural processes that shaped the worldview of this Mestiza/o healing system, and to provide direction for some culturally and spiritually sensitive therapeutic applications. To begin, it is necessary to define *religiousness* and *spirituality.* We do not intend to achieve absolute definitional clarity, but instead to find a common ground between these two constructs so we can refer to them with certain ease in our discussions of the sacred in curanderismo.

WORKING DEFINITIONS OF *RELIGIOUSNESS* AND *SPIRITUALITY*

It has become fashionable to make distinctions between religion and spirituality (Emmons, 1999). Zinnbauer, Pargament, and Scott (1999) have examined contemporary definitions of religiousness and spirituality and conclude that these two constructs are usually presented as polar opposites that reduce religion to a static and institutional entity and spirituality to a personal dynamic phenomenon. Instead of this polarized conceptualization, they propose an alternative integrative approach that defines both religion and spirituality in terms of dynamic search processes in which religion is seen as "a search for significance in ways related to the sacred," and spirituality "as a search for the sacred" (907). This search presupposes a proactive and goal-oriented view of human nature for ultimate purposes that are meaningful and significant. The final destination of the search is the sacred, which is defined as anything that is holy or set aside from the ordinary. A person may follow several pathways to reach the sacred; it is not only related to the divine, God, or higher powers, but encompasses anything associated or represented by it: time, places, events, materials, people, institutions, and roles. Whereas religion is oriented specifically for the search of many sacred objects of significance, spirituality focuses specifically and directly on the search for the sacred. Zinnbauer et al. (1997) have also found that although religiousness and spirituality appear to describe different concepts, they are not fully independent. They concluded that both religiousness and spirituality definitions commonly incorporate traditional concepts of the sacred (e.g., references to God, Christ, and the church). Richards and Bergin (1997) note that religious expressions tend to be denominational, external, cognitive, behavioral, ritualistic, and public, whereas spiritual experiences tend to be universal, ecumenical, internal, affective, spontaneous, and private. Moreover, they note that it is possible to be religious without being spiritual and spiritual without being religious.

Religious and spiritual beliefs define the worldview of believers in curanderismo, and psychotherapists and mental health professionals have noted the importance of understanding a person's worldview, or perspective on the world (Altman & Rogoff, 1987; Miller & West, 1993; Overton, 1984). A worldview (German *Weltanschauung*, which literally translates as "view of the world") is composed of beliefs a person holds about the universe and the nature of reality—metaphysical beliefs (Josephson & Peteet, 2004; Koltko-Rivera, 2004). Because of the ubiquitous status of the term *worldview* in this chapter, we adopt Naugle's definition, which proposes that

> a worldview might best be understood as a semiotic phenomenon... as a semiotic structure consists primarily of a network of narrative signs that offers an interpretation of reality and establishes an overarching framework of life... as a semiotic system of world-interpreting stories also provides a foundation or governing platform upon or by which people think, interpret, and know.... Semiotic has to do with signs and symbols, and how they convey meaning. Thus, a worldview uses a particular set of narrative signs to establish a symbolic universe, or a way of understanding reality. (2002, pp. 291)

In the following sections we examine the foundational beliefs, values, and assumptions embedded in curanderismo, a semiotic phenomenon that has resulted from the blending of two great narratives.

THE MESTIZA/O WORLDVIEW AND SYNCRETISM

A mestiza/o ("mixed-blood") worldview resulted from the mutual influence of the Iberian and Nahuatl cultures in the Americas through a continual process of interpenetration, transformation, and synthesis (Gruzinski, 2002; Ramirez, 1998). This complex and complicated process was facilitated by a similar cosmovision among the popular classes of both groups, which included belief in: (1) the supernatural; (2) the supernatural's activity in the natural world; (3) the resultant permeation of these two planes of reality; (4) access to the supernatural through religious rituals and spiritual leaders; and (5) that such supernatural activity in the natural world can be miraculous— that is, suspending the laws of nature, as in curing illness or disease that natural forces alone cannot cure (Pardo, 2004).

The traditional worldview that results from this encounter of cultures is a popular religion constitutive of mestizas/os and expressed through symbols and rituals that are adopted, exchanged, or integrated among both original cultures (Nygren, 1998). Greeley (1989, 2000) speaks of such a Catholic worldview as a sacramental or analogical imagination integral to the Catholic faith. A sacramental imagination is more than dogma or theology, it is a zeitgeist based on the conviction that since the incarnation (or God) became human, the divine becomes present in physical things; matter touches spirit (Tracy, 1982). Thus, the ubiquity and ordinariness of the sacred, the divine, or the extraordinary can be discovered in the quotidian (Rosenberg, 2002). This sacramental imagination includes, but is not limited to, the seven official sacraments of the Catholic Church.

Catholicism recognizes many "sacramentals" or sensual objects such as medals, statues, prayers, and holy cards that act as symbols. These sensual objects are symbolic (i.e., they bring together the natural and the supernatural) rather than diabolic (dividing the two planes) as well as superrational and somatic. Their efficacy depends on the devotion, faith, and love of the believer, often evoked through the blessings of particular objects (Stevens-Arroyo, 1998). Common sacramentals include making the sign of the cross (blessing ourselves), candles, holy water, images, scapulars, and blessed medals, all of which are intended to incite devotion and prayer. Believers renew the sacramental dimension in their lives through rituals—that is, relating to symbols through the senses. Such rituals both communicate and embody meaning, thereby directly shaping the character of the people involved (Cunningham, 1987).

Iberian Catholicism as well as Nahuatl religion understood that ritual environment communicates meaning by touching the senses of the believer. Statues, sculptures, crucifixes, posters, tapestries, mosaics, and incense, as well as music, dance, drama, and sacrifice or penance effectively incorporated into ritual to affectively engage the whole human, individual and community, body and soul (Davies, 1990; Pardo 2004). Burhart notes that the "intense ceremonialism" of the Nahuatl religion impressed the European Catholic friars and this was:

> a pervasive feature of Nahua religious life in central Mexico. For the Nahuas, contact with the sacred was established through ritual and the collective carrying out of certain actions at prescribed moments in a calendrical sequence of life cycle. Ritual acts produced, in the here and now, fleeting but authentic manifestations of the

sacred forces upon which all life depended. Through rituals, men and women laid themselves open to the power
of the gods; the frame of the ritual worked to channel
and limit this dangerous contact by directing the sacred
forces into persons, images, or other objects invested with
a god's regalia, which served as conduits for the sacred
manifestations. (Burkhart, 1998, p. 361)

Rituals express popular (from Latin *populus,* "the people") religion (from Latin *religare,* "to tie together") by enact-
ing a "shared worldview that constitutes a group of persons
as a people or community (Davis, 2005, p. 3). Through ritual,
a group normally divided by social status, economic class, or
political opinion becomes a community. This is the conclu-
sion of social scientists, theologians, and now the Catholic
bishops of Latin America, who, in their Third General Conference in Puebla, Mexico, have concluded that [the Liturgy
and the common people's piety cross-fertilize each other....
the religion of the people, with its symbolic and expressive
richness, can provide the Liturgy with creative dynamism]
(Conferencia Episcopal Latinoamerica, 1979, para. 465). Such
cross-fertilization is evident in the communion of saints as
well as in the folk healer or curandera/o. The communal and
highly symbolic and ritualistic character of popular mestiza/o
Catholicism "involves the whole person—intellect, will, emotion, and imagination. It affirms life by providing powerful
myths or stories with graphic imagery... it is more symbolic
than cognitive, more affective than rationalist, more practical
than speculative" (Figueroa-Deck, 2002, p. 14).

The Communion of Saints is a Catholic dogma that
expresses the felt extension of the mestiza/o community, and
refers to spiritual solidarity among the faithful on earth, the
souls of purgatory, and the saints in heaven (Kieckhefer &
Bond, 1988; Ryan, 2004). Their organic unity is experienced
through a constant supernatural interchange and interdependence among these planes. The belief in the efficacy of
intercession of the saints in Heaven for their fellow faithful
on earth is based on faith in that spiritual solidarity and fellowship (Brown, 1981). Though this spirituality of continuing bonds and interdependent relationships with others who
are believed to be in a supernatural plane is similarly found
in other religious and spiritual worldviews (e.g., in Japanese
Buddhism, Native American spirituality, and spiritualism;
see Klass & Goss, 1999), mestiza/o spirituality celebrates this

fellowship, and celebrations such as *Día de los Muertos* (Day of the Dead) become a vehicle for communication with ancestors (Rodriguez, 2004).

As the Communion of Saints gives a dogmatic label to a mestiza/o concept, so is *curandera/o* a mestiza/o label for the folk healer much influenced by the church's concept of saintliness (Orsi, 2005; Oktavec, 1995). Like the average Catholic saint, curanderas/os obey a call from God, live a simple life of dedication to the good of the community, and supercede normal gender as well as gender expectations and roles (Davis, 2004). Some curanderas/os believe that only certain people have a divine gift (*el don*) or vocation to work on the spiritual level and to communicate with God and the spirits (Hamburger, 1978; Lopez, 2005).

THE MESOAMERICAN WORLDVIEW

Curanderismo borrowed important anthropological, religious, ritualistic, and medical concepts from Mesoamerican cultures, primarily from the Nahuatl civilization (Carrasco, 1990, 1999). Ortiz de Montellano (1987) notes the existence of a pan-Mesoamerican religious system that represented a unified theological and cosmo-magical system. The human being was considered the *axis mundi*, or the center of the cosmos, and conceived by the convergence of the five components of the universe—that is, when the four terrestrial planes met in perfect equilibrium in time (on a fifth plane). Thus, the human was the result of perfect cosmic balance, and the Aztec cosmovisión was very mindful of factors that contribute to a lack of equilibrium in human existence: social inequalities, sex, animistic changes, temperament, and changes in health (Ingham, 1970). The human embodiment of balance and harmony mirrored the geometry and dynamics of the cosmos. In their locative view of the world, they depicted the universe as tightly ordered, a place where all of life is organized (Lopez Austin, 1988).

Mesoamerican civilizations believed in multiple souls that animated the body, gave humans their collective and individual traits, and survived after death (McKeever Furst, 1995). These souls were constituted of a subtle matter with animistic forces and physical features. The Nahuatl believed that three souls or "animistic entities" dwell in three areas of the body: the skull, the heart, and the liver (Guerra, 1971). Health was conceptualized as the balance, equilibrium, and harmony of these three life-giving entities: *Tonalli* (from Nahuatl *tona*, "to irradiate or make warm, to make sun"), *Ihiyotl* (luminous gas capable of attracting other beings), and *Teyolia* (from Nahuatl *yolia*, "he who animates," and *yol*, "life"). Tonalli is warmth derived from the sun, and is located in the head and in blood pulsing in the joints. Carrasco (1999) has listed nine characteristics of Tonalli: (1) it is the source of warmth, vigor, valor, and growth in the human body; (2) animals, plants, and gods all have Tonalli; (3) it comes from the celestial gods—first, from the dual god Ometeotl, who breathed Tonalli into the fetus, and second, from the sun, whose warmth and light provide Tonalli to humans; (4) newborn children accumulate more Tonalli when placed near the home fire, where the god Xiuhtecuhtli resides; (5) human blood generates Tonalli; (6) it has a physical nature—it is hot and luminous; (7) it can leave the body, causing disequilibrium during sexual intercourse, dreams, and sleep; (8) a warrior gains control over an enemy's Tonalli when grabbing the opponent by a tuft of hair on the front of the head; and (9) the loss of too much Tonalli results in death. The Nahuatl believed that the gods breathed life into the human body in utero because of the actual association between body warmth and the presence of life. The flight of Tonalli, or soul loss, is a realistic description of death because the disappearance of heat from the human body is a sure sign of the end of life. The very young and the very old alike are vulnerable to the flight of Tonalli because they actually have a lower body temperature (Carrasco, 1990).

Ihiyotl was believed to be an animistic entity that resided in the liver—the container of passion, vigor, and feeling. This animating soul is infused into infants through ritual in a bathing ceremony four days after their birth. It is associated with "night air" or "dead air," and is the source of either beneficent or malevolent energy. This energy can be supplied to the person by nourishment or through breathing air onto or within the person. The Nahuatl people believed that magicians or folk healers could externalize their Ihiyotl and inject it into people, animals, objects, or insects, with pathogenic or therapeutic effects.

The most important animistic entity was the heart, the place of equilibrium. In the Aztec cosmovision, the heart is ubiquitous: animals, lakes, plants, and even towns have a heart, called *altepeyollotl*. *Tepolia* was conceived in the mother's womb as a gift from the gods and is hot during life and cold during death. *Yolia* is associated with breath and with the heart. The Nahuatl believed that Yolia leaves the human body after death in the form of a bird, butterfly, or insect (Carrasco, 1999; Lopez Austin, 1988).

In addition to inheriting sophisticated anthropological notions from the Nahuatl culture, curanderismo also borrowed a wealth of herbal and medicinal concepts (Heinrich, Ankli, Frei, Weimann, & Sticher, 1998; Schendel, 1968). The use of plants for medical purposes and pharmacology were highly developed among the Aztecs and their predecessors (Hirschhorn, 1968; Rodriguez, 1959). The Spanish were astonished at the size and variety of the well-kept Mexican botanical gardens. Kidwell (1982) has found that herbal remedies were adopted by the Spanish colonists and thus constituted a case of "reverse acculturation," even though Aztec medicine was highly religious in nature and, essentially, supernaturalism with some rational elements, whereas European medicine was firmly rooted in the rational traditions of the Greeks. The *Badianus* manuscript illustrates and describes 204 medicinal herbs ranging from small rock plants to large trees, from aquatic to desert and tropical to alpine forms. Numerous Nahuatl manuscripts provide detailed descriptions of the pharmacological properties of plants, revealing an extensive botanical and medicinal knowledge. Plants with psychotropic pharmacological effects were often used as hallucinogens and for therapeutic, religious, and divinatory purposes (e.g., *peyotl*, *teonanacatl*, and *ololiuhqui*; see Del Pozo, 1966).

The medicine used by the Aztecs (*ticiotl*) is representative of all Mesoamerican medicine (Ortiz de Montellano, 1975). The medical history of the ticiotl was recovered in the years that followed the conquest from the works of Bernardino de Sahagun, Francisco Hernandez, and the *Badianus* manuscript (Peña, 1999). These documents include formulas for the preparation and application of herbal drugs, as well as the belief in the medicinal power of animal body parts and precious stones. The Aztec doctors (*titici*) possessed a relatively high level of sophistication in the classification and diagnosis of diseases, and they were excellent healers of wounds and fractures (Lopez Austin, 1988). These Nahuatl doctors used a complex and philosophically elaborated medical theory based on religion, astronomy, divination, and the polarity of cold and hot; this differs from the four-humor theory of Galenic medicine. The titici developed culture-specific notions of disease that modern science is beginning to appreciate for their uniqueness (and at times, comparability) with modern medical views

(Belsasso, 1969; Guerra, 1980). Nahuatl healers understood mental illness as the result of possession by evil spirits, a punishment for some immoral behavior, or an imbalance of the inner balance of a person (Guajardo, 1999).

CURANDERISMO AS A SPIRITUAL RESOURCE IN PSYCHOTHERAPY

Mental health professionals working with Latinas/os have observed that spirituality and religiosity can be an important component of psychotherapy (Paniagua, 1998). Curanderismo offers a viable complementary indigenous alternative, with religious and spiritual practices that have therapeutic value. A curandera/o utilizes culturally appropriate methods of working with a client; considers the religious and spiritual aspects of the healing process, including the client's faith and beliefs; incorporates methods that activate the natural support system within the community; and facilitates the healing through the use of culturally and ritually meaningful methods (Torres, 1983; Trotter & Chavira, 1997). This holistic system of healing addresses the communal, physical, psychological, and spiritual aspects of the ailment (Trotter & Chavira, 1980). Working on these multiple planes of reality, and especially on the interdependence of the natural and supernatural phenomena, are seen as integral, not separate, aspects in human experience (Weclew, 1975). Illness from natural causes can be cured by natural means such as herbs. Problems that precipitate from supernatural influence, such as a hex, require a spiritual cure (Scheffler, 1986).

Another culturally salient component of the curanderismo method of healing is ritual, which is formalized behavior that evokes specific emotions and gives symbolic expression to feelings and thoughts (Al-Krenawi, 1999). Ritual embodies a holistic form of healing that incorporates psychological issues, physical conditions, and spiritual and cultural patterns. These can provide safety and meaning to life, allowing some aspects of existence to be experienced. Frank and Frank (1991) highlight several functions of ritual in healing, including combating demoralization through the strengthening of the therapeutic relationship, instilling healing expectations, structuring new learning experiences, evoking affective experiences, enhancing both mastery and self-efficacy, and creating opportunities for rehearsal and practice. Rituals contain symbols that are enacted to perform, modulate, and transform. In the use of symbols, concerns can be externalized in physical or tangible form. People usually find consolation in their religious rituals. Ritual includes promise making, offerings to the church, prayer offerings, and votive promises (Guajardo, 1999; Nall & Speilberg, 1967).

Professionals in the mental health professions who want to become effective with Latinas/os must discover and become culturally competent in using some of these nontraditional therapeutic methods traditionally utilized by curanderas/os (Prieto, McNeill, & Gómez, 2001). Many segments of the Latina/o population hold a worldview that includes beliefs that illness and health are strongly influenced by spiritual and religious factors that may ultimately affect therapeutic outcomes. Many of these beliefs are part of complex medicine system that originated in Mesoamerican times and remains to this day present among some segments of the Latina/o population. When mental health professionals are not familiar with a worldview other than their own, they may encounter difficulties in understanding, treating, and communicating with Latinas/os. What follows are the main philosophical foundations derived from the mestiza/o worldview of curanderismo that can provide a theoretical basis for guiding culturally sensitive therapeutic practices with Latinas/os.

Theism and Spiritualism

Contrasting the empiricist and materialistic epistemology of traditional psychotherapeutic approaches, the worldview of curanderismo is both material and immaterial and healing practices are based on the premise of a mutual interdependence between these two planes of reality. Religion and spirituality permeate human experience. An individual's life is a spiritual phenomenon, and humans, animals, plants, and the natural world are interrelated, with God being the driving force. Spirits belong to the ontological realm of existence between human beings and God. Supernatural and magical elements play a crucial role in the etiology of natural and spiritual diseases. Sinful behavior can result in illness or disharmony and the interventions of spiritual and divine entities are invoked in therapeutic practices.

Animism and Vitalism

Curanderismo is founded on the belief in personalized, spiritual beings (or *animas*) endowed with intellect, reason, and volition. Animistic belief systems often believe that the spirit or soul can detach from the body and believe in the immortality of this spiritual entity. Animistic theories in curanderismo encourage the use of rituals to connect with spiritual entities. In some variations of curanderismo, the souls are seen as vital forces that animate and sustain the body through some force, energy, or essence. It is believed that loss or disruption of this vital energy can cause disease.

Holism and Pluralism

Curanderismo views the human person as a holistic unified being (Guajardo, 1999). It emphasizes the interconnectedness of body, mind, and spirit (Brady, 2001). Human beings are more than the sum of their parts, and they cannot be adequately understood by reducing or dividing them into smaller pieces. Reductionism, atomism, dualism, and elementism have traditionally defined the human person as a fragmented being, and these anthropological notions have served as the philosophical foundations of the behavioral sciences. In curanderismo and in other folk medical systems, physical ailments may result in emotional, psychological, and/or spiritual distress. Spiritual wellness and harmony are integral dimensions of health.

Experiential Sacramentalism

Curanderismo relies on ritual and sacramental expression to mediate healing and the experience of the sacred. Embodiment, physicality, sacramentality, and the involvement of the senses are highly valued. Tactile contact with healing and therapeutic elements and with representations of the divine is intrinsic to this sacramental way of perceiving the world. Linguistically, *tocar* means "to touch," but semantically and culturally it connotes more than its English translation. In Spanish, it is much more likely to connote a concrete effect. For instance, in Spanish one does not "play" a musical instrument, one "touches" it. But the effect is music. Thus, *touch* in Spanish is much more an action with a presumed effect. This may be influenced by cultural differences concerning interpersonal space. In general, an English speaker requires more personal space than a Spanish speaker. For the latter, physical proximity, like touch, implies some communion considered necessary to real communication. The lexicon of curanderismo contains a plethora of specifications about healing touch, such as *masaje* (massage), *barrida* (spiritual sweeping), *soba* (rubbing), and *ventosa* (cupping glass).

Scientific medicine is more high tech, but folk medicine is more "high touch." And the verb *tocar* is one of the essentials of a *naturalismo* ritual, perhaps because touch is the one human sense that is necessarily mutual. One can see without being seen and hear without being heard, but one cannot touch another without being touched oneself. While medical professionals are arguably better at curing biological contagion and physical injury, the human touch of an accepted folk healer may do more to cure the psychic fragmentation and social alienation that a sick person often suffers. Touch demonstrates acceptance to a person whose shame at personal weakness may endanger his integrity. Since it is necessarily a mutual interaction between two humans, touch bridges social isolation. Popular Hispanic Catholicism is tactile. Throngs turn out to feel the grit of ashes, grasp the sleekness of palm leaves, sense the warmth of candles, and heft the weight of statues. Images are caressed and kissed, and love notes are left behind. Beads are counted, crosses carried, breasts beaten, water sprinkled. People want to touch God and be touched by God.

The laying on of hands and anointing with oil are tactile symbols that recall the somatic quality of Hispanic popular Catholicism. The words of blessing and anointing also speak of comfort, consolation, fortitude, and protection. These are at the heart of the popular spirituality of this community, which finds God in the concrete, historic, ordinary experience of relationships both human and divine. For this community, health and disease are not just physical nor even only social realities; they also include humanknd and the world's relationship to God. And that is why this anthropology emphasizes healing as liberation from all personal and social oppression.

Culture-Related Syndromes

Culture-specific beliefs about health and illness are an important part of culture-bound syndromes, or indigenously defined illnesses (Guajardo, 1999). The American Psychiatric Association's *Diagnostic and Statistical Manual of Mental Disorders*, fourth edition, defines *culture-bound syndrome* as denoting:

> recurrent, locally, specific patterns of aberrant behavior and troubling experience that may or may not be linked to a particular DSM-IV diagnostic category. Many of these patterns are indigenously considered to be "illnesses," or at least afflictions, and most have local names... culture-bound syndromes are generally limited to specific soci-

eties or culture areas and are localized, folk, diagnostic categories that frame coherent meanings for certain repetitive, patterned, and troubling sets of experiences and observations. (American Psychiatric Association, 2000, p. 898)

Illnesses that are treatable by curanderas/os are as follows: *mal de ojo*, or *mal ojo*, (the "bad eye" or "evil eye"); *susto* (fright, or spirit loss); *caida de mollera* (fallen fontanel); *empacho* (indigestion); *mal aire* (upper respiratory illness and colds); *desasombro* (a more severe grade of susto, or spirit loss); *cólico* (colic), *espanto* (the most serious form of spirit loss); *bilis* (excessive bile); *muina* ("anger sickness"); *latido* (palpitation or throb), *embrujado* (being "hexed"), *envidia* (envy), and *mal puesto, salar,* or *maleficio* (a physical disorder caused by envy; see Mull & Mull, 1983). These syndromes suggest that spiritual beliefs and other cultural influences play an important role in symptom formation and the interpretation of perceptual experiences. The spiritual beliefs defining these culture-related syndromes classify ailments into two groups, the natural and the unnatural (*males naturales* and *males artificiales*, or *mal puesto*). Natural ailments are seen as being in the realm of God or good spirits, and unnatural ones as being the result of evil spirits or the devil (Gonzales, 1976). Moreover, consistent with a culture with a collectivistic orientation that values smooth interpersonal relationships, Gonzales (1976) notes that most of the folk illnesses are closely related to social relationships and are connected with faulty interpersonal relations.

The wide range of ailments and conditions parallels the diversified and eclectic specialization of curanderas/os. Folk medicine practitioners include herbalists (*yerberos*), bone and muscle therapists (*hueseros* and *sobadores*), and midwives (*parteras;* see Applewhite, 1995). Folk healing can be classified in either malevolent (witchcraft) or benevolent practices (curanderismo and spiritualism). Supernatural forces and beings can be accessed by spiritualists (*espiritualistas*), and witches (*brujas/os*). Specific treatments include home remedies and herbs, bone and muscle manipulation, midwifery, faith healing, spiritualism, tarot card reading, witchcraft, praying, and the use of religious icons and paraphernalia. In some cases, healing is facilitated through specific prescriptive magicoreligious or expiatory ritual practices such as promise making; visiting shrines; and offering medals, candles, and prayers (Gonzales, 1976). Applewhite (1995) has found that people who resort to curanderismo have a strong faith in God's will—for example, *si Dios quiere* (if God wishes), *la fé en Dios* (the faith in God), *lo que Dios mande* (that which God commands), *la voluntad de Dios* (the will of God). Gonzales (1976) has found that *primero Dios* (God first) is an axiom that consistently accompanies discussion of illness or injury. These verbal expressions of faith suggest a belief in divine will and providence.

In the following case study, we exemplify a case of a culture-related syndrome and illustrate some culturally relevant notions of indigenous folk traditions.

MARIA: A CASE STUDY

Maria is a 28-year-old Mexican woman who emigrated to the United States when she was 16. She currently lives with her parents and has a part-time job. Maria described herself as a very religious person, one who grew up Catholic and is presently active in various church activities.

She was referred to psychotherapy by her primary care physician. During the intake session Maria indicates that she has had three medical appointments, and expresses frustration and anger that her symptoms continue to affect her level of functioning in several areas of her life. She attributes the onset of her presenting problems to witnessing a relative's sudden and violent death while visiting Mexico during the holidays (two weeks prior to the intake). She appears sad and frightened, and states that she has been experiencing the following symptoms: anxiety, fear, worry, and irritability. Apparently, this is affecting her ability to sleep and to concentrate at work, and she is also feeling fatigued during the day. She mentions that the medical doctor does not seem to understand her problem, and she is thinking of not following up on future appointments at the hospital.

Maria and her family believe that she is suffering from susto. She notes that her family is originally from the state of Oaxaca, and that other family members had experienced susto in the past as the result of traumatic events. When asked to elaborate on susto, she states that in her indigenous Zapotec language the term is *es pir it gon sa we't* ("the spirit wanders outside") or, in Spanish, *asustado* [see Glazer, Baer, Weller, & Liebowitz, 2004], which translates as "frightened."

She states that she truly believes that her soul, her *alma*, has left her. She mentions that she and her family have prayed at her home altar, or *altarcito*. They spoke to the local priest, and he blessed several images, including a small statue of Saint Michael the Archangel, to protect her soul from evil spirits. They also asked for holy water to sprinkle on the area where she sleeps at night. At the altar, her mother has been calling the spirit back with the words, "Spirit of Maria, return here. You can't live without her." Her family is currently looking for a well-known curandera/o in the community who has a good reputation for curing susto.

She reported having faith in the ceremony known as *barrida*, or spiritual sweeping. Her family has told her that the curandera/o is going to ask her to recount the details of the frightening experience in Mexico and she is going to lie down on the floor on the axis of a crucifix. Then, the curandera/o is going to "sweep" her body with the fresh herbs basil and purple sage, and an egg. She mentions that she has faith that the curandera/o is going to persuade the frightened soul to return to her body.

ASSESSMENT, DIAGNOSIS, AND INTERVENTION

Assessment

The *DSM-IV* has included a new diagnostic category, "Religious or Spiritual Problems," under "Other Conditions that May Be a Focus of Clinical Attention." For the first time, there is acknowledgment of distressing religious and spiritual experiences as nonpathological problems (Turner, Lukoff, Barnhouse, & Lu, 1995). This category (V62.89) is usually used "when the focus of clinical attention is a religious or spiritual problem." Some examples include "distressing experiences that involve loss or questioning of faith," and "questioning of spiritual values" (American Psychiatric Association, 2000, p. 741) In the case study of Maria, above, the use of this label would be a misdiagnosis, because the distress is not directly associated with her religious beliefs. On the contrary, her religious and spiritual beliefs provide her with a frame of reference to attempt to make sense of what she has experienced.

Any theoretical orientation and intervention that respects Maria's internal frame of reference or worldview (Koltko-Rivera, 2004) and validates her experience of susto in a culturally sensitive therapeutic relationship would be effective (Glazer et al., 2004). Constructivist perspectives are especially helpful when working with culturally diverse clients who maintain a variety of spiritual and religious beliefs. Constructivist counseling practice emphasizes the meaning that develops in the ongoing narratives developed by the clients (Neimeyer & Mahoney, 1995). The implication of this perspective is that counseling should create a social context for reconstruction (Sexton & Griffin, 1997). The constructivist counselor attempts to provide a "holding environment" by acknowledging the client's reality and by supporting the client's effort to reconstruct that reality. An atmosphere of total acceptance for the client's multicultural frame of reference is important (Sue & Sue, 1990). Maria's personal perspective on susto is highly personal and carries strong cultural connotations. The counselor needs to develop an understanding of how the construction of the indigenous beliefs on susto is connected to the way Maria is responding to the loss. It is also crucial that the counselor understand Maria's cultural and spiritual context so that her presenting problems are not misinterpreted or overpathologized. Rather, Maria needs to reconstruct the narrative as a way of making sense of the traumatic experience. The counselor needs to be comfortable exploring the meaning that Maria attaches to her beliefs. Religious beliefs influence both the way in which clients construct the meanings of life events and the coping strategies they use to confront challenges.

For many individuals, spiritual beliefs are expressed through an organized religious community (Van Oss Marin, et al., 1983), and this seems to be the case with Maria. Religion may be an asset because it provides an indigenous social network for support and it supplies a system to make meaning of life. In order to help Maria, the counselor must first be willing to explore the spiritual and religious framework within which she is functioning. The existing framework of meaning, strengthened by family emotional and spiritual support, seems to be pretty significant in her life, and this can be validated.

Ritual is another important component of many spiritual belief systems, and in Maria's case it provides an important strategy for addressing her emotional and psychological issues. By engaging in rituals at home and at her church, she is able to integrate the meaning of the loss of her soul, and the traumatic event that facilitated it, into her personal narrative. Rituals offer assurance and guidance in a structured way that provides support and encourages positive coping.

SPIRITUALLY AND RELIGIOUSLY-ORIENTED PSYCHOTHERAPY

We propose a conceptual model that integrates specific therapeutic competencies and practices for counseling. We use the Multicultural Competencies Model (Sue, Arrendondo, & McDavis, 1992) that conceptualizes a competency as comprising self-awareness, knowledge, and skills. This heuristic framework is consistent with transtheoretical models (Prochaska & Norcross, 1999) that posit that no single theory or set of interventions can serve all client needs and problems. We have applied the dimensions of multicultural competencies to the integration of spiritual and religious aspects in counseling and added some indigenous components derived from the mestiza/o and Mesoamerican worldviews. The holistic, ritualistic, and sacramental (experiential) domains are three salient aspects of the spiritual and religious experience of mestizas/os that, in our view, can inform a culturally and spiritually sensitive approach to psychotherapy.

A Conceptual Framework for Spiritually and Religiously-Oriented Psychotherapy

Self-Awareness

> Be aware and sensitive to your own beliefs and assumptions concerning health and disease, as well as value-alternative worldviews.
>
> Monitor how your own experiences, attitudes, values, and biases may influence the therapeutic process.
>
> Be comfortable with differences that exist between yourself and clients in terms of religious and spiritual experiences.
>
> Include issues of spirituality, religion, culture, and language during intake, assessment, diagnosis, and treatment.

Knowledge

> Recognize the limits of your knowledge of indigenous concepts and worldviews.
>
> Acquire specific knowledge of personal worldviews on disease processes in your own culture and in other cultures.
>
> Establish consultative relationships with folk healers, cultural consultants (interpreters), and religious and spiritual leaders.

Skills

Learn metaphors and culture-specific or indigenous descriptors, and use them in the proper context to connect with the client's frame of reference.

Incorporate into your clinical practice and theoretical orientation the use of indigenous therapeutic practices.

Role-play, consult, and get feedback on the practice of ethically responsible therapeutic practices that use alternative modalities of treatment.

Holism

Use multidimensional conceptualization of issues that consider holistic approaches during assessment and treatment, with close consideration to multiple levels of human reality (body, mind, soul, and spirit) across multiple dimensions of existence (terrestrial, natural, supernatural, etc.).

Attend to the interplay of both internal and external factors contributing to the client's reported issues and determine the sense of balance and harmony in human reality and existence.

Appreciate the overlap and interrelation between internal subjective constructions (cognitions, emotions, beliefs, perceptions, values, attitudes, orientations, epistemologies, consciousness levels, expectations, and personhood) and external constructions of reality (artifacts, roles, institutions, social structures, and lifestyles).

Ritual

Discuss the use of symbols and ritual in the client's experience in both the domestic as well as organized/denominational spheres.

Explore the meanings attached to symbol and ritual, and how these relate to other levels of human reality and areas of functioning in the client's life.

Encourage rituals that are practical and proportional when they address relationships—either human or spiritual—that are healing.

Experiential/Sacramental Practices

Be receptive and sensitive to the client's sacramental imagination and experience of the divine in her life.

Identify any transformational, spiritual experience, or sacramental moment, and how this has impacted the client.

Facilitate the description and expression of the client's participation in sensual, visual, and communal practices related to the transcendent and divine. This may include client use/demonstration of material religion.[1]

We will now attempt to apply this model to the case study of Maria. It is of paramount importance that the counselor develop self-awareness regarding personal epistemologies of health and disease. Every culture endorses different and distinct notions of pathology and normalcy. There is a danger in operating from a purely Eurocentric or Western worldview, and thus the counselor needs to be sensitive to Maria's Zapotec and indigenous concept of distress. During the assessment of Maria's presentation and description of susto, the counselor needs to be aware not to dismiss or categorize her subjective experience of "soul loss" simply as pathological. Religious and spiritual experiences may reflect very individual core dimensions of one's identity, and the counselor needs to be comfortable with differences in the expression of religiosity and spirituality.

Some counselors avoid topics related to spirituality because they do not feel competent to address these issues in counseling. A counselor may not know how to proceed in a case like Maria's because curanderismo conceptualizes emotional and psychological experiences using culture-specific terms (e.g., *es pir it gon sa we't*). We suggest that the counselor make an effort to acquire specific knowledge by establishing collaborative relationships with cultural informants. This may include folk healers who understand the culture and can assist counselors through consultation and education. Maria reports that she is about to see a folk healer, and it may be helpful to discuss the possibility of the counselor's properly getting her authorization to consult with the folk healer.

Maria is using specific metaphors and culturally relevant descriptors (e.g., the spirit that "wanders outside," and the *barrida* "sweeping") to describe her traumatic experience. The counselor can learn the cultural meaning of these metaphors and use them correctly to relate to Maria's subjective world-view. Whether the counselor operates from a constructivist, cognitive, or interpersonal theoretical orientation, integration of these indigenous descriptors into therapeutic practices may be extremely helpful in establishing rapport and validating the client's experience. The client's metaphorical narratives and indigenous lexical explanations of symptoms encode salient cultural meanings that the counselor can theoretically integrate into the conceptualization of the presenting problems. Guajardo (1999) stresses the importance of *naming the illness*, and how that in itself is therapeutic for the client. This is a validation intervention in that it conveys to the individual seeking treatment that someone understands her experience. Naming the illness in a culturally meaningful manner instills hope for a possible cure in the client because the symptom or illness can be identified and located.

A basic assumption of spirituality and religiosity is the multidimensional nature of the human person as a whole. This is clearly illustrated in the practice of curanderismo, which addresses multiple levels of human reality. Maria will experience therapeutic interventions that touch upon cognitive or mental perceptions of her problem, her spiritual and religious awareness and physiological and sensory experiences. In her worldview, her spirit wanders on a supernatural and celestial plane while she reports dysphoric states of anxiety, worry, and fear. The counselor can broaden simplistic and reductionistic anthropological definitions derived from empiricist, dualistic, and materialistic epistemologies to include other dimensions of human existence when assessing and treating emotional and psychological problems. Traditionally, psychology has addressed the intrapsychic (internal) factors that contribute to a client's distress. Furthermore, the approach has been deficit based. We advocate an approach that attends to both internal and external factors that contribute to the client's problems and moves beyond deficits and purely remedial interventions to include strengths, wellness, and prevention.

The mestiza/o worldview is holistic, or organic, in character (Goizueta, 1994, p. 5). In contrast to Euro-American analytical psychotherapeutic notions, the very experience of *mestizaje*, or "mixedness," implies, by definition, an affirmation of human existence as "both/and" rather than "either/or" (Goinzueta, 1995, p. 5). Instead of focusing merely on cognitive schemata or emotional contributing factors to Maria's presenting problem, the counselor can conduct a thorough assessment of Maria's internal subjective constructions and how these correspond or interact with external realities. Cultures are both internally and externally represented, and cultural expressions shape our realities (i.e., they contribute to our worldviews, perceptions, and orientations), although some cultural components may be pathogenic and/or salutogenic. Our model posits that, in counseling, the interrelations of these components should be part of the assessment and treatment of the client's issues.

Ritual both externalizes and internalizes one's religious and spiritual experience. Maria engages in institutional and personal ritualistic devotions that externalize her devotion and faith, through which she incorporates and integrates meaning and values in her life. The counselor can explore the meanings associated with such symbols and rituals and how these relieve some of Maria's anxiety and worry. The counselor may validate her participation in indigenous institutions (e.g., church activities) and further encourage the reasonable participation in rituals that strengthen her relationships with her family, her soul, and her God.

The practice of psychotherapy has traditionally emphasized the assessment and treatment of observable phenomena, but such an approach has left little room for the exploration of the experience of the supernatural. In indigenous religious traditions (e.g., the Mesoamerican worldview) and in Catholicism, the whole natural order is sacred because it is a visible sign of the invisible reality of the divine. Maria lives in a world of statues and holy water, of votive candles and prayers. In her life the supernatural is enmeshed with the natural, and the counselor needs to be receptive and sensitive to this sacramental imagination. Gently and sensitively facilitating the expression of her participation in the recalling of her soul, as well as her communal religious and spiritual practices, can have positive therapeutic effects.

CONCLUSION

An understanding of the worldview of curanderismo is essential for the appreciation of spirituality and religiousness among Latinas/os. Some scholars have advocated the integration of curanderismo's therapeutic practices and psychotherapeutic techniques (Kreisman, 1975; Slesinger & Richards, 1981). We propose a paradigm for this type of spiritually and religiously oriented psychotherapy derived from the main cultural dimensions of the mestiza/o worldview. Our hope is that healing professionals should not only have theoretical, diagnostic, and professional knowledge in the exercise of their therapeutic professions, but tools of consciousness and multicultural sensitivity at their disposal that enable them to touch and connect with the hearts, minds, and souls of the people they treat. A reductionistic medicalization of the healing process ultimately dehumanizes the client, but a holistic integration of the therapeutic approach creatively dignifies the human person. In curanderismo the whole person heals, and this includes the multidimensionality of the individual.

Mental health professionals must exercise sound clinical judgment in the ethically responsible integration of indigenous healing practices. In the case of referrals to indigenous folk healers, clients need to be thoroughly informed regarding treatment interventions, including herbal remedies and any other folk indigenous healing methods, in order to prevent misunderstanding about the possible interactions and dangers. Risks associated with the misuse of indigenous folk methods of healing include misdiagnosis of symptoms that lead to an ineffective treatment plan. It is necessary to practice culturally competent care, but it is also imperative that clinicians not sacrifice an accurate psychiatric diagnosis in favor of a culturally defined syndrome such as susto. Clinicians need to be familiar with the syndromes discussed in this chapter, as well as those covered herein.

NOTE

1. This conceptual framework for spiritually and religiously oriented psychotherapy was adapted from Sue, Arrendondo, & McDavis (1992).

REFERENCES

Abbot, N. C., White, A. R, & Ernst, E. (1996). Complimentary medicine. *Nature, 30*, 361, 381.

Al-Krenawi, A. (1999). An overview of rituals in Western therapies and intervention: Argument for their use in cross-cultural therapy. *International Journal for the Advancement of Counseling, 21*, 3–17.

Altman, I., & Rogoff, B. (1987). World views in psychology: Trait, interactional, organismic, and transactional perspectives. In D. Stokols & I. Altman (Eds.), *Handbook of environmental psychology* (Vol. 1, pp. 7–40). New York: Wiley.

American Psychiatric Association (2000). *Diagnostic and statistical manual of mental disorders* (4th ed.). Washington, DC: Author.

Applewhite, S. L. (1995). Curanderismo: Demystifying the health beliefs and practices of elderly Mexican Americans. *Health and Social Work, 20,* 247–253.

Arenas, S., Cross, H., & Willard, W. (1980). Curanderos and mental health professionals: A comparative study on perceptions of psychopathology. *Hispanic Journal of Behavioral Sciences, 2,* 407–442.

Astin, J. A. (1998). Why patients use alternative medicine: Results of a national study. *Journal of the American Medical Association, 20,* 1548–1553.

Belsasso, G. (1969). The history of psychiatry in Mexico. *Hospital and Community Psychiatry, 20,* 342–344.

Brady, E. (2001). *Healing logics: Culture and medicine in modern health belief systems.* Logan: Utah State University Press.

Brown, P. (1981). *The cult of the saints: Its rise and function in Latin Christianity.* Chicago: University of Chicago Press.

Burkhart, L., M. (1992). Pious performances: Christian pageantry and native identity in early colonial Mexico. In E. H. Boone & T. Cummins (Eds.), *Native traditions in the postconquest world* (pp. 361–379). Washington, DC: Dumbarton Oaks Research Library and Collection.

Campion, E. W. (1993). Why unconventional medicine? *New England Journal of Medicine, 328,* , 282–283.

Carrasco, D. (1990). *Religions of Mesoamerica: Cosmovision and ceremonial centers.* San Francisco: Harper and Row.

Carrasco, D. (1999). Uttered from the heart: Guilty rhetoric among the Aztecs. *History of Religions, 39,* 1–31.

Conferencia Episcopal Latinoamerica. (1979). *Conferencia Episcopal Latinoamerica: Tercera Conferencia General* [Latin American Episcopal Conference: Third General Conference]. Puebla, Mexico: Author.

Cunningham, L .S. (1987). *The Catholic faith: An introduction.* New York: Paulist Press.

Davies, N. (1990). *The ancient kingdoms of Mexico.* London: Penguin Books.

Davis, K. G. (2004). Annoying the sick? Cultural considerations for the celebration of a sacrament. *Worship, 78,* 35–50.

Davis, K. G. (2005). Hispanic popular Catholicism. *Pastoral Life, 54,* 3.

Del Pozo, E. C. (1966). Aztec pharmacology. *Annual Review of Pharmacology, 6*, 9–18.

Emmons, R. A. (1999). Religion in the psychology of personality: An introduction. *Journal of Personality, 67*, 873–888.

Figueroa-Deck, A. (2002). The Latino Catholic ethos: Ancient history or future promise? *Journal of Hispanic Latino Theology, 9*, 5–21.

Frank, J. D., & Frank, J. B. (1991). *Persuasion and healing.* Baltimore: Johns Hopkins University Press.

Glannon, W. (2004). Transcendence and healing. *Medical Humanities, 30*, 70–73.

Glazer, M., Baer, R. D., Weller, S. C., & Liebowitz, S. W. (2004). Susto and soul loss in Mexicans and Mexican Americans. *Cross-Cultural Research, 38*, 270–288.

Goizueta, R. S. (1994). La raza cósmica? La visión of José Vasconcelos [The cosmic race? The vision of José Vasconcelos]. *Journal of Hispanic/Latino Theology, 1*, 5–27.

Gonzales, E. (1976). The role of Chicano folk beliefs and practices in mental health. In C. A. Hernández, M. J. Haug, & N. N. Wagner (Eds.), *Chicanos: Social and psychological perspectives* (2nd ed., pp. 263–281). St. Louis, MO: Mosby.

Greeley, A. M. (1989). Protestant and Catholic: Is the analogical imagination extinct? *American Sociological Review, 54*, 485–502.

Greeley, A. M. (2000). *The Catholic imagination.* Berkeley: University of California Press.

Gruzinski, S. (2002). *The mestizo mind: The intellectual dynamics of colonization and globalization.* New York: Routledge.

Guajardo, K. A. (1999). *Spirituality and curanderismo in Mexican-American culture: A psychospiritual model of conjoint treatment.* Berkeley, CA: Unpublished doctoral dissertation, California School of Professional Psychology.

Guerra, F. (1971). *The Pre-Columbian mind.* New York: Seminar Press.

Guerra, F. (1980). Medical Folklore in Spanish America. In W. D. Hand (Ed.), *American folk medicine.* Berkeley: University of California Press.

Hamburger, S. (1978). Profile of curandero/as: A study of Mexican folk practitioners. *International Journal of Social Psychiatry, 24*, 19–25.

Heinrich, M., Ankli, A., Frei, B., Weimann, C., & Sticher, O. (1998). Medicinal plants in Mexico: Healers' consensus and cultural importance. *Social Science and Medicine, 47*(11), 1859–1871.

Hirschhorn, H. H. (1968). Botanical remedies of South America and the Caribbean. An archival analysis, part 1. *Journal of Ethnopharmacology, 3*, 83–91.

Ingham, J. M. (1970). On Mexican folk medicine. *American Anthropologist, 72*, 76–87.

Josephson, A. J., & Peteet, J. R. (2004) *Handbook of spirituality and world view in clinical practice.* Washington, DC: American Psychiatric Press.

Kidwell, S. C. (1982). Aztec and European Medicine in the New World, 1521–1600. In L. R. Ross, D. Moerman, L. Tancredi, & S. Hadley (Eds.), *Anthropology of medicine* (pp. 19–30). Westport, CT: J. F. Bergin.

Kieckhefer, R., & Bond, G. D. (1988). *Sainthood: Its manifestations in world religions.* Berkeley: University of California Press.

Kiev, A. (1968). *Curanderismo: Mexican American folk psychiatry.* New York: Free Press.

Klass, D., & Goss, R. (1999). Spiritual bonds to the dead in cross-cultural and historical perspective: Comparative religion and modern grief. *Death Studies, 23*, 547–567.

Koltko-Rivera, M. (2004). The psychology of worldviews. *Review of General Psychology, 8*, 3–58.

Kreisman, J. J. (1975). The curandero's apprentice: A therapeutic integration of folk and medical healing. *American Journal of Psychiatry, 132*, 81–83.

Lopez, R. A. (2005). Use of alternative folk medicine by Mexican American women. *Journal of Immigrant Health, 7*, 23–31.

Lopez Austin, A. (1988). *The human body and ideology: Concepts of the ancient Nahuas* (B. Ortiz de Montellano & T. Ortiz de Montellano, Trans.). Salt Lake City: University of Utah Press.

McKeever Furst, J. L. (1995). *The natural history of the soul in ancient Mexico.* New Haven, CT: Yale University Press.

Miller, M. E., & West, A. N. (1993). Influences of world view on personality, epistemology, and choice of profession. In J. Demick & P. M. Miller (Eds.), *Development in the workplace* (pp. 3–19). Hillsdale, NJ: Erlbaum.

Mull, J. D., & Mull, D. S. (1983). A visit with a curandero: Cross-cultural medicine. *Western Journal of Medicine, 139,* 730–736.

Nall, F. C., & Speilberg, J. (1967). Social and cultural factors in the responses of Mexican-Americans to medical treatment. *Journal of Health and Social Behavior, 8,* 299–308.

Naugle, D. K. (2002). *Wordview: The history of a concept.* Grand Rapids, MI: Eerdmans.

Neimeyer, R. A., & Mahoney, M. J. (Eds.). (1995). *Constructivism in psychotherapy.* Washington, DC: American Psychological Association.

Nygren, A. (1998). Struggle over meanings: Reconstruction of indigenous mythology, cultural identity, and social representation. *Ethnohistory, 45,* 31–63.

Oktavec, E. (1995). *Answered prayers: Miracles and milagros along the border.* Tucson: University of Arizona Press.

Orsi, R. A. (2005). The cult of the saints and the reimagination of the space and time of sickness in twentieth-century American Catholicism. In L. L. Barnes & S. S. Sered (Eds.), *Religion and healing in America* (pp. 28–47). Oxford: Oxford University Press.

Ortiz de Montellano, B. R. (1975). Empirical Aztec medicine. *Science, 188,* 215–220.

Ortiz de Montellano, B. R. (1987). *Aztec medicine, health, and nutrition.* New Brunswick, NJ: Rutgers University Press.

Overton, W. F. (1984). World views and their influence on psychological theory and research: Kuhn–Lakatos–Laudan. *Advances in Child Development and Behavior, 18,* 191–226.

Pal, S. K. (2002). Complementary and alternative medicine: An overview. *Current Science, 82,* 518–521.

Paniagua, F. A. (1998). *Assessing and treating culturally diverse clients: A practical guide.* Thousand Oaks, CA: Sage.

Pardo, O. F. (2004). *The origins of Mexican Catholicism: Nahua rituals and Christian sacraments in sixteenth-century Mexico.* Ann Arbor: University of Michigan Press.

Pargament, K. I. (1997). *The psychology of religion and coping: Theory, research, and practice.* New York: Guilford Press.

Peña, J. C. (1999). Pre-Columbian medicine and the kidney. *American Journal of Nephrology, 19,* 148–154.

Prieto, L. R., McNeill, B. W., Walls, R. G., & Gómez, S. P. (2001). Chicanas/os and mental health services: An overview of utilization, counselor preference, and assessment issues. *Counseling Psychologist, 29*, 18–54.

Prochaska, J. O., & Norcross, J. C. (1999). *Systems of psychotherapy: A transtheoretical approach.* Pacific Grove, CA: Brooks/Cole.

Ramirez. M. (1998). *Multicultural/Multiracial psychology: Mestizo perspectives in personality and mental health.* Northvale, NJ: Aronson.

Real Academia Española (2001). *Diccionario de la Real Academia Española.* Mexico City, Mexico: Espasa Calpe Mexicana.

Richards, P. S., & Bergin, A. E. (1997). A spiritual strategy for counseling and psychotherapy. Washington, DC: American Psychological Association.

Rosenberg, R. S. (2002). The religious dimensions of life: Can we discover the extraordinary in the quotidian? The spiritual in conscious experience. *America, 187*, 19.

Rodriguez, J. (2004). Mestiza spirituality: Community, ritual and justice. *Theological Studies, 65*, 317–339.

Rodrigues, L. A. (1959). *La ciencia medica de los Aztecas* [The medical science of the Aztecs]. Mexico City, Mexico: Editorial Hispano Mexicana.

Ruesch, J. (1963). The healing traditions: Some assumptions made by physicians. In I. Galdston (Ed.), *Man's image in medicine and anthropology* (pp. 502–520). New York: International Universities Press.

Ruiz, P., & Langrod, J. (1976). Psychiatry and folk healing: A dichotomy? *American Journal of Psychiatry, 133*, 95–97.

Ryan, J. D. (2004). Missionary saints of the High Middle Ages: Martyrdom, popular veneration, and canonization. *Catholic Historical Review, 40*, 1–28.

Scheffler, L. (1986). *Magia y brujeriá en México* [Magic and Witchcraft in Mexico]. Mexico City, Mexico: Panorama Editorial.

Schendel, G. (1968). *Medicine in Mexico: From Aztec herb to betatrons.* Austin: University of Texas Press.

Sexton, T. L., & Griffin, B. G. (1997). *Constructivist thinking in counseling research, practice and training.* New York: Teachers College Press.

Slesinger, D. P., & Richards, M. (1981). Folk and clinical medical utilization patterns among Mejicano migrant farmworkers. *Hispanic Journal of Behavioral Sciences, 3*, 59–73.

Snow, L. (1974). Folk medical beliefs and their implications for care of patients. *Annals of Internal Medicine, 81*, 82–96.

Steiner, R. P. (1986). *Folk medicine: The art and the science.* Washington, DC: American Chemical Society.

Stevens-Arroyo, A. M. (1998). The evolution of Marian devotionalism within Christianity and the Ibero-Mediterranean polity. *Journal for the Scientific Study of Religion, 37*, 50–73.

Sue, D. W. (1990). The change of multiculturalism: The road less traveled. *American Counselor, 1*, 6–10, 12–14.

Sue, D. W., Arrendondo, P., & McDavis, R. J. (1992). Multicultural counseling competencies: A call to the profession. *Journal of Counseling and Development, 70*, 477–486.

Sue, D. W., & Sue, D. (1990). *Counseling the culturally different: Theory and practice* (2nd ed.). New York: Wiley.

Tan, M. L. (1988). Primary health care and indigenous medicine. *Cultural Survival Quarterly, 12*, 1, 8–10.

Torres, E. (1983). *The folk healer: The Mexican-American tradition of curanderismo.* Kingsville, TX: Nieves Press.

Torrey, E. F. (1972). *The mind game: Witchdoctors and psychiatrists.* New York: Bantam Books.

Tracy, D. (1982). *The analogical imagination.* New York: Seabury.

Trotter, R. T., & Chavira, J. A. (1997). *Curanderismo: Mexican American folk healing* (2nd ed). Athens: University of Georgia Press.

Turner, R. P., Lukoff, D., Barnhouse, R. T., & Lu, F. G. (1995). Religious or spiritual problem: A culturally sensitive diagnostic category in the *DSM-IV. Journal of Nervous and Mental Disorders, 185*, 435–444.

Van Oss Marin, B., Marin, G., Padilla, A. M., & De La Rocha, C. (1983). Utilization of traditional and nontraditional sources of health care among Hispanics. *Hispanic Journal of Behavioral Sciences, 5*(1), 65–80.

Viesca-Treviño, C. (2001). Curanderismo in Mexico and Guatemala: Its historical evolution from the sixteenth to the nineteenth century. In B. R. Huber & A. R. Sandstrom (Eds.), *Mesoamerican healers* (pp. 47–65). Austin: University of Texas Press.

Weclew, R. V. (1975). The nature, prevalence, and level of awareness of "curanderismo" and some of its implications for community mental health. *Community Mental Health Journal, 11*, 145–54.

Zinnbauer, B. J., Pargament, K. I., Cole, B., Rye, M. S., Butter, E. M., Belavich, T. G., et al. (1997). Religion and spirituality: Unfuzzing the fuzzy. *Journal for the Scientific Study of Religion, 36,* 549–564.

Zinnbauer, B. J., Pargament, K. I., & Scott, A. B. (1999). The emerging meanings of religiousness and spirituality: Problems and prospects. *Journal of Personality, 67,* 889–919.

Part Four

EPILOGUE

Epilogue
Summary and Future Research and Practice Agendas

JOSEPH M. CERVANTES AND BRIAN W. MCNEILL

Latina/o populations have increased such that this diverse, ethnic/cultural grouping is now the largest minority group in the United States, and projections are for a continued increase in both immigrant and native-born populations (U.S. Census Bureau, 2006). Consequently, it is vitally important for both practitioners and researchers to become educated regarding not only the mental health needs of the Latina/o population, but also, as this volume argues, their religious and spiritual belief systems. As such, the writings in this volume have provided a necessary foundation for a dialogue about how an indigenous spirituality for mestiza/o and Latina/o populations is a relevant dimension to psychological well-being. Trujillo (2000) and others (Carrillo & Tello, 1998; Duran, 2006; Falicov, 1999; Matovina & Riebe-Estrella, 2002) have underscored the importance of understanding and accepting the role of religion and spirituality as an essential step toward recognizing that a Christian-based spirituality is only one of other perspectives that impact the psychological functioning of individuals.

Systems of healing, both traditional and alternative, have evolved in communities across the world for thousands of years (Frank & Frank, 1991). Yet, as Cohen (2001) asserts, Western psychotherapists continue to struggle with an ethnocentric point of view and fail to benefit from alternative systems that are present in all world cultures. It is only recently that researchers and practitioners have started to acknowledge the importance of a sense of religiosity or spirituality in the lives of people (e.g., Kleinman, 1980; Krippner & Welch,

1992, Gielen, Fish, & Draguns, 2004). For example, two recent writings (Baruss, 2003; Cardena, Lynn, & Kripner, 2000) lend additional theoretical support and scientific validity to the study of altered consciousness and the exploration of extraordinary and unexplained human experiences and encounters. These types of experiences have often become the foundation for healing traditions and paradigms that have historically challenged mainstream views of reality and, by association, the dominant healing system of the period (Wampold, 2001). Consequently, conventional medicine and folk medicine traditions have had difficulty existing side by side with only narrow margins of validity credited to folk traditions that are often discredited and defined as irrelevant, unscientific, and dangerous (Cohen, 2001).

As noted by Karen V. Holiday in this volume (chapter 9), so-called folk medicine has provided alternative conceptualizations of health, illness, and the process of healing. A relevant definition has been noted by Finkler (1994) in her differentiation between conventional medicine and folk medicine traditions. She writes, "Spiritualism is embedded in a sacred world while biomedicine is sanctioned by secular science" (p. 179). Each of these concepts emphasize a distinct shaping of a healing paradigm that is critical toward an understanding of how the healing process is understood between the professional and the patient. In essence, folk/spiritual healing places emphasis exclusively on the patient such that the cause of the disease is identified and guided by the healer so that the patient can feel mentally and emotionally prepared to allow her internal system to proceed accordingly. In contrast, with biomedicine, the focus of the patient's healing is on the practitioner, which typically includes his personality, knowledge base, and reputation. Consequently, the appearance of nonspecific factors (e.g., expectations) may play a more active role in the healing process. There have been numerous debates about the advantages and disadvantages of each of these healing systems. Consequently, the important distinction is that for folk traditions, the advantage of the healing process is maximized with the patient.

All too often, however, definitions of spirituality are limited to mainstream Christianity. While the sense of spiritualism addressed in its many forms in this volume is a product of the traditions passed down through generations of *la gente* (our people; see Ramirez, 1983, 1998), it is extremely important that the spirituality that exits with Latina/o peoples not be confused with the pejorative connotations often associated with the term *folk beliefs* (Matovina & Riebe-Estrella, 2002). Consequently, the spiritual systems of culturally diverse peoples should not be marginalized because they are not as well known and recognized as those of traditional Christian-based religions. Instead, mestiza/o- and indigenous-based spiritual systems need to be viewed as equal to traditional Christianity or religiosity, with the expected outcome that the healing /psychotherapy paradigm develops as a necessary therapeutic consequence.

Krippner's (1995) article on the comparison of four healing models is an important backdrop to the emerging fact that a non-Christian—based spirituality involves a series of healing traditions that are each unique in their own right. These healing traditions—whether they are Native American, *curanderismo*, or beliefs relevant to other parts of the world—are important facets to the understanding of individuals. It is a salient and immediate consequence that these healing traditions need to be considered in any useful clinical dialogue with a diverse client population. An interesting article by Cole (2003) highlights healing principles for use in psychotherapy. The emergence of these types of articles in more mainstream journals are being published with growing frequency, which again emphasizes the increased relevance of integrating these unique spiritual traditions in counseling practice.

FUTURE RESEARCH DIRECTIONS

A significant consideration in any integration of alternative perspectives in medicine and counseling is the observation that while empirically validated treatments show promise for generalizing to some minority groups, they have not expanded enough into nonmainstream client populations (Miranda et al., 2005). Consequently, as Miranda et al. conclude, more research is needed, especially in designing and evaluating evidence-based interventions tailored to be sensitive to the culture of the individual in order to guide the practitioner to provide clear and consensual assessment and treatment. Fortunately, there is an emerging literature base that has been forming in the last few years that is starting to provide important sources of knowledge for a dialogue about these issues (see, e.g., Gielen, Fish, & Draguns, 2004; Koss-Chionino & Hefner, 2006; Moodley & West, 2005).

In addition, recent literature is beginning to support the critical importance of spirituality in mental health (Koss-Chioino & Hefner, 2006; Paloutzian & Park, 2005). However, what is not known is specifically how the healing traditions in a given population assist with the emotional and psychological wellness of individuals. First, how does spirituality impact the worldview of Latina/o communities? Second, how might mental health professionals integrate their learning within the increased era of empirically validated treatments when adopting a perspective of spirituality? Third, how does spirituality impact resilience in coping with Latina/o populations? Some of these issues have been addressed within African American and some Asian American populations (Parham, White, & Ajamu, 2000). However, the literature is very sparse and there remains little information to guide practitioners with Latina/o families and communities.

There is significant room for the exploration of spirituality in psychological wellness for Latina/o populations. As previously articulated, spirituality has had minimal dialogue in the professional literature, even though historically it has been at the hub of the interrelationships and psychological backdrop of Latina/o families. Related areas of research may include the role of prayer, the ethics of Spanish-language consultation in integrating spirituality with psychological wellness, and the role of ritual where this process is deemed to be appropriate in working with Latina/o populations. Further, there exists a diversity of traditional and indigenous belief systems in Central America, Mexico, and the United States. As such, how does a researcher begin to catalog these belief systems consistent with psychological practice? Indeed, there are many research agendas and implications for professional practice issues that are being introduced with the advent of this volume.

IMPLICATIONS FOR FUTURE PRACTICE

The writings that have been included in this volume emphasize some relevant implications for clinical and counseling practice. The first is that the role of anomalous and transpersonal experience is an important event with Latina/o clients. Inclusion of spirituality, use of prayer, devotion to other deities, and belief in a higher healing source is a relevant and important backdrop to the understanding of this client population (Matovina & Riebe-Estrella, 2002). One of the most distinguishing features of practice with Latina/o families is that the worldview is symbolic as evidenced through the role of transpersonal experience, intercessory prayer, and intervention through other saints and deities. Consequently, a belief in the constant presence of the sacred in daily life is a signifying characteristic that underscores psychospiritual concerns and forms of coping with this population (Cervantes, 2004; Matovina & Riebe-Estrella, 2002).

The chapters in this volume highlight the fact that Latina/o clients may emphasize a strong folk tradition and significant belief system in their worldview and that this perspective is not to be taken lightly. These folk traditions are background to salient spiritual and healing systems that impact an individual's cultural, familial, and interpersonal framework. In addition to the folk traditions relevant with Latina/o groups, the writings in this edited volume emphasize the fact that the inclusion of spirituality as a relevant parameter has come to bridge an important gap in professional work for mental health professionals. In brief, the role of spirituality and the importance of this experience for Latina/o clients is a commonly validated observation that needs to be entertained and supported in mental health consultation with this community (Finkler, 1994; Koss-Chioino & Hefner, 2006). It is promising to see that the language of evidence-based psychology practice (American Psychological Association, 2005) emphasizes the integration of the best available research with clinical expertise in the context of patient characteristics, culture, and preferences including ethnicity, race, religion, beliefs, and worldviews.

As noted previously in this epilogue, there are a few practice guidelines that assist counselors with the incorporation of spirituality while recognizing the ethical imperative of expected practice. However, there have been a handful of published articles and books that now address these issues even though they are not assembled into a collective group of guidelines (e.g., Cervantes & Parham, 2005; Duran, 2006; Matovina & Riebe-Estrella, 2004; Yeh, Hunter, Madan-Bahell, Chang, & Arora, 2004). The essence of this writing provides awareness, practice skills, and interventions that are specific to Native American and other indigenous populations. These authors also underscore the fact that the dimension of spirituality is the foundation to psychological behavior, which indicates that practitioners have an ethical and professional responsibility to acknowledge and be educated about these concerns. Cervantes and Parham (2005) further highlight the fact that it is an ethical violation for failing to provide culturally appropriate professional care in working with people of color.

Similar considerations should guide any process of psychological assessment. Both López and Weisman (2004) and Velásquez, Garrido, Castellanos, and Burton (2004), provide guidelines for culturally competent test development and use. While it is generally accepted that variables such as acculturation, enculturation, and/or ethnic identity should be routinely assessed along with the variety of psychological variables in the process of a psychological evaluation, it is also necessary that we include an assessment of spirituality as a component of worldview in any psychological evaluation of Latina/o individuals. Such variables as degree and level of involvement in a spiritual tradition or religion should be evaluated (Zea, Mason, & Murguía, 2000). This element should provide additional information that compliments the psychological concerns noted in the clients presenting problems.

Nonetheless, much progress needs to be made in regard to the treatment effects of both mainstream therapies and culturally sensitive adaptations that reflect Latina/o ways of coping, resilience, and hardiness. Krippner (1995) provides a useful discussion in his comparison of four healing models wherein he highlights specific dimensions of mainstream or allopathic medicine with Native American, curanderismo, and Chinese healing traditions. It is important to note that there are a variety of traditions that emphasize wellness and opportunities for personal, emotional, and spiritual growth. The list of these approaches is endless. For example, a collection of healing practices documented by Carlson and Shield (1989) highlight unique approaches, belief systems, and healing energy paradigms where each practitioner claims a particular usefulness and ethics of treatment. Each of these healing models emphasizes distinct differences in the roles that practitioners play regarding diagnosis, cause of disease, treatment, prognosis, and goals. Perhaps what is being argued and detailed in this volume is that there are two coexisting models of psychological care. The model understood in this volume emphasizes a healing tradition (Cohen, 2001; Duran, 2006; Koss-Chionino & Hefner, 2006), which then implies a distinct paradigm in the alleviation of emotional, psychological, and psychospiritual maladies with individuals.

Cervantes and Parham (2005) provide some relevant lessons for the counseling practitioner. These guidelines include the recognition of multidimensional manifestations of spiritualism, religiousness, and respect for the diversity of belief systems, along with recognition of one's role as a healer, and not simply a therapist in the eyes of mestiza/o peoples. Additionally, we need to realize the sense of interconnectedness and extended family systems where emotional reliance, interdependency, and community responsibility define the mestiza/o worldview in order to manage the spiritual aspects of a clients life. Perhaps the most important aspect, however, is that the practitioner recognize her own role in spirituality and that there be some resolution with how practitioners and counselors acknowledge and explore their own spiritual essence and how their energy and life force manifests in their lives.

A REDEFINITION OF ETHICS IN CLINICAL AND COUNSELING PRACTICE

The ethical practice of counseling and psychotherapy has had a long history of recognition in directing the practicing clinician and professional counselor. However, there is little to no information relative to ethical practice within mestiza/o and indigenous populations regarding psychological care and wellness. While Trimble and Fisher (2005) have recently incorporated a cultural perspective in the conduct of research with multicultural populations, a similar level of dialogue does not yet exist for clinical work with diverse populations in general, or for work within the spiritual realm with Latina/o peoples. When working in the barrio/neighborhood or community, it may not be possible to always avoid what we mandate against in the form of dual role relationships. When addressing spiritual needs, it may not be possible to always meet within the confines of the confidential office or work only in the 50-minute hour (Parham, 1997). The most current guidelines for professional psychology (American Psychological Association, 2003), provide minimal guidance regarding the appropriate professional care of cultural populations. While these guidelines address important aspects relevant to practice with U.S. ethnic and racial minority groups inclusive of individuals, children, and families from biracial, multiethnic, and multiracial backgrounds, they do not provide the specific examples relevant to the issues addressed in this volume. Relevant practice concerns that should be considered include several distinct arenas. Initially, how does a practitioner integrate Western training with indigenous spirituality as it applies to psychological care? Secondly, what guidelines can be provided about using nontraditional methods of healing that are not considered empirically validated treatments but are typically not even part of the mainstream? Some of these practices may include the use of sage for purification, initiating a cleansing (i.e., a *limpia*) for the clearing of negative emotional and mental energy, and utilizing more spiritual metaphors that are consistent with the worldview of a client. Duran (2005) provides a reiteration of healing and wellness categories originally described by Clements (1932). These categories are not consistent with traditional diagnostic frameworks such as the American Psychiatric Association's *Diagnostic and Statistical Manual of Mental Disorders* and may include: object intrusion, loss of soul, spirit intrusion, breech of taboo, and sorcery. These classifications bridge a psychospiritual framework that is distinct from traditional mainstream practice, and impact how these beliefs affect wellness and behavior.

What is being suggested by this volume is that as practitioners, researchers, and program administrators, we are being challenged to recognize the diversity of indigenous spiritual frameworks as a significant dimension in the lives of many Latina/o families. In addition, this recognition will require that in the provision of psychological services there be conceptual room to consider culturally appropriate interventions that are consistent with the psychological wellness of Latina/o populations. In brief, the writings in this book are a call to lay a foundation for acknowledging the need to develop new ideas and professional practices relevant to appropriate ethical treatment with this population.

IMPLICATIONS FOR TRAINING

The field of applied psychology, while making some progress, has not recruited enough Latina/o and culturally diverse practitioners who are more likely to share the experiences and worldviews of diverse mestiza/o populations (Bernal, 2004). Thus, it becomes incumbent on mental health training programs to implement policies to recruit and train practitioners who are open to issues of diversity and/or have similar experiences and who are able to understand or educate others in their workplaces (McNeill, Prieto, Ortiz, and Yamokoski, 2004).

The training of professionals to understand distinct worldviews and accompanying spiritualities is an important aspect to working with Latina/o communities. In addition, it is important to highlight an emerging subdiscipline called *clinical spirituality*, a conceptual base that provides useful counseling guidance and intervention in working with distinct populations relevant to healing traditions. It is the intent of this volume to influence mental health professionals to view the inclusion of a spiritual framework as not only another dimension to understanding a client, but a necessary and ethical one when evaluating and treating Latina/o families. It is further the intent of this volume to provide an overarching perspective to the conceptual and clinical foundation that underscores the belief system, socialization experiences, and inherent thought process evident with this population. It is our deep hope that the knowledge, detailed skills, and prescribed interventions will be useful to practitioners as we meaningfully explore the integration of culture, practice, and healing traditions with Latina/o communities.

REFERENCES

Achterberg, J., Dossey, B., & Kolkmeier, K. (1994). *Rituals of healing: Using imagery for health and wellness.* New York: Bantam Books.

American Psychological Association. (2003). Guidelines on multicultural education, training, research, practice, and organizational change for psychologists. *American Psychologist, 58,* 377– 402.

American Psychological Association. (2005). *Report of the 2005 Presidential Task Force on evidence-based practice.* Washington, DC: Author.

Baruss, I. (2003). *Alterations of consciousness: An empirical analysis for the social scientist.* Washington, D.C.: American Psychological Association.

Bernal, M. (2004). Epilogue: Challenges and opportunities for Chicana/o psychologists: Past, present, and future. In R. Velasquez, L. Arrellano, & B. W. McNeill (Eds.). *Handbook of Chicana/o psychology and mental health* (pp. 469–482). Mahwah, NJ: Erlbaum.

Cardena, E., Lynn, S. J., & Kripper, S. N. (Eds.). (2000). *Varieties of anomalous experience: Examining the scientific evidence.* Washington, DC: American Psychological Association.

Carlson, R., & Shield, B. (Eds.). (1989). *Healers on healing.* Los Angeles: Tarcher.

Carrillo, R., & Tello, J. (Eds.). (1998). *Family violence and men of color: Healing the wounded male spirit.* New York: Springer.

Cervantes, J. M. (2004). *Mestizo spirituality: A Mesoamerican counseling epistemology and model for psychological intervention.* Unpublished manuscript.

Cervantes, J. M. & Parham, T. A. (2005). Toward a meaningful spirituality for people of color: Lessons for the counseling practitioner. *Cultural Diversity and Ethnic Minority Psychology, 2,* 69–81.

Clements, F. E. (1932). *Primitive concepts of disease* (University of California Publications in Archeology and Ethnography, No. 32). Berkeley: University of California Press.

Cohen, D. (2001). Cultural variation: Consideration and implications. *Psychological Bulletin, 127,* 451–471.

Cole, V. L. (2003). Healing principles: A model for the use of ritual in psychotherapy. *Counseling and Values, 47,* 184–194.

Duran, E. (2006). *Healing the soul wound: Counseling with American Indians and other native peoples.* New York: Teachers College Press.

Falicov, C. J. (1999). *Religion and spiritual folk traditions in immigrant families: Therapeutic resources in family therapy.* New York: Guilford Press.

Finkler, K. (1994). *Spiritualist healers in Mexico.* Salem, WI: Sheffield.

Frank, J. D., & Frank, J. B. (1991). *Persuasion and healing: A comparative study of psychotherapy* (3rd ed.). Baltimore: Johns Hopkins University Press.

Gielen, U. P., Fish, J. M., & Draguns, J. G. (Eds.). (2002). *Handbook of culture, therapy, and healing.* Mahwah, NJ: Lawrence Erlbaum Associates.

Goldsmith, J. S. (1992). *The art of spiritual healing.* San Francisco: HarperCollins.

Hastings, A. (1991). *With the tongues of men and angels: A study of channeling.* Orlando, FL: Holt, Rinehart and Winston.

Kleinman, A. (1980). *Patients and Healers in the Context of Culture: An Exploration of the Borders between Anthropology, Medicine, and Psychiatry.* Berkeley: University of California Press.

Koss-Chioino, J. D., & Hefner, P. (2006). *Spiritual transformation and healing: Anthropological, theological, neuroscientific, and clinical perspectives.* New York: Altamira Press.

Krippner, S. (1995). A cross-cultural comparison of four healing models. *Alternative Therapies, 1,* 21–29.

Krippner, S. & Welch, R. (1992). *Spiritual Dimensions of Healing*. New York: Irvington.

López, S., & Weisman, A. (2004). Integrating a cultural perspective in psychological test development. In R. Velasquez, L. Arrellano, & B. W. McNeill (Eds.), *Handbook of Chicana/o psychology and mental* health (pp. 129–152). Mahwah, NJ: Erlbaum.

Matovina, T. & Riebe-Estrella, G. (Eds.). (2002). *Horizons of the sacred: Mexican Traditions in U.S. Catholicism*. Ithaca, NY: Cornell University Press.

McNeill, B. W., Prieto, L. P., & Ortiz, F., & Yamokoski, C. A. (2004). Cultural competency: Teaching, training, and the delivery of services for chicana/os. In R. Velasquez, L. Arrellano, & B. W. McNeill (Eds.), *Handbook of Chicana/o psychology and mental health* (pp. 427–454). Mahwah, NJ: Lawrence Erlbaum Associates.

Miranda, J., Bernal, G., Lau, A., Kohn, L., Hwang, W. C., & Lafromboise, T. (2005). State of the science on psychosocial interventions for ethnic minorities. *Annual Review of Clinical Psychology, 1*, 113–142.

Moodley, R., & West, W. (Eds.) (2005). *Integrating traditional healing practices into counseling and psychotherapy*. Thousand Oaks, CA: Sage.

Paloutzian, R. F., & Park, C. L. (Eds.). (2005). *Handbook of the psychology of religion and spirituality*. New York: Guilford Press.

Parham, T. A. (1997). An African-centered view of dual relationships. In B. Herlihy & G. Corey (Eds.), *Boundary issues in counseling: Multiple roles and responsibilities* (pp. 109–111). Alexandria, VA: American Counseling Association.

Parham, T. A., White, J. L., & Ajamu, A. (2000). *The psychology of blacks: An African centered perspective*. Upper Saddle River, NJ: Prentice Hall.

Ramirez, M., III. (1983). *Psychology of the Americas: Mestizo perspectives on personality and mental health*. New York: Pergamon Press.

Ramirez, M., III. (1998). *Multicultural/multiracial psychology: Mestizo perspectives on personality and mental health*. Northvale, NJ: Aronson,.

Torrey, E. F. (1972). What Western psychotherapists can learn from witchdoctors. *American Journal of Orthopsychiatry, 42*, 69–76.

Trimble, J. E., and Fisher, C. B. (2005). *The handbook of ethical research with ethnocultural populations and communities.* Thousand Oaks, CA: Sage.

Trujillo, A. (2000). Psychotherapy with Native Americans: A view into the role of religion and spirituality. In A. E. Bergin & P. S. Richards (Eds.), *Psychotherapy and religious diversity: A guide for mental health professionals* (pp. 445–466). Washington, DC: American Psychological Association.

U.S. Census Bureau. (2006). *Nation's population one-third minority.* Retrived October 12, 2006, from http:www.census.gov/Press-Release/www/releases/archives/population/006808.html.

Velásquez, R. J., Garrido, M., Castellanos, J., & Burton, P. (2004). Culturally competent assessment of Chicana/os with the Minnesota Multiphasic Personality Inventory-2. In R. J. Velasquez, L. M. Arrellano, & B. W. McNeill (Eds.), *Handbook of Chicana/o psychology and mental health* (pp. 153–174). Mahwah, NJ: Erlbaum.

Wampold, B. E. (2001). Contextualizing psychotherapy as a healing practice: Culture history and methods. *Applied and Preventative Psychology, 10,* 69–86.

Yeh, C. J, Hunter, C. D., Madan-Bahel, A., Chiang, L., & Arora, A. (2004). Indigenous and interdependent perspectives of healing: Implications for counseling and research. *Journal of Counseling and Development, 82,* 410–419.

Zea, M. C., Mason, M. A., & Murguia, A. (2000). Psychotherapy with members of Latino/Latina religions and spiritual traditions. In A. E. Bergin & P. S. Richards (Eds.), *Psychotherapy and religious diversity: A guide for mental health professionals* (pp. 397–419). Washington, DC: American Psychological Association.

Index

Psychotherapy
  and ceremony, 19–20
  Cuban perspective, 73
  and folk healing, 256
  holistic approach, 280, 293
  indigenous perspectives,
    19–21
  nontraditional methods,
    19–20
  ritual in, 19–20
  spiritually-oriented, 20,
    288–290
  traditional, 292
  visionary experiences, 20–21
Puberty rites, 241
Puerto Rican Espiritismo, 64

R

Readings
  of coffee grounds, 235
  of seashells, 65, 67
  tarot cards, 284
Registro (reading), 65, 67
Regla de Ocha, see Santería
Reincarnation, 153, 155, 182
Relational consciousness, 6, 13
Religion
  rationalized versus popular,
    39
  versus science, 255
Religious awe, 43, 47
Religiousness, 273
Rites of revitalization, 45
Ritual cleansing, 67, 175; see
    also La Limpia de San
    Lazaro
Rituals, 275, 281; see also
    Ceremonies
  communal performance, 185
  for coping, 287
  in curanderismo, 280–281
  forming communities, 276
  healing function, 280
  performance benefits,
    184–185, 292
  in psychotherapy, 289

  role in therapy, 19–20
  for the senses, 275
Rosemary, 88
Rue, 88
Ruta chalepensis, 89

S

Sacramentality, 41, 275,
    282–283
Sacrifice, 41
  animal, 65, 67, 253
Saint Barbara, 249
Saint-John's-Wort
  active constituents, 91
  contraindications, 95–96
  effectiveness, 92–94
  history, 90–91
  mechanism of action, 91–92
  side effects, 95
  toxicity, 94–95
  usage, 85
Saints, see Catholic saints; Folk
    saints
Saint veneration, 29, 30, 31, 44
  devotion orientations, 44–49,
    50–51
  expressions of, 39–40
  and intercession, 41, 42, 44
  and miraculous healing, 42,
    51–52
  reasons for, 41–42
  sensory involvement, 40
  through relics, 41
San Lazaro, 176, 177, 185, 186
Santeras/os, 66, 251, 261
  ability to diagnose, 75
  communication with spirits,
    69
  as healers, 69–70
  interviews with, 70–72
  meaning of psychological
    health, 73–74
  response to help-seeking,
    74–75
  seeking counsel from, 67,
    251–252